WINTER
SPORTS
MEDICINE
HANDBOOK

Notice

Medicine is an ever-changing science. As new research and clinical experience broaden our knowledge, changes in treatment and drug therapy are required. The authors and the publisher of this work have checked with sources believed to be reliable in their efforts to provide information that is complete and generally in accord with the standards accepted at the time of publication. However, in view of the possibility of human error or changes in medical sciences, neither the authors nor the publisher nor any other party who has been involved in the preparation or publication of this work warrants that the information contained herein is in every respect accurate or complete, and they disclaim all responsibility for any errors or omissions or for the results obtained from use of the information contained in this work. Readers are encouraged to confirm the information contained herein with other sources. For example and in particular, readers are advised to check the product information sheet included in the package of each drug they plan to administer to be certain that the information contained in this work is accurate and that changes have not been made in the recommended dose or in the contraindications for administration. This recommendation is of particular importance in connection with new or infrequently used drugs.

WINTER SPORTS MEDICINE

HANDBOOK

James L. Moeller, MD, FACSM

Sports Medicine Associates, PLC
Auburn Hills, Michigan
Chief, Division of Sports Medicine
William Beaumont Hospital
Troy, Michigan

Sami F. Rifat, MD, FACSM

Sports Medicine Associates, PLC
Auburn Hills, Michigan
Clinical Associate Professor
School of Health Sciences
Oakland University
Head Team Physician
Oakland University
Rochester, Michigan

McGraw-Hill
Medical Publishing Division

New York   Chicago   San Francisco   Lisbon   London
Madrid   Mexico City   Milan   New Delhi   San Juan
Seoul   Singapore   Sydney   Toronto

Winter Sports Medicine Handbook

1 2 3 4 5 6 7 8 9 0   DOC/DOC 0 9 8 7 6 5 4

ISBN   0-07-141209-3

This book was set in New Aster by International Typesetting and
    Composition.
The editors were Darlene Cooke and James F. Shanahan.
The production supervisor was Richard Ruzycka.
Project management was provided by Andover Publishing Services.
The index was prepared by Andover Publishing Services.
RR Donnelley was printer and binder.
This book was printed on acid-free paper.

Library of Congress Cataloging-in-Publication Data

Winter sports injuries / edited by James L. Moeller and Sami F. Rifat.
    p. cm.
  Includes bibliographical references and index.
  ISBN 0-07-141209-3
    1. Winter sports injuries. 2. Sports medicine. I. Moeller, James L.
II. Rifat, Sami F.

  RC1220.W55W555 2004
  617.1'027–dc22

                                                    2003065132

To my wife Marlo and my beautiful daughters Lindsay, Hannah, and Kelsey–daddy's "hat trick"–for your understanding, support, and love throughout the creation of this book and always.

JAMES L. MOELLER

To my wife Dana and my wonderful children Alex and Chloe. You make it all possible.

SAMI F. RIFAT

CONTENTS

CONTRIBUTORS

Michael R. Bracko, EdD, CSCS, FACSM

Director, Institute for Hockey Research
Calgary, Alberta
Canada

Eugene Byrne, MD

Lake Placid Sports Medicine Center
Orthopaedic Consultant
United States Olympic Training Center
Lake Placid, New York

Janus D. Butcher, MD

Chief Flight Surgeon, 179th Fighter Squadron
Duluth, Minnesota
Head Physician, Cross-Country Team
U.S. Ski and Snowboard Association
SMDC Department of Orthopedics
Duluth, Minnesota

Jim Carrabre, MD, MPE, FACSM

Chairman
Medical Committee of the International Biathlon Union
Watertown, Minnesota

Adam deJong, MA

Assistant Director
Preventative Cardiology and Rehabilitation
William Beaumont Hospital
Royal Oak, Michigan

Jos J. deKoning, PhD, FACSM

Assistant Professor, IFKB Faculty of Human Movement Studies
Vrije Universiteit Amsterdam
Amsterdam
The Netherlands

Carol S. Federiuk, MD, PhD

Sports Medicine Fellow
Department of Family Medicine/Sports Medicine
Thomas Jefferson University
Philadelphia, Pennsylvania
Clinical Associate Professor
Department of Emergency Medicine
Oregon Health and Science University
Portland, Oregon

Carl Foster, PhD, FACSM

Professor, Department of Exercise and Sport Science
University of Wisconsin-La Crosse
LaCrosse, Wisconsin

Barry Franklin, PhD, FACSM

Director, Cardiac Rehabilitation and Exercise Laboratories
William Beaumont Hospital
Royal Oak, Michigan

Eric A. Heiden, MD

Team Physician, U.S. Speedskating
Assistant Professor, Arthroscopy and Sports Medicine
Department of Orthopaedic Surgery
University of California, Davis, Health System
Davis, California

Scott M. Koehler, MD

Team Physician, U.S. Snowboarding
Medical Director, Allina Medical Clinic
Center for Sports Medicine and Rehabilitation
Head Team Physician, Carleton and St. Olaf Colleges
Northfield, Minnesota

James Macintyre, MD, MPE, FACSM

Team Physician, U.S. Speedskating, U.S. Ski and Snowboarding
Advanced Orthopedics and Sports Medicine
Associate Director, Primary Care Sports Medicine Fellowship
Clinical Assistant Professor
Department of Family and Preventive Medicine
University of Utah

William O. Roberts, MD, MS, FACSM

Phalen Village Clinic
Department of Family Practice and Community Health
University of Minnesota Medical School
St. Paul, Minnesota

Kenneth W. Rundell, PhD, FACSM

Professor of Health Science
Marywood University
Director of the Human Performance Laboratory
Keith J. O'Neill Center for Healthy Families
Scranton, Pennsylvania

Ann Snyder, PhD, FACSM

Professor and Director of Human Performance Laboratory
Department of Human Movement Sciences
University of Wisconsin-Milwaukee
Milwaukee, Wisconsin

Bradford A. Stephens, MD

Medical Director
Lake Placid Sports Medicine Center
Orthopaedic Consultant
United States Olympic Training Center
Lake Placid, New York

FOREWORD

Most professionals involved in sports medicine either have a basic interest in sport or have had the experience of overcoming a sports injury. Sometimes it is both. For me, breaking a leg as a young skater was, at the time, a catastrophe. How was I going to stay in shape? Would I be able to salvage the season? With hindsight, it was this experience that influenced my decision to pursue sports medicine and has brought me to where I am today.

Most sports physicians have a formal education in either orthopaedic surgery or sports medicine. As a whole, we are comfortable treating musculoskeletal injuries, and there is an abundance of texts written on the diagnosis and treatment of such injuries. There is a plethora of literature on the biology of healing bones, ligaments, tendons, articular cartilage, and so forth, and there is no substitute for having extensive knowledge of these basic principles. In recent years our knowledge of the medical aspects of athlete care has grown tremendously. How physicians incorporate this vast array of knowledge in treating athletes is when the science of sports medicine becomes a true art.

To be involved in sports as a physician today means being part of a comprehensive team, including physicians, trainers, physical therapists, physiologists, biomechanists, kinesiologists, psychologists, nutritionists, and equipment designers. It also requires a broad understanding of the sport, its demands, and current trends. We can prescribe a treatment plan, but for that plan to be followed, an athlete must have confidence in our understanding of their sport. Where are they in their season? At what level do they compete? Can they take time off? Answers to these questions must be known if we are to implement a sound treatment plan for the aspiring athlete. It is from these ideas that Drs. Jim Moeller and Sami Rifat found the inspiration to write *Winter Sports Medicine Handbook*. The "sports medicine team" concept is evidenced in this book by the diversity of the contributing authors who have lent their expertise.

Winter Sports Medicine Handbook is a unique and interesting book that will be an excellent addition to the library of physicians, trainers, therapists, and sports scientists involved in the training and care of winter sport athletes. Coaches and the athletes themselves can also benefit from its information.

The focus of the book, winter sports, is an area of sports medicine that is often overlooked in other texts. The sport-by-sport organization of the book, which includes the history, physiology, and mechanics of the sport as well as the medical and musculoskeletal problems encountered, allows for a more comprehensive understanding of the medical issues involved in the various winter sports. The quick reference guides in the front of the book are a unique feature that allows the busy practitioner an opportunity to rapidly learn the key aspects of an injury or disease process that is discussed in greater detail in the text.

That brings me back to where I am today, providing care for and traveling with the U.S. Speedskating Team. We recently found ourselves living in a small town (population of about 1,000 people, plus or minus a couple of moose) high in the mountains of Norway. Despite a treacherous, hair-raising, two-hour drive to the rink (which had a nice hotel right next door) we lived in the mountains to maximize the physiologic benefits of altitude. My formal education had left me inept regarding the physiologic benefits and risks of altitude exposure and how it affects performance. Years of experience have educated me in this area. Traveling with the team has made me aware of the importance of a well-rounded knowledge base that physicians must possess in order to provide appropriate care for their athletes.

ERIC A. HEIDEN, MD

Team Physician, U.S. Speedskating
Assistant Professor Arthroscopy and Sports Medicine
Department of Orthopaedic Surgery
University of California, Davis, Health System

PREFACE

Winter Sports Medicine Handbook is written based on the premise that the most effective sports medicine practitioners not only understand the medical problems encountered in active people but understand their sport as well. The book exclusively uses this sports-centered approach.

Each winter sport is addressed individually, with experts examining its physiology and biomechanics as they relate to commonly encountered injuries and illnesses. Physicians, biomechanists, and exercise scientists with expertise in working with winter sport athletes have contributed to this unique format. We are proud to have many National Team Physicians, International Sport Committee members, and other nationally recognized authors contributing to the book.

Winter Sports Medicine Handbook is designed for physicians, physical therapists, and athletic trainers. We feel the book will also be helpful for coaches and athletes. The book is written in an "expanded outline" format to help the reader find important points easily. For the practitioner who needs to learn the "bare bones" of an injury or disease process rapidly, there is a quick reference section as well. The book is not intended to cover all sports medicine topics, but rather only those common or particular to winter sport athletes.

For many people, certain winter sports are nothing more than a curiosity, something that peaks an interest every four years during the Olympic Games. For others, winter sports are a part of everyday life. For sports medicine practitioners to appropriately care for winter sport athletes, they must learn and understand as much about the different sports as possible. We are very pleased to bring you this information and hope that it assists you in your interaction with these athletes.

JAMES L. MOELLER
SAMI F. RIFAT

ACKNOWLEDGMENTS

The idea for this book grew from our interest in winter sports and the belief that an appreciation of the sport is essential to understanding the athlete. We thank all of those physicians involved in our sports medicine training who made us aware of this. We would also like to thank the residents and fellows we have worked with through the years. Teaching these young physicians motivates us to stay up-to-date and rekindles our professional enthusiasm.

We appreciate McGraw-Hill for believing in this concept, and we thank Darlene Cooke, Michelle Watt, and Jim Shanahan for their support and encouragement during this project. We would also like to acknowledge Niels Buessem of Andover Publishing Services for his editorial support.

We greatly appreciate the excellent work of all of our contributing authors. Their experience in the research and medical care of winter sport athletes is unsurpassed, and their enthusiasm for this project made them all a pleasure to work with. Thanks, too, to Dr. Eric Heiden for his contributions to this book, including writing the Foreword.

We also thank the athletic trainers, coaches, and parents we have worked with through the years. Finally, we want to express our appreciation to all the athletes who have trusted us with their medical care, for they are the greatest teachers of all.

QUICK REFERENCE GUIDE

MUSCULOSKELETAL ISSUES

Injury	Diagnosis	Management	Chapter
1st metatarsophalangeal joint injury (skier's toe)	• Pain, swelling, and decreased motion at 1st MTP joint • More common with classic skiing technique • Local tenderness • May be signs of degeneration on examination and/or radiographs	• Relative rest • Analgesics/NSAIDs • Supportive footwear • Surgery sometimes necessary	9. Cross-Country Skiing
Achilles tendon rupture	• Acute posterior ankle pain • "Pop" often heard • Inability to actively plantar flex foot • Local tenderness • Palpable defect may be present • Positive Thompson's test	• Analgesics • Surgery is usually indicated for young healthy athletes • Equine cast for those who are not surgical candidates	7. Freestyle Skiing
Acromioclavicular pseudo-sprain	• Mainly in young athletes • AC pain after trauma • Swelling may be present • AC and distal clavicle tenderness • Initial x-rays usually normal	• Ice • Analgesics • Sling for comfort	11. Ice Hockey

continued

(Continued)

Injury	Diagnosis	Management	Chapter
Acromioclavicular sprain	• AC pain after trauma • Swelling and/or deformity • AC tenderness • Positive crossover test	• General measures include: sling for comfort, ice, and analgesics • Definitive treatment varies depending on severity	11. Ice Hockey
Ankle tendinopathies	• Aggravated by activity • Localized swelling • Localized tenderness	• Relative rest • Ice • Analgesics/NSAIDs • Rehabilitation	12. Figure Skating
Anterior cruciate ligament injury	• Acute knee pain associated with injury • Effusion • Feeling of instability • Positive Lachman	• Control swelling • Analgesics • Physical therapy • Surgical reconstruction for those in high demand sports	5. Alpine Skiing
Apophyseal injuries	• Skeletally immature athlete • Pain and weakness of involved muscle • Apophyseal tenderness • X-rays usually reveal avulsion	• Rest • Crutches if necessary • Ice • Analgesics • Flexibility and strength training when sufficiently healed • Surgical fixation for widely displaced fractures	12. Figure Skating
Calcaneus stress fracture	• Heel pain • Symptoms worse with loading • Tenderness • Pain with squeeze test • X-rays usually negative • Bone scan usually confirms diagnosis	• Relative rest • Analgesics • Immobilization sometimes necessary	7. Freestyle Skiing
Cervical spine injury	• Neck/head trauma • Neck pain • Possible loss of consciousness • Cervical injury should be assumed in all unconscious athletes • Local tenderness • Neurologic signs may be present	• Follow BLS guidelines • Stabilize cervical spine • Do NOT remove helmet • Immobilize cervical spine and place athlete on backboard • Prompt transport to hospital	11. Ice Hockey

Injury	Diagnosis	Management	Chapter
Cervical strain	• Posterior neck pain • Usually neurologic symptoms absent • Tender paracervical and trapezius muscles • Decreased range of motion	• Relative rest • Ice/heat • Analgesics/NSAIDs • ROM exercises • Strengthening	14. Sliding Sports
Clavicle fracture	• Clavicle pain after trauma • Swelling and gross deformity • Local tenderness • Decreased ROM shoulder	• Treatment is generally conservative • Ice • Analgesics • Sling for comfort • Reduction for severe angulation • Surgery if open or severely angulated and if neurovascular status is compromised	11. Ice Hockey
Common peroneal nerve injury	• Usually secondary to trauma • Weakness ankle dorsiflexors and evertors • Sensory changes anterolateral leg and dorsum of foot	• Recovery from blunt trauma is typically complete, but may take up to 6 months • Lacerations typically lead to long-term deficit	11. Ice Hockey
Compression fracture thoracolumbar spine	• Pain after trauma • Midline pain without radiation • Midline tenderness • Usually no neurologic symptoms • X-rays usually confirm diagnosis	• Varies depending on severity • Simple fractures are treated with rest, analgesics, ice, and a thoracolumbar orthosis • "Burst" fractures should be referred to a specialist	5. Alpine Skiing
DeQuervain's tenosynovitis	• Radial wrist pain • Occasional swelling • Tenderness proximal to the radial syloid • Positive Finkelstein test	• Activity modification • Ice • Analgesics/NSAIDs • Immobilization may be necessary • Rehabilitation • Corticosteroid injection • Surgery is the last resort	15. Curling

continued

(Continued)

Injury	Diagnosis	Management	Chapter
Distal radius fracture	• Typically occurs as a result of a fall onto an outstretched hand • Wrist pain • Distal radius tenderness • Deformity may or may not be present • Confirmed by X-ray	• Treatment depends on severity • Nondisplaced fractures are treated with cast immobilization for 4–6 weeks • Displaced, angulated, and comminuted fractures should be treated by an orthopedic surgeon	6. Snowboarding
Elbow dislocation	• Usually caused by a fall onto outstretched arm • Immediate pain • Gross deformity • Inability to move elbow • Neurovascular status may be affected • X-rays confirm diagnosis and may reveal fracture	• If neurovascular status is affected, on-field reduction may be attempted by qualified personnel • If neurovascularly intact, stabilize and transport to hospital • Reduce	6. Snowboarding
Chronic exertional compartment syndrome	• Leg pain worse with exercise • Relieved by rest • Weakness may or may not be present • Examination may be normal • Diagnosis confirmed with compartment pressure measurement	• Rest, ice, massage • Conservative treatment often ineffective • Fasciotomy is the definitive treatment	13. Speed Skating
Extensor carpi ulnaris tendonitis	• Ulnar wrist pain • Aggravated by wrist extension and ulnar deviation • Tender ulnar wrist • Pain with resisted wrist extension and ulnar deviation	• Activity modification • Ice • Analgesics/NSAIDs • Immobilization sometimes necessary • Physical therapy • Corticosteroid injection	9. Cross-Country Skiing
Femur fracture	• Immediate thigh pain after trauma • Inability to bear weight • Femoral tenderness • Swelling may be present • Gross deformity may be present • X-ray confirms diagnosis	• Stabilize and transport to hospital • Should be referred to orthopedic surgery for definitive treatment	7. Freestyle Skiing

Injury	Diagnosis	Management	Chapter
Fibula stress fracture	• Lateral lower leg pain • Focal tenderness • X-rays usually negative • Bone scan confirms diagnosis	• Relative rest • Ice • Analgesics • Address predisposing factors	12. Figure Skating
Forearm periostitis	• Forearm pain • Symptoms worse with activity (e.g., slapshot) • Ulnar tenderness • X-rays usually negative • Bone scan can confirm diagnosis	• Relative rest • Ice • Analgesics	11. Ice Hockey
Greater trochanteric bursitis	• Deep aching lateral hip pain • May radiate down toward knee • Local tenderness • Pain with resisted hip abduction and external rotation	• Activity modification • Ice • Analgesics/NSAIDs • Address flexibility deficits • Corticosteroid injection	9. Cross-Country Skiing
Hamate fracture	• Tenderness over the hypothenar eminence/hamate bone • X-ray with carpal tunnel views • CT scan may be necessary	• Nondisplaced fractures treated with cast • Displaced fractures are usually treated surgically	11. Ice Hockey
Hamstring strain	• Acute pain often accompanied by a pop or tear in posterior thigh • Bruising often present • Limp • Tenderness sometimes accompanied by a palpable defect	• Relative rest • Ice • Analgesic/NSAIDs • ROM exercise • Physical therapy • Surgery if tendinous avulsion	14. Sliding Sports
Hand contusion	• Pain after trauma • Swelling • Bruising • Local tenderness • X-rays negative	• Relative rest • Ice • Analgesics/NSAIDs	14. Sliding Sports
Hip dislocation	• Usually caused by a hard fall • Immediate pain • Unable to bear weight • Pain with any attempted movement • The hip may appear shortened, internally rotated, and adducted • X-rays confirm diagnosis	• Stabilize and transport to hospital • Refer to orthopedic surgery	7. Freestyle Skiing

continued

(Continued)

Injury	Diagnosis	Management	Chapter
Hip flexor strain	• Anterior hip pain • Worse with activity • Local tenderness • Pain with passive hip flexor stretch • Pain with resisted hip flexion • Weakness may be present	• Ice • Analgesics/NSAIDs • Relative rest • ROM exercises advancing to strength training • Physical therapy is often required	13. Speed Skating
Iliotibial band friction syndrome	• Lateral knee pain • Usually seen in runners or cross-country skiers using the skate technique • Tender distal IT band and lateral epicondyle of knee • Tight IT band • Positive Ober's test	• Analgesic/NSAIDs • Ice • Relative rest • Address flexibility deficits • Physical therapy • Corticosteroid injection	9. Cross-Country Skiing
Intersection syndrome	• Distal forearm pain aggravated by movement • Tenderness dorsal radial forearm	• Relative rest • Ice • Analgesics/NSAIDs • Thumb spica splint/ cast • Physical therapy • Corticosteroid injection	15. Curling
Lateral ankle sprain	• History of inversion ankle trauma • Lateral ankle pain and swelling • Lateral ligamentous tenderness • Lateral ligamentous laxity • Normal X-rays	• Relative rest • Ice • Compression • Elevation • Analgesics/NSAIDs • Brace • Rehabilitation	6. Snowboarding
Lateral epicondylitis	• Lateral elbow pain • Symptoms aggravated by active wrist extension • Tender lateral epicondyle/ lateral elbow • Pain with resisted wrist extension	• Relative rest • Ice • Analgesics/NSAIDs • Rehabilitation • Corticosteroid injection	9. Cross-Country Skiing
Lumbar strain	• Low back pain • Decreased range of motion • Local tenderness • Neurological exam normal	• Activity as tolerated • Ice/ice massage • Analgesics/NSAIDs • Rehabilitation	10. Biathlon

Injury	Diagnosis	Management	Chapter
Malleolar bursitis	• No history of trauma • No or minimal pain • Fluctuant swelling over malleolus • Usually not tender	• Asses skate for proper fit • Ice • Iontophoresis • Aspiration/injection	12. Figure Skating
Mechanical low back pain	• Low back pain without radiation • Usually atraumatic • Worse with activity • Decreased range of motion • Local tenderness may or may not be present • No neurological findings	• Activity as tolerated • Ice • Analgesics • Address strength and flexibility deficiencies	13. Speed Skating
Medial collateral ligament injury	• Acute onset of medial knee pain after trauma • Minimal or no joint effusion • Instability with lateral movement • Tender MCL • Pain and possible laxity with valgus stress • X-rays usually negative	• Varies depending on severity • Relative rest • Ice • Analgesics/NSAIDs • Brace • Immobilization for Grade III injury • Rehabilitation	5. Alpine Skiing
Meniscus injury	• Usually a twisting or squatting mechanism • Joint line pain • Effusion • Joint line tenderness • Pain with meniscal testing • X-rays usually negative • MRI often identifies injury	• May try initial conservative management • Relative rest • Ice • Analgesics/NSAIDs • Range of motion exercises • Physical therapy • Surgery if conservative treatment fails	5. Alpine Skiing
Metatarsal fracture	• History of trauma • Pain and swelling • Local tenderness • Usually visualized on X-ray	• Varies from simple immobilization with rigid sole shoe/cast to surgical fixation depending on location and severity of injury	14. Sliding Sports

continued

(Continued)

Injury	Diagnosis	Management	Chapter
Metatarsal stress fracture	• Pain without trauma • History of change in activity level, frequency, or intensity • Swelling and local tenderness • X-rays often do not visualize fracture • Bone scan can confirm diagnosis	• Depends on location • 2nd through 4th metatarsal stress fractures are usually treated conservatively • Ice • Relative rest • Supportive or wooden sole shoe • Analgesics • Surgical fixation for 5th metatarsal stress fracture should be considered due to high risk of non/delayed union	10. Biathlon
Olecranon bursitis	• Localized swelling at tip of elbow after trauma • X-rays should be obtained to rule out fracture	• Aspiration should be considered • Compression wrap • Ice • NSAIDs • Corticosteroid injection considered if no signs of infection present	12. Figure Skating
Olecranon fracture	• Pain after fall onto elbow • Tender over olecranon, sulcus may be noted • Neurovascular status typically intact • X-ray confirms diagnosis	• Long-arm cast for nondisplaced fractures • Displaced fractures should be treated surgically	12. Figure Skating
Osteochondral injury (knee)	• Insidious onset of medial knee pain • Tender over medial femoral condyle • Effusion may be present • X-rays (include notch view) confirm diagnosis • MRI used for grading of injury	• Nonoperative if lesion is stable • Short course of non-weight bearing • Discontinue impact loading activities • Surgical treatment for unstable fractures or failed nonoperative treatment	12. Figure Skating
Patella tendon rupture	• Acute anterior knee pain associated with a pop or tearing sensation • Unable to extend knee • Patella located superiorly, palpable gap in patellar tendon • X-ray reveals patella alta	• Initially ice, immobilize, crutch ambulation, analgesics • Referral to orthopedic surgery for repair	7. Freestyle Skiing

Injury	Diagnosis	Management	Chapter
Patellar dislocation	• Acute knee pain usually associated with a fall • A pop and instability at the time of injury may be described • Positive apprehension test • X-rays may reveal signs of effusion but are usually otherwise negative	• If still dislocated, reduce the patella • Immobilize • Ice • Elevate • NSAID/analgesic • Begin active rehabilitation when pain and swelling under good control	8. Telemark Skiing
Patellar tendinopathy	• Insidious onset anterior knee pain • Tender over patellar tendon	• Activity modification • Ice • NSAID or analgesic • Quadriceps stretching • Eccentric loading program • Bracing may be helpful	13. Speed Skating
Patellofemoral pain syndrome	• Insidious onset anterior knee pain • Positive grind test • X-rays typically negative	• VMO strengthening • Ice • Analgesics • Patellar taping may be helpful	13. Speed Skating
Peroneus tendon injury	• Mechanism may be acute (tear or sublux) or overuse • Tender posterior to the lateral malleolus • Pain with resisted foot/ankle eversion	• Tears often require surgery • Ice • NSAID • Stretching • Eccentric load exercises	9. Cross-Country Skiing
Posterior cruciate ligament injury	• Acute knee pain associated with injury • Effusion • Feeling of instability • Positive Lachman	• Control swelling • Analgesics • Physical therapy • Bracing • Surgical reconstruction for severe laxity or chronic symptoms	5. Alpine Skiing
Prepatellar bursitis	• Swollen, sometimes painful anterior knee • Localized swelling of the prepatellar bursa	• Aspiration should be considered • Compression wrap • Ice • NSAIDs • Corticosteroid injection considered if no signs of infection present	15. Curling

continued

(Continued)

Injury	Diagnosis	Management	Chapter
Pyriformis syndrome	• Mechanism may be acute or overuse • Buttock pain and/or sciatica symptoms • Tender over gluteal prominence • Pain with passive internal hip rotation	• PRICEMM • Deep tissue massage	9. Cross-Country Skiing
Quad contusion	• Acute pain in anterior thigh after direct (e.g., knee vs. thigh) impact • Tender over anterior thigh • Swelling and/or palpable hematoma may be present	• Stop the bleeding with ice, compression, elevation, and knee flexion • ROME/stretch • Massage • Strengthening	11. Ice Hockey
Quadriceps strain	• Acute pain often accompanied by a pop or tearing sensation in anterior thigh • Bruising often present • Limp • Tenderness sometimes accompanied by a palpable defect	• Relative rest • Ice • Analgesic/NSAIDs • ROM exercise • Physical therapy	14. Sliding Sports
Quadriceps tendinopathy	• Anterior knee pain • Malalignment commonly seen • Tender over quadriceps tendon	• Ice • NSAID • Eccentric loading exercises • Stretching	
Rotator cuff tear	• Anterolateral pain usually after a fall onto an outstretched arm • Decreased, painful range of motion • Profound weakness and pain with resisted strength testing • MRI not necessary for initiation of treatment in most cases	• Initial treatment is similar to rotator cuff tendinopathy (see below) • Corticosteroid injection • Surgery considered if conservative measures fail	5. Alpine Skiing
Rotator cuff tendinopathy	• Insidious onset shoulder pain • Often present along with impingement syndrome • Resisted strength testing causes pain and may reveal slight weakness • Consider X-rays, MRI occasionally needed	• Ice • NSAID • Rotator cuff strengthening • Shoulder stabilization • Activity and/or equipment modifications	9. Cross-Country Skiing

Injury	Diagnosis	Management	Chapter
Sacroiliitis	• Most common cause of low back pain in cross country • Back or hip pain complaints • Tender over SI joint • Positive FABER	• Ice • Massage • Stretching • Manipulation • Core conditioning • Technique and equipment adjustments	9. Cross-Country Skiing
Scaphoid fracture	• Pain in radial side of wrist after fall on out-stretched hand or using hand to brace for impact with boards • Tender in anatomical snuff box • X-rays may be negative initially • Bone scan or CT scan may be needed to confirm diagnosis	• Nondisplaced fractures treated with thumb spica casting • Surgical consulta-tion for treatment of displaced or proximal pole fractures	13. Speed Skating
Scapholunate dissociation	• Dorsal wrist pain after fall on outstretched hand • Tender on palpation of scapholunate joint • Positive Watson test • X-rays reveal widening of scapholunate junction	• Surgical treatment recommended for displacement	6. Snowboarding
Shoulder contusion	• Pain after a direct blow (usually a fall) to the shoulder • Tender to palpation, motion and strength testing • X-rays negative	• Ice • NSAID • Active rehabilitation	5. Alpine Skiing
Shoulder dislocation/subluxation	• Anterior dislocation is most common • Spontaneous reduction may occur • Abduction/external rotation of arm is the "dislocation position" • Gross deformity may be noted • Axillary nerve paresthesias may be present • X-rays to assess for associated fracture	• Reduce the joint if still dislocated • Sling • Analgesics • Protected ROM • Dynamic stabiliza-tion program • Risk of re-dislocation is high • Surgery considered for recurrent instability	6. Snowboarding

continued

(Continued)

Injury	Diagnosis	Management	Chapter
Shoulder impingement syndrome	• Insidious onset shoulder pain • Often present along with rotator cuff tendinosis • Positive Hawkins and/or Neer test • Resisted strength testing causes pain and may reveal slight weaknesss • Consider X-rays, MRI occasionally needed	• Ice • NSAID • Rotator cuff strengthening • Shoulder stabilization • Corticosteroid injection • Activity and/or equipment modifications	9. Cross-Country Skiing
Spondylolisthesis	• Anterior slip of superior vertebral body in relation to adjacent inferior segment • More common in females • History and physical findings similar to spondylolysis • Lateral radiographs reveal degree of slip	• Symptomatic for low-grade injury • TLSO brace for larger degrees of slip • Surgical stabilization for unstable injuries or those with neurologic compromise	12. Figure Skating
Spondylolysis	• Stress fracture of the pars interarticularis • Most common cause of back pain in adolescent athletes who seek medical care for their pain • Insidious onset pain, worse with spine extension activities • Tender to palpation • Positive stork test • X-rays may be normal • Bone scan with SPECT confirms acute injury	• Remove from impact loading, particularly spine hyperextension activities • Analgesics • Core flexibility and strength training • Bracing and surgery occasionally necessary	12. Figure Skating
Talus lateral process fracture	• "Snowboarder's fracture" represents 15% of ankle injuries in this sport • Pain in lateral ankle after fall • Point tender over lateral process of talus • X-rays may not show the fracture • CT scan	• Surgical fixation for large or displaced fractures • Smaller, non-displaced fractures can be treated with cast immobilization	6. Snowboarding

Injury	Diagnosis	Management	Chapter
Thumb ulnar collateral ligament sprain	• Most common upper extremity injury in skiing • Due to fall on outstretched hand while holding ski pole • Pain along ulnar aspect of 1st MCP joint • Valgus stress testing causes pain and may reveal instability • X-ray to assess for associated fracture	• Incomplete tears can be treated with thumb spica immobilization • Complete tears typically require surgical repair	5. Alpine Skiing
Tibia fracture	• Incidence greatly decreased due to equipment changes • Severe leg pain after trauma	• Stabilize extremity • Prompt transport to hospital • X-rays confirm diagnosis • Stable fractures may be treated with cast immobilization • Unstable fractures require surgical fixation	5. Alpine Skiing
Tibia stress fracture	• Most commonly due to repeated hard landings during dry-land training • Tender to direct palpation of tibia • May be tender with percussion hammer or tuning fork testing • X-rays usually negative • Bone scan or MRI often needed to confirm diagnosis	• Protect from further injury • Discontinue impact loading activities • Correct underlying mechanical issues • Nonimpact conditioning	7. Freestyle Skiing
Trochanteric bursitis	• Lateral hip pain • Pain on direct palpation over trochanteric bursa	• Ice • NSAID • Stretching of gluteal muscles and ITB • Corticosteroid injection	9. Cross-Country Skiing

MEDICAL ISSUES

Medical Issue	Diagnosis	Management	Chapter
Abdominal injury hollow viscera	• Persistent abdominal pain with signs of bacterial or chemical peritonitis • Referred pain to the shoulder • Localized abdominal pain with guarding • Plain radiographs may reveal free air • CT scanning if often useful	• Laparotomy is often necessary for definitive treatment	5. Alpine Skiing
Abdominal wall contusion	• Pain with trunk flexion or rotation • Localized tenderness and ecchymosis	• Usually self-limited • Relative rest, ice, and analgesics • Rehabilitation sometimes necessary	5. Alpine Skiing
Altitude sickness	• Acute mountain sickness is most common type • High-altitude cerebral edema • High-altitude pulmonary edema	• Descend from altitude • Supplemental oxygen • Hyperbaric oxygen considered for severe illness • Diuretics can be prophylactic or therapeutic	6. Snowboarding
Blister	• Fluid filled vesicles in skin • Found in areas subject to increased shearing forces	• Try to keep intact • Hydrocolloid gel if epidermal layer has been removed • Prevention is the best treatment	15. Curling
Calluses	• Thickened area of skin over bony prominence	• Treatment only if painful • Pare down with pumice stone or file	15. Curling
Carcinogen exposure (inhalation)	• Fluorocarbon-based ski wax exposure • Symptoms vary from cough to full-blown ARDS	• Prevention of exposure is best treatment • Adequate ventilation and respiratory protection	10. Biathlon
Chillblains	• Chronic vasculitis of the dermis • Most commonly affects the face, shins, hands, and feet	• Prevention is key	3. Cold Injury

Medical Issue	Diagnosis	Management	Chapter
Commotio cordis	• Sudden cardiac death due to blunt, nonpenetrating chest trauma • Impact during T-wave repolarization causes ventricular fibrillation • Over 80% of cases are fatal	• Currently approved chest protection may not prevent • Prompt defibrillation/ resuscitation (< 3 minutes) leads to a 25% chance of survival	11. Ice Hockey
Concussion	• Traumatic brain injury typically due to direct contact • Symptoms and clinical evaluation variable • Incidence appears to be increasing	• Remove from play • Full neurological and mental status evaluations performed serially • Return to play considered when the athlete is completely asymptomatic and has normal neuropsychologic testing and clinical evaluation	11. Ice Hockey
Dental injury	• Less common with consistent use of mouth guards and full facial protection	• Save the injured tooth • Immediate dental referral	11. Ice Hockey
Depression	• Dysphoria, hopelessness, decreased appetite • Suicidal thoughts • Altered sleep habits, lack of energy	• Psychotherapy • Pharmacotherapy	10. Biathlon

Eating disorders	Anorexia nervosa
	  • Hallmark: refusal to maintain body weight despite extreme thinness
	Bulimia nervosa
	  • Hallmark: binge/purge pattern of eating
		• Both types of primary eating disorders should be considered as poten- tially life-threatening
		• Treatment is multi- factorial: medical, behavioral, nutritional
			12. Figure Skating

Exercise-induced bronchospasm (EIB)	• Incidence of 4–20% of general population • Defined as a post-exercise decrease in FEV1 $\geq$ 10% • History and symptom complex are not adequate to make diagnosis • Clinical evaluation is usually negative	• After appropriate diagnosis made, pre- exercise treatment with inhaled β_2-ago- nist • Other medications may be effective options	2. Pulmonary Pathophysiology

continued

(Continued)

Medical Issue	Diagnosis	Management	Chapter
Eye trauma	• Less common with consistent use of half-shield or full facial protection • Corneal abrasion is most common injury encountered • Other injury types include hyphema and traumatic iritis	• Low threshold for referral to ophthalmologist	11. Ice Hockey
Facial laceration	• Less common with consistent use of full facial protection	• Many repair options available	11. Ice Hockey
Female athlete triad	• Disordered eating • Menstrual irregularities • Osteoporosis	• Multifaceted including behavioral, nutritional, and medical intervention	12. Figure Skating
Frostbite	• Freezing of tissues including intracellular contents • Occurs at 28–31°F • White, cold, hard tissue	• Protect and insulate until rewarming can be properly initiated • Rapid rewarming in water bath • Surgical debridement of nonviable tissue • Prevention is the key	3. Cold Injury
Frozen cornea	• Symptoms similar to corneal abrasion • Pain, blurred vision, foreign body sensaation	• Similar to corneal abrasion • Prevention with eye protection and frequent blinking	10. Biathlon
Hepatic injury	• Right upper quadrant pain with radiation to the shoulder • Tender RUQ • CT scan can confirm	• Prompt transport to hospital • Nonoperative management if hemodynamically stable • Emergent laparotomy if hemodynamically unstable	5. Alpine Skiing
Hypothermia	• Core temperature < 36.5°C (97°F) • Clinical picture can be quite variable • Many cardiac and metabolic problems may develop	• Transfer, then treat • Active external and internal rewarming techniques need to be considered • Cardiac monitoring recommended during rewarming • Be prepared for complications • Prevention is the key	3. Cold Injury

Medical Issue	Diagnosis	Management	Chapter
Menstrual irregularities	• Primary amenorrhea is common • Secondary amenorrhea also common and may be due in part to increased training, reduced body fat, poor nutrition, or stress • Not a common presenting complaint • Physical examination typically normal	• Laboratory workup for metabolic causes • Progestin challenge • Treatment may require progesterone or estrogen/progesterone medications • May require alterations in training and nutrition patterns	12. Figure Skating
Mononucleosis	• Self-limited illness caused by EBV • Fatigue, sore throat, myalgias, headache • Enlarged tonsils with/without exudates, generalized lymphadenopathy, splenomegaly	• Laboratory diagnosis: CBC with differential, mono spot • Supportive treatment • No sports activities for at least 3–4 weeks (not even light activities) and must be asymptomatic • Hold return to more vigorous activities for additional week	11. Ice Hockey
Overtraining syndrome	• Fatigue, irritability, lack of concentration, decreased motivation • Poor sleep and decreased appetite • "Heavy legs," muscle soreness • Increased resting heart rate	• Proper coaching and training can prevent • Short periods of relative rest for weeks to months • Absolute rest is sometimes necessary	10. Biathlon
Pneumothorax	• Dyspnea, pleuritic chest pain, cough • Appears anxious • Tachypnea, tachycardia • Absent or reduced breath sounds on affected side • Tracheal shift is a dangerous sign (tension pneumothorax) requiring immediate intervention	• Prompt transportation to hospital • X-ray confirms diagnosis and severity of lung collapse • Treatment is supportive for small pneumothorax. • Chest tube required for larger injuries	7. Freestyle Skiing
Rectus sheath hematoma	• Can mimic acute abdomen • Sudden abdominal pain and swelling • Relieved with supported flexion, pain with active flexion • Tender palpable mass • May be seen on CT scan or ultrasound	• Relative rest • Ice • Analgesics • Large hematomas may require surgery	5. Alpine Skiing

continued

(Continued)

Medical Issue	Diagnosis	Management	Chapter
Rifle safety	• Risk of accidental shooting is exceedingly low	• Rules of the sport are designed with safety as a priority	10. Biathlon
Skin abrasion	• Painful wound with serous exudate	• Clean wound • Topical antibiotics • Oral antibiotics if signs of more serious infection	10. Biathlon
Snow blindness	• Pain, foreign body sensation, blurred vision • Photophobia • Corneal injection • Sometimes corneal opacification	• Protect from further UV exposure • Patch eye • Emergent ophthalmology evaluation	10. Biathlon
Snow immersion death	• Typically occurs when snowboarder is trapped upside-down in the soft snow in a tree well	• Always snowboard with a partner particularly on deep powder or forest runs	6. Snowboarding
Splenic injury	• Abdominal pain with radiation to the shoulder • LUQ tenderness though tenderness may be generalized • Be suspicious of delayed rupture • CT scan confirms diagnosis	• Prompt transportation to hospital • Splenic preservation is preferred if hemodynamically stable • Splenectomy if injury is extensive or hemodynamically unstable	5. Alpine Skiing
Sportsman's hernia	• It's very existence is controversial • Lower abdominal/groin pain caused by posterior inguinal wall weakness without the presence of a frank hernia • Diagnosis of exclusion	• Conservative treatments rarely successful • Surgical repair recommended	11. Ice Hockey
Subdural hematoma	• Seems to occur from rotational and shear forces that tear the subdural bridging veins perpendicular to the force of the blow to the head • Be suspicious if there is deteriorating mental function after a lucent period	• Prompt transportation to hospital if suspected • Neurosurgery consultation • May require evacuation of hematoma and ligation of bleeding vessels	6. Snowboarding

Medical Issue	Diagnosis	Management	Chapter
Transient quadriparesis	• Numbness, tingling, and/or paralysis of all four limbs after axial load trauma to the neck • In most cases, symptoms resolve within 15 minutes • Examination may reveal focal neurological deficits	• Prompt transportation to hospital with full spinal immobilization • X-ray to rule out fracture • MRI to look for cord injury, spinal stenosis • If spinal stenosis present, athlete is disqualified from further contact, collision, and other high-risk activities	7. Freestyle Skiing
Viral upper respiratory infection	• Fever, chills, myalgias, cough, sore throat, congestion, and fatigue	• Rest, fluids • Symptomatic treatment • No participation if temp > 38°C	10. Biathlon
Vulvar injuries	• Usually due to fall onto one's bindings • Typically occurs when unloading the chair lift	• Prevention is the key • Nearly 70% of cases require surgical intervention	6. Snowboarding

WINTER
SPORTS
MEDICINE
HANDBOOK

1

CARDIAC PHYSIOLOGY

Adam deJong
Barry Franklin

ENERGY SYSTEMS

Anaerobic Metabolism

A. The process by which energy, in the form of adenosine triphosphate (ATP; Figure 1-1), is provided to active muscles, when energy demands exceed the available ATP supplied via aerobic metabolism.

    1. Expedited form of energy production (2 molecules of ATP/glucose molecule) only available through carbohydrate utilization.

    2. ATP is synthesized from the splitting of phosphate molecules from creatine phosphate and through the chemical breakdown of carbohydrates via glycolysis.

    3. Anaerobic glycolysis results in increased levels of lactic acid, which is derived from pyruvic acid degradation in the absence of oxygen.

Aerobic Pathway

A. The process by which glycogen, fats, and proteins can be used, in combination with oxygen, to produce ATP.

B. Krebs citric acid cycle and the electron transport chain.

    1. Oxidative process which complements glycolysis to provide additional ATP for energy production (Table 1-1).

    2. These processes, which occur in the mitochondria, combine acetyl-coenzyme A and oxaloacetic acid to form citric acid.

1

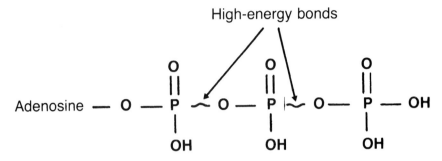

FIGURE 1-1   Simplified structure of an ATP molecule.

The subsequent removal of hydrogen atoms produces ATP for energy.
3. Results in the production of 36 ATP, or ~95% of the potential energy production, when a glucose molecule is completely degraded to carbon dioxide and water.

TABLE 1-1

Characteristics of the two mechanisms by which ATP is formed.

Mechanism	Food or Chemical Fuel	Oxygen Required?	Relative ATP Yield
I. Anaerobic			
1. Phosphocreatine	Phosphocreatine	No	Extremely limited
2. Glycolysis	Glycogen (glucose)	No	Extremely limited
II. Aerobic Krebs cycle and electron transport system	Glycogen, fats, proteins	Yes	Large

Adapted from Mathews DK, Fox EL. *The Physiological Basis of Physical Education and Athletics*, 2nd ed. Philadelphia: Saunders; 1976.

Muscle Types

A. Muscle fiber type determines the capacity at which a particular muscle can work.

B. Factors influencing the speed of contraction and fatigability are determined by the fiber composition.

C. Muscle can be comprised of varied fiber types, which is largely determined by genetics.

D. Muscle fiber types.

    1. Slow-twitch or type I (slow, oxidative).

    2. Fast-twitch or type II (fast, glycolytic).

        a. Several subdivisions of properties (types IIa, IIab, IIb).

OXYGEN CONSUMPTION AND HEMODYNAMIC DETERMINANTS

Metabolic Equivalent (MET)

A. A term used to quantify the energy expenditure required for any given activity.

B. Resting metabolism is defined as 1 MET, which is equal to approximately 3.5 mL of oxygen consumed per kilogram of body weight per minute (mL/kg/min).

C. Increases in energy expenditure during physical activity can be expressed as multiples of the resting metabolic rate (e.g., 5 METs equals 5 times the resting energy expenditure). Table 1-2 illustrates the approximate metabolic cost of various recreational and training activities.

Somatic Oxygen Consumption

Somatic oxygen consumption can be calculated using heart rate (HR), stroke volume (SV), and arteriovenous oxygen difference (a-vDo$_2$).

A. Heart rate generally increases in a linear fashion relative to workload.

    1. The progressive increase in heart rate tends to plateau at maximal effort.

    2. Maximum heart rate decreases with age, but may also be influenced by body position, fitness, disease state, activity, and environment, including temperature and humidity.

B. SV is the volume of blood pumped from the left ventricle (LV) with each beat, calculated as the difference between end diastolic volume (EDV) and end systolic volume (ESV).

TABLE 1-2

Approximate metabolic cost of various recreational and training activities. *

	Metabolic Cost	
Activity	**METs**	**kcal/min**†
Walking (1 mph)	1.5–2.0	2.0–2.5
Walking (2 mph), bicycling (5 mph), billiards, bowling, golf (power cart)	2.0–3.0	2.5–4.0
Walking (3 mph), bicycling (6 mph), volleyball, golf (pulling bag cart), archery, badminton (social doubles)	3.0–4.0	4.0–5.0
Walking (3.5 mph), bicycling (8 mph), table tennis, golf (carrying clubs), badminton (singles), tennis (doubles), many calisthenics	4.0–5.0	5.0–6.0
Walking (4 mph), bicycling (10 mph), ice skating, roller skating	5.0–6.0	6.0–7.0
Walking (5 mph), bicycling (11 mph), badminton (competitive), tennis (singles), square dancing, light downhill skiing, water skiing	6.0–7.0	7.0–8.0
Jogging (5 mph), bicycling (12 mph), vigorous downhill skiing, basketball, ice hockey, touch football, paddleball	7.0–8.0	8.0–10.0
Running (5.5 mph), bicycling (13 mph), squash racquets (social), handball (social), fencing, basketball (vigorous)	8.0–9.0	10.0–11.0
Running (6.0 mph), handball (competitive), squash (competitive)	10.0 plus	11.0 plus

* Adapted from Fox SM, Naughton JP, Gorman PA. Physical activity and cardiovascular health. III. The exercise prescription; frequency and type of activity. *Mod Concepts Cardiovasc Dis* 1972; 41:21–24.

† Represents gross caloric expenditure (i.e., includes the resting metabolic needs). Caloric requirements have been calculated for a 70-kg person and must be decreased or increased for lighter or heavier weights, respectively.

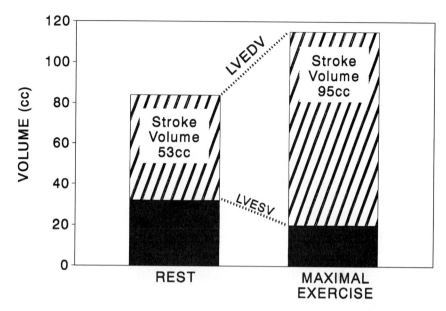

FIGURE 1-2 Increase in stroke volume from rest to maximal upright exercise in young, healthy men. Adapted from Poliner et al. (1980).

    1. Resting stroke volume generally approximates 50–100 mL/beat.

    2. During exercise, SV increases in a curvilinear fashion until approximately 50% of the individual's aerobic capacity is achieved.

        a. The augmented SV with exercise is due to increases and decreases in LVEDV and LVESV, respectively (Figure 1-2).

C. Ejection fraction (EF) is determined by venous return and myocardial contractility and can be estimated by the equation:

$$EF = (SV/EDV) \times 100$$

    1. Normal resting ejection fraction approximates 65 ± 8%; however, this variable can be largely affected by coronary artery disease, ventricular function, medications, and body position.

D. Cardiac output is a product of HR and SV, with resting values approximating 5 L/min.

    1. Cardiac output generally shows a fourfold increase from rest to maximal exercise; however, the incremental response is influenced by several variables, including body size and fitness level.

    2. Cardiac output generally increases linearly during exercise; it is influenced by HR and SV up to ~50% of maximal oxygen consumption and primarily by HR thereafter.

E. Arteriovenous oxygen difference is the difference in oxygen content between arterial and venous blood.
  1. Arterial and mixed venous oxygen content at rest approximate 20 and 15 mL of oxygen per dL blood, respectively.
  2. During maximal exercise, mixed venous blood decreases to approximately 5 mL of oxygen per dL blood, widening the arteriovenous oxygen difference to 15 mL per dL blood.
    a. Accordingly, the utilization coefficient typically increases from 25% at rest to 75% at maximal exercise.
  3. Increases in submaximal and maximal arteriovenous oxygen difference are noted in trained individuals as the oxidative capacity of skeletal muscle improves.

Blood Pressure

A. Systolic blood pressure, the pressure exerted by the heart during each contraction, increases linearly with increases in exercise intensity.
B. Diastolic blood pressure, the pressure in the blood vessels between heart contractions, generally remains constant or decreases slightly.
C. Pulse pressure, that is, systolic minus diastolic blood pressure, generally increases in direct proportion to the exercise intensity.

BLOOD FLOW DISTRIBUTION

Resting Blood Flow

A. Approximately 15–20% is distributed to skeletal muscles.
B. Remaining 80–85% is distributed to the heart, brain, and visceral organs.

Blood Flow During Exercise

A. Approximately 85–90% of the cardiac output is shunted to exercising muscles.
B. Increase in blood flow distribution to myocardium.
  1. Proportionally increased relative to cardiac demands.
C. Blood flow to the brain remains comparable to resting levels due to autoregulation.
D. Blood flow to skin increases with exercise to propagate heat loss.
  1. Maximal exercise causes a decrease in cutaneous circulation in an effort to meet increasing work demands.

PULMONARY VENTILATION

Minute Ventilation

Minute ventilation (V_E) is the volume of air moved per minute.
A. Resting values approximate 6 L/min.
B. Exercise values in healthy, fit adults may approximate or even exceed 75 L/min.
C. Increases in V_E are due to increases in respiratory rate and tidal volume.
  1. Tidal volume is largely responsible for the rise in V_E during mild to moderate exertion, and approximates 50–60% of the vital capacity.
  2. Respiratory rate, the number of breaths per minute, increases proportionately with exercise intensity and is primarily responsible for the rise in V_E during vigorous physical exertion.
  3. There is a one to threefold increase in respiratory rate during exercise; however, a five to sevenfold increase may occur in fit individuals.

Pulmonary Ventilation Regulation

A. Pulmonary ventilation is proportionately regulated by increases in somatic oxygen consumption and carbon dioxide production.
B. Disproportionate increases are noted in V_E during heavy exertion.
C. Proportionate rise in V_E relative to carbon dioxide production suggests that the potential regulating factor of pulmonary ventilation is the need for carbon dioxide removal more than the need for oxygen consumption.
  1. This suggests that carbon dioxide removal is the primary facilitator of pulmonary regulation and that minute ventilation is not normally a limiting factor to aerobic capacity.

MAXIMAL OXYGEN CONSUMPTION

$\dot{V}O_2$ max

$\dot{V}O_2$ max remains the most widely recognized measure of cardiovascular fitness.
A. $\dot{V}O_2$ increases linearly with progressive, incremental effort and is signified by a plateau in oxygen consumption despite a further increase in workload. This value is designated as the $\dot{V}O_2$ max.

1. Increases in $\dot{V}o_2$ during exercise typically approximate 10 to 12 times the normal resting aerobic requirement as determined by the relative increases in heart rate, stroke volume, and arteriovenous oxygen difference.

Determinants of Oxygen Consumption

A. Central and peripheral regulatory mechanisms affect the measurement of oxygen consumption and can be expressed by a rearrangement of the Fick equation:

$$\dot{V}o_2 = HR \times SV \times (a\text{-}vDo_2)$$

Where: $\dot{V}o_2$ = oxygen consumption in mL/min
     HR = heart rate in beats per minute
     SV = stroke volume in mL per beat
     $a\text{-}vDo_2$ = difference in oxygen content between arterial and venous blood, expressed as mL of oxygen per dL of blood

1. Oxygen consumption may be expressed relative to body weight (mL/kg/min) or as an absolute measure (L/min or kcal, where 1 L approximates 5 kcal).

B. Measurement of the volume and oxygen content of expired air, when corrected to standard temperature, pressure, and saturation, can also be used to determine oxygen consumption, using the equation:

$$\dot{V}o_2 = V_E \,(FIo_2 - FEo_2)$$

Where: V_E = minute ventilation in L/min
     FIo_2 = the directly measured concentration of inspired oxygen (normally 20.93%)
     FEo_2 = the directly measured concentration of expired oxygen

Estimating the $\dot{V}o_2$ max

A. Direct measurement of oxygen consumption is associated with several limitations.
1. Specialized equipment is required.
   a. Equipment is expensive.
   b. Specially trained staff is needed for operation of the equipment.
   c. Frequent calibration of the equipment is needed.
2. Verbal communication with the subject is difficult.

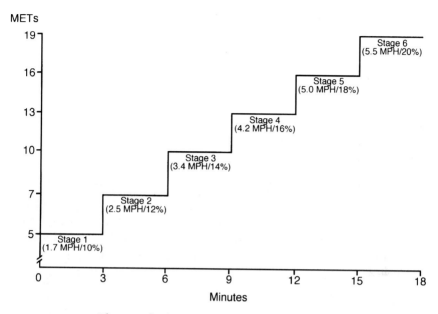

FIGURE 1-3 The standard Bruce treadmill protocol showing progressive stages (speed, percentage grade) and the estimated aerobic requirement (assuming completion of the stage), expressed as metabolic equivalents or METs.

    B. Consequently, clinicians have increasingly sought to estimate oxygen consumption during exercise testing.
        1. Because treadmill or cycle ergometer testing has been shown to be relatively constant in regard to mechanical efficiency, researchers have demonstrated that the oxygen consumption can be reasonably predicted based on exercise time or the peak workload achieved (Figure 1-3).
        a. $\dot{V}o_2$ max is often overestimated.
    C. Possible explanations for the disparity between measured and estimated $\dot{V}o_2$ max values include:
        1. Population differences in energy expenditure.
        2. Differences in level of physical fitness.
        3. Inappropriate extrapolation of steady-state aerobic requirements to non-steady-state work.
        4. Differences in exercise protocol intensity increments.
        5. Methodological variables.
    D. Recent advances in ramping protocols have increased the validity of estimating oxygen consumption due to the uniform increases in demand, which allows for a steady rise in cardiopulmonary responses.

Functional Aerobic Impairment (FAI)

A. Concept developed by Bruce et al. which utilizes the estimated or measured $\dot{V}o_2$ max and compares it with values expected for a healthy person matched for age, gender, and habitual physical activity (Table 1-3).

TABLE 1-3

$\dot{V}o_2$ max of healthy active and sedentary men and women.[*]

Age (years)	Men		Women	
	Active 69.7–0.612 years	Sedentary[†] 57.8–0.445 years	Active 42.9–0.312 years	Sedentary[†] 42.3–0.356 years
20	57.5	48.9	36.7	35.2
22	56.2	48.0	36.0	34.5
24	55.0	47.1	35.4	33.8
26	53.8	46.2	34.8	33.0
28	52.6	45.3	34.2	32.3
30	51.3	44.5	33.5	31.6
32	50.1	43.6	32.9	30.9
34	48.9	42.7	32.3	30.2
36	47.7	41.8	31.7	29.5
38	46.4	40.9	31.0	28.8
40	45.2	40.0	30.4	28.1
42	44.0	39.1	29.8	27.3
44	42.8	38.2	29.2	26.6
46	41.5	37.3	28.5	25.9
48	40.3	36.4	27.9	25.2
50	39.1	35.6	27.3	24.5
52	37.9	34.7	26.7	23.8
54	36.7	33.8	26.1	23.1
56	35.4	32.9	25.4	22.4
58	34.2	32.0	24.8	21.7
60	33.0	31.1	24.2	20.9
62	31.8	30.2	23.6	20.2
64	30.5	29.3	22.9	19.5
66	29.3	28.4	22.3	18.8
68	28.1	27.5	21.7	18.1
70	26.9	26.7	21.1	17.4

[*] Adapted from Bruce et al., 1973.

[†] Subjects who do not exert themselves sufficiently to develop sweating at least once per week.

B. FAI is calculated using the following formula:

$$\%FAI = \frac{\text{Predicted } \dot{V}o_2 \text{ max} - \text{Observed } \dot{V}o_2 \text{ max} \times 100}{\text{Predicted } \dot{V}o_2 \text{ max}}$$

C. The normal value for FAI is 0%, indicating a fitness level that equals that expected in a person of the same age, gender, and activity status.
   1. Negative values of FAI indicate an above-average fitness level.
   2. Positive values of FAI (indicating below-average fitness) are separated into four categories, indicating progressive functional impairment.
      a. 27 to 40%:   Mild FAI.
      b. 41 to 54%:   Moderate FAI.
      c. 55 to 68%:   Marked FAI.
      d. >68%:   Extreme FAI.
   3. The concept of FAI is useful in comparing serial test results, particularly after varied interventions (e.g., exercise training, coronary revascularization, cardiovascular medications).

Physiologic Variations

A. Body size, muscle mass, age, gender, habitual physical activity, and aerobic conditioning (Figure 1-4) can account for individual variations in $\dot{V}o_2$ max.
B. Body size and muscle mass.
   1. Lean body tissue exerts the greatest influence on $\dot{V}o_2$ max when it is expressed in absolute terms (i.e., L/min).
      a. Because of the influence of muscle mass, large individuals generally have higher absolute levels of $\dot{V}o_2$ max.
      b. To more accurately compare individual fitness data, $\dot{V}o_2$ max should be expressed in mL of oxygen/kg body weight/minute.
      c. Increase in muscle mass recruitment (i.e., combined arm/leg exercise) will also raise somatic oxygen consumption.
   2. Arm versus leg exercise.
      a. At any given submaximal workload, heart rate, rate-pressure product (Figure 1-5), and $\dot{V}o_2$ are higher during arm exercise as compared with leg exercise.
      b. Arm crank ergometry generally approximates 64–80% of the maximal $\dot{V}o_2$ achieved during lower extremity exercise.
      c. A weak correlation exists in determining leg $\dot{V}o_2$ max from arm exercise, and vice versa.

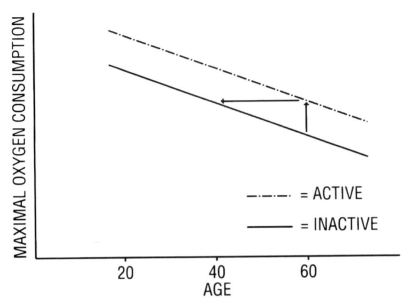

FIGURE 1-4   Influence of endurance exercise training on an inactive 60-year-old. The typical increase in maximal oxygen consumption (~20%) transforms the individual's aerobic fitness to what it was at the age of 40—corresponding to a 20-year functional rejuvenation.

C. Age and gender variables.
   1. Aging leads to a decline in aerobic capacity at an average rate of approximately 1% per year after age 20.
      a. Although $\dot{V}o_2$ max decreases as a result of biological aging, habitually sedentary individuals exhibit an accelerated deterioration in functional capacity.
      b. Following adolescence, $\dot{V}o_2$ max values in women are approximately 15–25% lower than those in men (Figure 1-6).
         i. This may be attributed to increased relative body fat, a lower stroke volume, reduced hemoglobin levels, decreased physical activity, or combinations thereof.
D. Physical conditioning.
   1. Regular physical exercise results in an estimated 10–25% increase in $\dot{V}o_2$ max values, due predominantly to increased stroke volume.
   2. $\dot{V}o_2$ max demonstrates a positive correlation with the intensity, frequency, and duration of physical activity.
   3. Nevertheless, the $\dot{V}o_2$ max is predominantly determined by genetic factors.

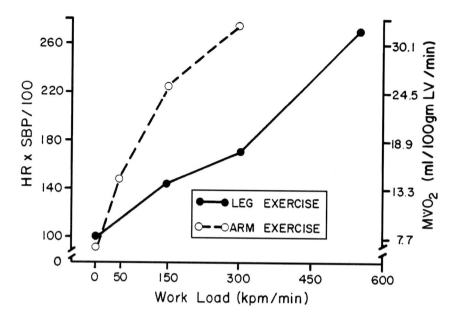

FIGURE 1-5 Rate-pressure product and estimated myocardial aerobic requirements (MVo_2) during submaximal arm and leg exercise. At any given workrate (kpm/min) the cardiac demands are considerably higher during arm exercise. Adapted from Schwade J, Blomqvist CG, Shapiro W. A comparison of the response to arm and leg work in patients with ischemic heart disease. Am Heart J 1977; 94:203–8.

Respiratory Exchange Ratio (RER)

A. Delineates the relative contribution from fat and carbohydrate utilized to provide energy (ATP) at rest and during exercise.

B. Derived from the volume of carbon dioxide expired per minute (Vco_2) divided by the amount of oxygen consumed during the same interval.

   1. $RER = Vco_2/\dot{V}o_2$.

C. RER values at rest.

   1. Carbohydrate utilization is signified by an RER of 1.0.

   2. The RER for fat approximates 0.7.

   3. Values that fall between 0.7 and 1.0 indicate a relative, proportional utilization of both fuel sources.

      a. Resting substrate utilization, when consuming a varied diet, typically approximates 0.83, indicating a homogenous mix of fat and carbohydrate contribution to energy production.

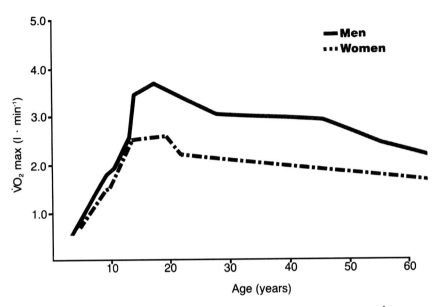

FIGURE 1-6 Influence of age on maximal oxygen consumption ($\dot{V}o_2$ max) in males and females. Before the age of 12, the values for boys and girls are comparable. A peak in $\dot{V}o_2$ max occurs between 15 and 20 years of age, followed by a gradual decline with advancing age. The average $\dot{V}o_2$ max of a 60-year-old adult is approximately 70% of the mean value at the age of 20. Adapted from Åstrand PO. *Health and Fitness*. Stockholm: Universaltryck; 1973: 12.

    4. Protein metabolism is associated with an RER of 0.8; however, protein is generally disregarded with respect to energy production.

D. RER values during exercise.

    1. Submaximal exercise.

        a. Fuel usage is largely determined by the percentage of maximal oxygen uptake that is employed.

        b. Carbohydrate utilization increases with incremental exercise intensity, thus raising the RER value.

    2. Maximal exercise.

        a. Carbon dioxide production exceeds oxygen consumption.

        b. RER values generally exceed 1.0, indicating exclusive carbohydrate usage.

        c. RER values ≥ 1.15 generally reflect a true maximal effort.

            i. RER values at maximal exercise have been found to range from 1.0 to 2.1.

            ii. In nonathletic individuals, peak values seldom exceed 1.30.

Anaerobic Threshold (AT)

A. The AT occurs with the onset of metabolic acidosis during exercise, traditionally determined by serial measurements of blood lactate.

B. Subsequent increases in the anaerobic production of energy or ATP occur, resulting in increased lactic acid accumulation.

    1. AT can also be estimated by observing the increase in ventilatory equivalent of oxygen ($V_E/\dot{V}O_2$) without a corresponding change in the ventilatory equivalent for carbon dioxide ($V_E/\dot{V}CO_2$).

        a. Accordingly, the AT is signified by the breakpoint in linearity for V_E or $\dot{V}CO_2$ (Figure 1-7).

    2. AT is typically expressed as a percentage of the maximal oxygen consumption.

        a. This percentage identifies the relative exercise intensity that can be maintained primarily via aerobic metabolism, minimizing the potential for lactic acid accumulation and the development of muscle fatigue.

        b. Common AT values.

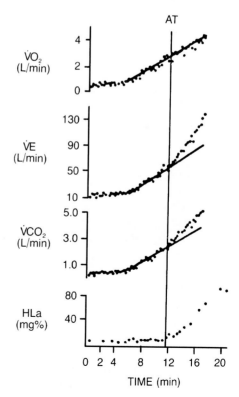

FIGURE 1-7 Relationship between intensity of exercise (oxygen consumption, $\dot{V}O_2$) and simultaneous, abrupt nonlinear increases in serum lactate (HLa), CO_2 production ($\dot{V}CO_2$), and minute ventilation (VE) occurring at the anaerobic threshold (AT). Modified from Figure 1 in Davis JA, Vodak P, Wilmore JH, et al. Anaerobic threshold and maximal aerobic power for three modes of exercise. *J Appl Physiol* 1976; 41:544–50.

    i. 55 ± 8% of $\dot{V}o_2$ max in sedentary persons.

    ii. 70 to 90% of $\dot{V}o_2$ max in aerobically trained individuals.

  c. The ability to maintain exercise at a high percentage of $\dot{V}o_2$ max (i.e., just below the AT) has been shown to be a better predictor of endurance performance than $\dot{V}o_2$ max.

FITNESS LEVELS FOR WINTER SPORT ATHLETES

Cross-Country Skiers and Biathletes

A. $\dot{V}o_2$ max values (mL/kg/min) in elite cross-country skiers are among the highest recorded (Figure 1-8).

B. Testing methods.

  1. Traditional performance evaluations have used treadmill or cycle ergometer testing.

  2. The perceived benefit of combined arm and leg testing in determining $\dot{V}o_2$ max has not been shown in recent investigations.

    a. Declines in $\dot{V}o_2$ max have been found when comparing combined arm and leg measurements to those determined from treadmill testing.

    b. Most investigations have shown no significant differences in $\dot{V}o_2$ max between testing methods.

    c. Recent investigations have determined a significant, inverse correlation ($r = -0.74$ to -0.79) between skiing performance time and upper body $\dot{V}o_2$ peak.

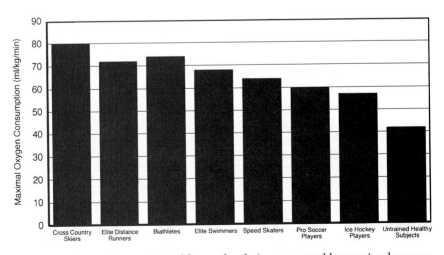

FIGURE 1-8 Comparison of fitness levels (as measured by maximal oxygen consumption) in various athletic groups versus untrained, healthy subjects.

  i. This may be attributed to the large upper body musculature involved in traditional skiing maneuvers, but not
  during treadmill testing.
 3. Field testing of $\dot{V}O_2$ peak utilizing roller skiing can be used to
 estimate the performance potential of skiers and biathletes.
  a. Values of $\dot{V}O_2$ max, expressed as $mL/kg^{2/3}/min$, have been
  found to be predictive of skiing performance.
C. In biathletes, significant additional aerobic requirements are
attributed to the associated rifle carriage.
 1. The relative percentage of body mass represented by the rifle
 weight during carriage has been shown to influence the percentage of $\dot{V}O_2$ peak achieved during testing.
 2. The percentage increase in $\dot{V}O_2$ peak is higher among women
 biathletes as the rifle comprises a greater percentage of their
 total body mass.

Speed Skaters

A. $\dot{V}O_2$ max in speed skaters has been reported to approximate
62–64 mL/kg/min when measured using both traditional treadmill
running and in-line skating protocols, respectively.
 1. In-line skating values are posture-dependent; however, there is
 a significant attenuation of $\dot{V}O_2$ max noted in the seated (speed
 skating) position.
  a. The lower $\dot{V}O_2$ max is believed to be due, at least in part, to
  the static sitting posture often employed during speed skating, which may decrease venous return and oxygen delivery,
  thus reducing the aerobic potential of the active muscles.
B. There is a significant negative correlation between $\dot{V}O_2$ max values
and speed-skating performance, particularly at the longer distances.
 1. $\dot{V}O_2$ max in the sitting position is highly negatively correlated
 with short-track speed-skating performance.

Ice Hockey Players

A. Ice hockey cannot be classified as a truly aerobic or anaerobic
sport, as the game is broken into multiple, short-duration exercise
bouts, often lasting 30 seconds to 2 minutes.
B. $\dot{V}O_2$ max values for well-trained ice hockey players have been
found to average 57 mL/kg/min.
 1. These values are lower (10–15%) than those traditionally
 observed in highly trained endurance athletes.

    a. Anaerobic capacity in ice hockey players is fairly high, approximating values found in sprinters and swimmers.

    b. $\dot{V}o_2$ max does not appear to be appreciably altered during high-volume seasonal practices, indicating that this training regimen does not further augment oxygen transport and utilization.

    c. On-ice performance in hockey players is more closely associated with the ability to work anaerobically rather than with $\dot{V}o_2$ max.

ALTITUDE TRAINING

Oxygen Saturation

A. Oxygen saturation is determined by the partial pressure of oxygen in ambient air.

B. The progressive decrease in barometric pressure with increased altitude causes a reduction in the partial pressure of oxygen, decreasing oxygen saturation.

Acute Physiological Responses to Altitude

A. Pulmonary ventilation increases at rest and during exercise.
    1. Due primarily to increases in tidal volume.
    2. Respiratory rates increase with prolonged exposure.
       a. Respiratory alkalosis causes a leftward shift of the oxygen-hemoglobin dissociation curve, increasing arterial oxygen saturation.

B. Supplemental increase in cardiac output is due primarily to increases in heart rate and stroke volume.

C. Blood oxygen saturation is directly related to altitude and exercise intensity.
    1. Desaturation that occurs with increasing exercise intensity is typically related to limited alveolar end capillary diffusion.
       a. This results in a linear decrease in maximal oxygen consumption at altitudes above 1524 m.

Physiological Adaptations to Long-Term Altitude Exposure

A. Acclimation occurs following days or weeks of altitude exposure leading to physiological changes to enhance functional status.
    1. Exercise ventilation rate stabilizes.
    2. Hematocrit levels increase by 4–12%.

   a. Due primarily to polycythemia resulting from a substantial increase in erythropoietin levels.
   b. Hematocrit (and blood viscosity) also increases due to decreases in plasma volume.
3. Stroke volume decreases, resulting in a concomitant reduction in cardiac output.
   a. The decrease in maximal stroke volume is attributed to:
      i. An increase in blood viscosity.
      ii. A decrease in venous return.
4. Heart rate remains elevated during submaximal exercise; however, chronic hypoxia tends to decrease the maximal heart rate.
5. Improvements in peripheral oxygen utilization may be secondary to enhanced capillary density and increased mitochondria and tissue myoglobin concentration.
B. Physiological adaptations acquired during acclimation are reversible upon return to sea level.

CARDIOVASCULAR RISK OF PHYSICAL EXERTION IN THE COLD

Reasons for Increased Risk

Increased risk for cardiovascular complications is attributed to structural cardiovascular abnormalities or underlying coronary artery disease and superimposed environmental stressors, associated cardiac and metabolic demands, and clothing.

A. Recent studies have shown that strenuous physical activity may precipitate acute cardiac events, especially in habitually sedentary individuals with known or occult coronary artery disease.
   1. Exercise-related cardiovascular complications may be triggered by:
      a. Abrupt increases in heart rate and blood pressure.
      b. Coronary artery spasm.
      c. Plaque rupture causing thrombus formation.
   2. The risk of myocardial ischemia:
      a. May be elevated during or immediately after physical exertion, especially when considering:
         i. The potential for venous pooling.
         ii. The abrupt initiation and cessation of exercise.
         iii. Decreased coronary perfusion.
      b. Increases the likelihood of malignant ventricular arrhythmias, including ventricular tachycardia and fibrillation.

Snow Shoveling

A. Significant cardiovascular risk is associated with a single bout of snow shoveling, likely due to the associated increases in cardiorespiratory and hemodynamic responses in the presence of underlying coronary artery disease.

   1. Somatic oxygen consumption increases only moderately during snow shoveling.

   2. Snow shoveling causes significant increases in heart rate, systolic blood pressure, and rate-pressure product, often rivaling those reported during maximal treadmill exercise testing (Table 1-4).

      a. Heart rate reaches the upper limit of prescribed exercise (85% of maximum heart rate) within 2 minutes of snow shoveling.

      b. Heart rate fails to plateau with increasing work.

      c. Aerobic fitness is inversely related to heart rate during shoveling.

         i. Persons with higher fitness levels demonstrate a more attenuated heart rate response.

   3. Five physiologic factors contribute to the demands placed on the heart.

TABLE 1-4

Cardiorespiratory measurements during treadmill testing and snow shoveling (mean ± SD).

Variable	Treadmill Testing	Snow Shoveling*
Heart rate (beats/min)	179 ± 17	175 ± 15
Systolic blood pressure (mm Hg)	181 ± 25	198 ± 17
Rate-pressure product (mm Hg × beats/min × 10^{-2})	322 ± 40	342 ± 34
Oxygen consumption (METs)[‡]	9.3 ± 1.8[†]	5.7 ± 0.8
Rating of perceived exertion (6–20 scale)	17.9 ± 1.5	16.7 ± 1.7

* Shoveling rates were self-paced and averaged 12 ± 2 loads/min during a 10-minute bout of work.

[†] $p < 0.003$ versus snow shoveling.

[‡] METs = metabolic equivalents: 1 MET = 3.5 mL/kg/min.

Adapted from Franklin et al., 1995.

    a. Arm exercise is less efficient when compared with leg exercise.
    b. Upright exercise combined with little or no leg movement may fail to adequately promote venous return to the heart.
    c. Isometric exertion is an integral component of the activity.
    d. Valsalva maneuver (expiratory strain) is often performed during the act of lifting and throwing the snow.
    e. Exposure to the environment, including the inhalation of cold air.

4. Snow shoveling during the early morning hours may be compounded by circadian surges, heightening the risk of cardiovascular events.
    a. Catecholamine levels.
    b. Blood pressure.
    c. Platelet aggregability.

The Effects of Windchill

The evaluation of cold during outdoor activity in the winter months should consider more than ambient temperature alone.

A. Wind augments heat loss (see Table 3-2), increasing the body's capacity to cool itself.

B. Exercising into the wind increases the effective cooling in direct proportion to the velocity at which the exerciser is moving; in contrast, a hind wind decreases the direct effects of the wind velocity.

Suggested Readings

Andersen KL, Shephard RJ, Denolin H, et al. *Fundamentals of Exercise Testing.* Belgium: World Health Organization; 1971:16.

Åstrand PO, Rodahl K. *Textbook of Work Physiology: Physiological Bases of Exercise.* Chicago: McGraw-Hill; 1986.

Åstrand PO, Saltin B. Maximal oxygen uptake and heart rate in various types of muscle activity. *J Appl Physiol* 1961; 16:977–81.

Åstrand PO. Exercise physiology and its role in disease prevention and in rehabilitation. *Arch Phys Med Rehabil* 1987; 68:305–9.

Bar-Or O, Zwiren LD. Maximal oxygen consumption test during arm exercise: Reliability and validity. *J Appl Physiol* 1975; 38:424–26.

Berg U, Forsberg A. Influence of body mass on cross-country ski racing performance. *Med Sci Sports Exerc* 1992; 24:1033–39.

Berg U, Kanstrup IL, Ekblom B. Maximal oxygen uptake during exercise with various combinations of arm and leg work. *J Appl Physiol* 1976; 41:191–96.

Berg U. The influence of body mass in cross-country skiing. *Med Sci Sports Exerc* 1987; 19:324–31.

Berglund B. High-altitude training: Aspects of hematological adaptation. *Sports Med* 1992; 14:289–303.

Bigard AX, Brunet A, Guezennec CY, et al. Skeletal muscle changes after endurance training at high altitude. *J Appl Physiol* 1991; 71:2114–21.

Blackie SP, Fairbarn MS, McElvaney NG, et al. Normal values and ranges for ventilation and breathing pattern at maximal exercise. *Chest* 1991; 100:136–42.

Bruce RA, Kusumi F, Hosmer D. Maximal oxygen intake and nomographic assessment of functional aerobic impairment in cardiovascular disease. *Am Heart J* 1973; 85:546–62.

Bruce RA. Principles of exercise testing. In: Naughton JP, Hellerstein HK, Mohler IC, eds. *Exercise Testing and Exercise Training in Coronary Heart Disease.* New York: Academic Press; 1973:53.

Buskirk E, Taylor HL. Maximal oxygen consumption, with special reference to chronic physical activity and obesity. *J Appl Physiol* 1957; 2:72–78.

Buskirk ER, Kollias J, Akers RF, et al. Maximal performance at altitude and on return from altitude in conditioned runners. *J Appl Physiol* 1967; 23: 259–66.

Consolazio CF, Johnson RE, Pecora LJ. *Physiological Measurements of Metabolic Functions in Man.* New York: McGraw-Hill; 1963.

Costill DL, Thomason H, Roberts E. Fractional utilization of the aerobic capacity during distance running. *Med Sci Sports* 1973; 5:248–52.

Costill DL. Physiology of marathon running. *JAMA* 1972; 221:1024–29.

Daub WB, Green HJ, Houston ME, et al. Specificity of physiologic adaptations resulting from ice-hockey training. *Med Sci Sports Exerc* 1983; 15:290–94.

Davis JA, Frank MH, Whipp BJ, et al. Anaerobic threshold alterations caused by endurance training in middle-aged men. *J Appl Physiol: Respirat Environ Exercise Physiol* 1979; 46:1039–46.

Davis JA, Vodak P, Wilmore JH, et al. Anaerobic threshold and maximal aerobic power for three modes of exercise. *J Appl Physiol* 1976; 41:544–50.

DeBoer RW, Ettema GC, Faessen BM, et al. Specific characteristics of speed skating: Implications for summer training. *Med Sci Sports Exerc* 1987; 19:504–10.

Degroot G, Van Ingen Schenau GJ, DeBoer RW. Evaluation of speed skating capacity on the basis of tests. In: Rispens P and Lamberts R, eds. *Physiological, Biomechanical, and Technical Aspects of Speed Skating.* Gronigen: Private Press; 1985:39–48.

Dehn MM, Bruce RA. Longitudinal variations in maximal oxygen intake with age and activity. *J Appl Physiol* 1972; 33:805–7.

DeVries HA. *Physiology of Exercise,* 3rd ed. Dubuque: William C Brown Publishers; 1980.

Foster C, Thompson NN, Snyder AC. Ergometric studies with speed skaters: Evolution of laboratory methods. *J Strength Cond Res* 1993; 7:193–200.

Franklin BA, Gordon S, Timmis GC. Fundamentals of exercise physiology: Implications for exercise testing and prescription. In: Franklin BA, Gordon S, Timmis GC, eds. *Exercise in Modern Medicine.* Baltimore: Williams and Wilkins; 1989:10.

Franklin BA, Hogan P, Bonzheim K, et al. Cardiac demands of heavy snow shoveling. *JAMA* 1995; 273:880–82.

Franklin BA, Kaimal KP, Moir TW, et al. Characteristics of national-class race walkers. *Phys Sportsmed* 1981; 9:101–9.

Franklin BA, Vander L, Wrisley D, et al. Aerobic requirements of arm ergometry: Implications for exercise testing and training. *Phys Sportsmed* 1983; 11:81–90.

Franklin BA, Wrisley D, Johnson S, et al. Chronic adaptations to physical conditioning in cardiac patients: Implications regarding exercise trainability. In: Franklin BA, Rubenfire M, eds. *Cardiac Rehabilitation (Clinics in Sports Medicine)*. Philadelphia: WB Saunders; 1984:495.

Franklin BA. Heart smart: To shovel or not to shovel? In: *Encyclopedia Britannica, Medical and Health Annual*. Chicago: Encyclopedia Britannica, Inc; 1997:192–96.

Franklin BA. Normal cardiorespiratory responses to acute aerobic exercise. In: Roitman JL, ed. *ACSM's Resource Manual for Guidelines for Exercise Testing and Prescription*, 4th ed. Baltimore: Lippincott Williams & Wilkins; 2001:144.

Franklin BA. Snow shoveling: A potentially hazardous winter workout. *Amer J Med and Sports* 2001; 3:339–42.

Franklin BA. Exercise testing, training, and arm ergometry. *Sportsmed* 1985; 2:100–19.

Geysel JM, Bomhoff G, Van Velzen G, et al. Bicycle ergometry and speed skating performance. *Int J Sports Med* 1984; 5:241–45.

Giri S, Thompson PD, Kiernan FJ, et al. Clinical and angiographic characteristics of exertion-related acute myocardial infarction. *JAMA* 1999; 282:1731–36.

Havenith G, Holewijn M. Exercise and the environment: Altitude and air pollution. In: Roitman JL, ed. *ACSM's Resource Manual for Guidelines for Exercise Testing and Prescription*, 4th ed. Baltimore: Lippincott Williams & Wilkins; 2001:217.

Ingjer F. Maximal oxygen uptake as a predictor of performance ability in women and men elite cross-country skiers. *Scand J Med Sci Sports* 1991; 1:25–30.

Issekutz B, Birkhead NC, Rodahl K. Use of respiratory quotients in assessment of aerobic work capacity. *J Appl Physiol* 1962; 17:47–50.

Issekutz B, Rodahl K. Respiratory quotient during exercise. *J Appl Physiology* 1961; 16:606–10.

Johnson BD, Saupe KW, Dempsey JA. Mechanical constraints on exercise in hyperpnea in endurance athletes. *J Appl Physiol* 1992; 73:874–86.

Kelly JM. Physiology of cross-country skiing. In: Casey MJ, Foster C, Hixson EG, eds. *Winter Sports Medicine*. Philadelphia: FA Davis; 1991:277–83.

Mahood NV, Kenefick RW, Kertzer R, et al. Physiological determinants of cross-country ski racing performance. *Med Sci Sports Exerc* 2001; 33:1379–84.

McArdle WD, Katch FI, Katch VL. *Exercise Physiology: Energy, Nutrition, and Human Performance*, 4th ed. Philadelphia: Lea & Febiger; 1996.

Millerhagen JO, Kelly M, Murphy RJ. A study of combined arm and leg exercise with application to Nordic skiing. *Can J Appl Sport Sci* 1983; 8:92–97.

Minkoff J. Evaluating parameters of a professional hockey team. *Am J Sports Med* 1982; 10:285–92.

Mitchell JH, Blomqvist G. Maximal oxygen uptake. *N Engl J Med* 1971; 284:1018–22.

Mitchell JH, Sproule BJ, Chapman CB. The physiological meaning of the maximal oxygen intake test. *J Clin Invest* 1958; 37:538–47.

Mittleman MA, Maclure M, Tofler GH, et al. Triggering of acute myocardial infarction by heavy physical exertion. *N Engl J Med* 1993; 329:1677–83.

Myers J, Buchanan N, Smith D, et al. Individual ramp treadmill: Observations on a new protocol. *Chest* 1992; 101:236S–241S.

Myers J, Buchanan N, Walsh D, et al. Comparison of the ramp versus standard exercise protocols. *J Am Coll Cardiol* 1991; 17:1334–42.

Niinimaa V, Shephard RJ, Dyon M. Determinations of performance and mechanical efficiency in Nordic skiing. *Br J Sports Med* 1979; 13:62–65.

Novich MM. Research in the physiology of exercise and sports. *J Med Soc NJ* 1985; 82:295–99.

Poliner LR, Dehmer GJ, Lewis SE, et al. Left ventricular performance in normal subjects: A comparison of the responses to exercise in the upright and supine position. *Circulation* 1980; 62:528–34.

Richardson PD, Davies MJ, Born GV. Influence of plaque configuration and stress distribution on fissuring of coronary atherosclerotic plaques. *Lancet* 1989; 2:941–44.

Rowell LB. Circulation. *Med Sci Sports* 1969; 1:15–22.

Rundell KW, Szmedra L. Energy cost of rifle carriage in biathlon skiing. *Med Sci Sports Exerc* 1998; 30:570–76.

Rundell KW. Compromised oxygen uptake in speed skaters during treadmill in-line skating. *Med Sci Sports Exerc* 1996; 28:120–27.

Rundell KW. Treadmill roller ski test predicts biathlon roller ski race results of elite U.S. biathlon women. *Med Sci Sports Exerc* 1995; 27:1677–85.

Savard GK, Areskog NH, Saltin B. Cardiovascular response to exercise in humans following acclimatization to extreme altitude. *Acta Physiol Scand* 1995; 154:499–509.

Shephard RJ. *Endurance Fitness*. Toronto: University of Toronto Press; 1969.

Sim FH, Simonet WT, Melton LJ, et al. Ice hockey injuries. *Am J Sports Med* 1987; 15:30–40.

Snyder AC, Foster C. Physiology and nutrition for skating. In: Lamb DR, Knuttgen HG, Murray R, eds. *Perspectives in Exercise Science and Sports Medicine*, Vol 7. Carmel: Cooper Publishing Group; 1994:181–219.

Staib JL, Im J, Caldwell Z, et al. Cross-country ski racing performance predicted by aerobic and anaerobic double poling power. *J Strength Cond Res* 2000; 14:282–88.

Taylor HL, Buskirk E, Henschel A. Maximal oxygen intake as an objective measure of cardiorespiratory performance. *J Appl Physiol* 1955; 8:73–80.

Thompson PD. The cardiovascular complications of vigorous physical activity. *Arch Intern Med* 1996; 156:2297–2302.

Von Dobeln W. Human standard and maximal metabolic rate in relation to fat-free body mass. *Acta Physiol Scand* 1956; 37:126S.

Willich SN, Lewis M, Lowel H, et al. Physical exertion as a trigger of acute myocardial infarction. *N Engl J Med* 1993; 329:1684–90.

Willich SN, Maclure M, Mittleman MA, et al. Sudden cardiac death: Support for a role of triggering in causation. *Circulation* 1993; 87:1442–50.

Wilmore JH, Norton AC. *The Heart and Lungs at Work: A Primer of Exercise Physiology*. Schiller Park: Beckman Instruments; 1973:2.

Young A, Young PA, Young AJ, et al. Human acclimatization to high terrestrial altitude. In: Pandolf KB, Sawka MN, Gonzalez RR, eds. *Human Performance Physiology and Environmental Medicine at Terrestrial Extremes*. Indianapolis: Benchmark; 1988:497–545.

2

PULMONARY PATHOPHYSIOLOGY

Kenneth W. Rundell

OVERVIEW

Airway Hyperreactivity and Chronic Inflammation

These are the most common airway dysfunctions among cold-weather athletes.

Exercise-Induced Bronchospasm (EIB)

A. Refers to the hyperreactive response of the airways to the stimulus of exercise; describes the transient narrowing of the airways that occurs most often after vigorous exercise, but sometimes during exercise.

  1. Flow limitation is typically measured by spirometry.
   a. A common diagnostic procedure is to compare pre- and post-measurements of maximal expiratory flows (Figure 2-1).
   b. A $\geq 10\%$ post-exercise fall in forced expiratory volume in the first second of an exhalation maneuver (FEV_1) is the "gold standard for diagnosis of EIB."
   c. Post-exercise falls in forced vital capacity (FVC), mid-expiratory flows ($FEF_{25-75\%}$, $FEF_{50\%}$), and peak expiratory flow (PEF) are also used.

  2. Symptoms.
   a. Cough, wheeze, shortness of breath, chest tightness, excess mucus, and climate-related performance issues.

  3. History of allergies and seasonal variation in symptom presentation.

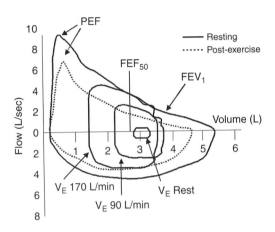

FIGURE 2-1 Flow-volume loops showing resting (baseline) and post-exercise maximal maneuvers of an individual with hyperreactive airways. Tidal volume loops at maximal exercise, at anaerobic threshold exercise, and at rest are shown. Note the overlap of the exercising tidal volumes on the maximal flow-volume loops, indicating exercise flow limitation.

   4. Disease chronicity.
      a. Chronic cough.
      b. Night symptoms.
   5. Edema.
   6. Mucous plug formation.
   7. Airway wall remodeling.
B. Complex multifaceted airway dysfunction that is multimediated.
C. Prevalent in the cold-weather athlete population.
D. EIB is more prevalent than asthma, but occurs in upward of 90% of asthmatics.
E. Other terms used to describe EIB.
   1. Airway hyperreactivity (AHR).
   2. Exercise-induced asthma (EIA).
   3. Cold-induced asthma.
   4. Skier asthma.
   5. Skier cough.
   6. Hockey hack.

Chronic Inflammation in Cold-Weather Athletes

A. Is it really asthma?
B. Chronic asthma-like condition in otherwise healthy athletes.
C. May result from prolonged high ventilation of cold, dry air or air pollutants (from volatized fluorocarbons in waxing rooms or exhaust from ice resurfacing machines in ice arenas).
D. Evidence that airway wall remodeling found in cold-weather athletes is pathologically different from asthma.

1. May or may not present symptoms.
2. Remodeling may or may not respond to pharmacological intervention.
3. Cellular profiles are different from those of frank asthmatics.

Other Respiratory Disorders of the Cold-Weather Athlete

A. Upper respiratory tract viral infections.
B. Reflex tracheal smooth-muscle contraction evoked by airway cooling.
C. Vocal cord dysfunction.

PREVALENCE OF AIRWAY DYSFUNCTION IN COLD-WEATHER ATHLETES

Asthma Prevalence

A. Probably 10–12% in the United States (not different from that found in the general population).

EIB Prevalence

A. 50–90% of all asthmatics are hyperresponsive to exercise (EIB+).
B. Estimates for EIB in the general population are 4–20%.
C. 8–20% of warm-weather athletes are estimated to suffer from EIB.
   1. 11% of 1984 U.S. Summer Olympians were found EIB+ by survey at Olympic athlete processing.
   2. 17% of 1996 U.S. Summer Olympians were identified as EIB+ by survey at Olympic athlete processing.
D. 11–50% of cold-weather athletic populations have been identified as EIB+ by various researchers.
E. Overall, across 1998 U.S. Winter Olympians, about 25% of the athletes were EIB+.
   1. 28% of the 1998 U.S. Winter Olympians were identified as EIB+ by survey at Olympic athlete processing.
   2. 23% of the 1998 U.S. Winter Olympians were found to suffer from EIB, measured by quantitative spirometry prior to the Nagano Olympic Games.
F. Nordic skiers 30–50% by various research groups.
G. U.S. short-track speed skaters: 43%.
H. U.S. figure skaters: 30–40%.
   1. Mannix et al. (1996): N = 124; 35%.
   2. Provost-Craig et al. (1996): N = 100; 30%.

I. U.S. ice hockey players: 20–35%.
  1. Judelson et al. (2001): N = 64, U.S. National Team men and women; 20%.
  2. Rundell (2003): N = 22, 2002 Olympic Team women; 32%.

Vocal Cord Dysfunction

A. Female-predominance
B. Rundell and Spiering (2003): N = 370, 174 females, 196 males.
  1. 5.1% VCD positive by presence of inspiratory stridor.
    a. 18 females (10.3%) and 1 male (0.5%).
  2. EIB was comorbid with 10 (53%) of VCD positive athletes.
  3. 8 of 9 VCD+/EIB– athletes were previously misdiagnosed as EIB+ and treated with a β_2 agonist.

AIRWAY FUNCTION DURING AND AFTER EXERCISE

Bronchodilation and Bronchoconstriction during Exercise

A. Normal response during exercise in meeting the demands for oxygen by the working muscle.
B. Airways of asthmatics and individuals with EIB:
  1. Show variable response during exercise and in part response depends on the type of exercise.
    a. Interval type exercise appears to affect the dilatory status of exercise more than ramp or steady state exercise (Figure 2-2).
    b. A simulated cross-country ski race demonstrated individual variability in airway response during exercise (Figure 2-3).
  2. Some individuals bronchodilate normally during exercise but bronchoconstrict after exercise.
  3. Others brochoconstrict during exercise.
C. Control of airway function during exercise.
  1. Mechanisms proposed for the improved airway function during exercise.
    a. Reduction in airway temperature inhibits bronchoconstricting mediator release in dogs.
    b. Bronchodilating mediator.
      i. Prostaglandin PGE_2 causes bronchodilation and is released by airway mast cells and epithelial cells.
    c. Circulating catecholamines are unlikely candidates for bronchodilation mediation.

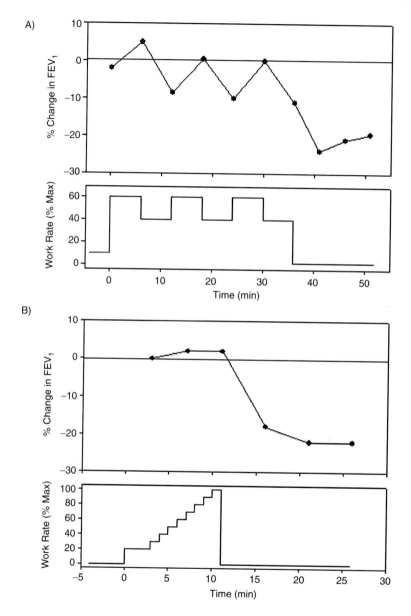

FIGURE 2-2 Changes in FEV_1 during interval (A) and progressive incremental exercise to maximum (B). Note the dynamic flow during interval exercise and the progressive bronchodilation during progressive exercise. Redrawn from Beck et al. (1994).

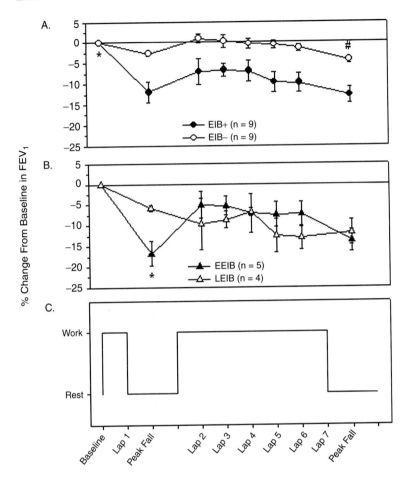

FIGURE 2-3 Airway response (FEV_1) during a simulated cross-country ski race by EIB+ and normal athletes (A). EIB+ athletes could be divided into early (EEIB) responders, those who were hyperreactive within 15 minutes after the first lap, and late (LEIB) responders, those who were hyperreactive during or after laps 2–7. Redrawn from Rundell et al. (2003).

 d. Withdrawal of vagal tone during exercise should relax airway smooth muscle, but research has shown it is not important to exercise bronchodilation.

 e. Mechanical balance between bronchoconstriction and bronchodilation can be altered rapidly by exercise intensity.

  i. Suggests that the interaction between airways and lung connective tissue keeps airways open.

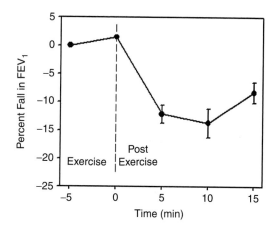

FIGURE 2-4 The typical EIB response to exercise is defined by a maximal fall in FEV_1 5–15 minutes after the cessation of exercise.

    ii. Bronchodilator influence (of exercise) is proportional to minute ventilation (e.g., greater VE = greater dilation), which provides support for this concept.

Bronchoconstriction after Exercise

A. EIB or EIA refers to a transient airway narrowing after vigorous exercise (Figure 2-4).
    1. EIB is used as a descriptor in individuals without a clinical diagnosis of asthma but who demonstrate bronchoconstriction from exercise.
    2. EIA is used to describe the post-exercise occurrence of airway narrowing in asthmatics.
    3. These definitions are quantitatively defined by a reduction in lung function and not on the basis of symptoms.
B. Symptoms may or may not accompany the bronchoconstriction.
C. Physiological changes that can accompany the airway narrowing of EIB include:
    1. Arterial hypoxemia.
    2. Gas trapping.
    3. Hyperinflation.
    4. These imply small airway involvement.
D. The response usually reaches peak between 5 and 20 minutes after exercise is stopped and generally spontaneously resolves within an hour or is reversed within minutes by administration of a β_2-receptor agonist.

EIB: PATHOPHYSIOLOGY

Symptoms Are the Tip of the Iceberg

A. May reflect airway inflammation or airway wall remodeling.

Severity of EIB

A. The major determinant is the level of ventilation reached and sustained during exercise and the water content of the inspired air.
  1. Cold air is dry air.
B. Airborne pollutants and allergens also play a role in initiation and severity of the hyperreactive response.
  1. Volatized fluorocarbons in ski wax rooms have been found to cause airway inflammation and hyperreactivity.
  2. CO, NO_2, and ultrafine and fine particulate matter (PM_1) are emitted at high levels from ice resurfacing machines in indoor ice rinks and are suspect in the high prevalence of airway dysfunction in ice rink athletes.
  3. Indoor allergens, either in the home or in the indoor training facility, may be responsible for airway dysfunction.
C. The presence of inflammatory cells in the airway mucosa is reflected in the severity of the response.
  1. Mast cells, eosinophils, macrophages, epithelial cells, and sensory nerves release inflammatory mediators.
    a. Histamine, leukotrienes, prostaglandins, neuropeptides.
    b. Other products of cyclooxygenation of arachidonic acid.

Mechanism of EIB

A. The stimulus is thought to result from the conditioning of inspired air.
B. Inspired air is heated and humidified to 37°C, 99% RH.
C. Warming and humidifying large volumes of air in relatively short periods (e.g., exercising at high ventilation rates in cold, dry air) is thought to dry airways, changing osmolarity in resident cells.
  1. This in turn leads to a cascade of inflammatory events in susceptible individuals.
D. Breathing room temperature air at 30% RH, 60 L/min would require 10–12 generations of airways to fully condition the air.
  1. Since each liter of air requires ~ 44 mg of water to humidify at body temperature, the 1 mL of water that is available from the airway surface would be used quickly if not replenished, even

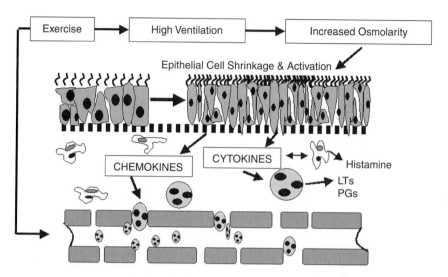

FIGURE 2-5 The high ventilation rates of exercise combined with cold/dry air remove water from the airway surface liquid, causing shrinkage of epithelial cells, increased osmolarity, and release of chemokines and cytokines. This results in an infiltration of inflammatory cells to the airways and release of inflammatory mediators.

    though it is thought that 70% of the water for conditioning comes from above the pharynx.
    a. Note that the burning throat sensation when breathing hot, dry air results because hot air requires immediate humidification, and this process occurs in the upper airways.
  2. The humidification process is thought to cause a change in resident cell osmolarity that results in the initiation of mediator release (Figure 2-5).
E. The osmotic theory.
  1. Water loss occurs through epithelium and mucosa during the conditioning of inspired air.
    a. This results in a change in osmolarity, pH, and temperature.
    b. Subsequently, resident cells are activated and release cytokines and chemokines.
    c. This causes an influx of proinflammatory cells that are poised for the release of mediators and proinflammatory cytokines.
  2. The influx of water to restore osmolarity when ventilation (exercise intensity) is reduced is thought to stimulate the release of inflammatory mediators.

    a. Mediators act by causing bronchial smooth-muscle constriction, mucus formation, and/or edema.

  3. The remodeling of the subepithelial basement membrane identified in cross-country skiers and asthmatics diminishes the capacity to respond to airway surface water loss.

    a. This results in recruitment of the deeper airways for the humidification process and enhances the hyperreactive response.

  4. No scientific evidence to reject the osmotic theory.

    a. Airways of asthmatics (but not normals) are very responsive to changes in airway osmolarity.

    b. The response to osmotic stimuli is inhibited by mast cell stabilizers and leukotriene antagonists.

F. The respiratory heat exchange theory.

  1. EIB results from heat transfer from bronchiolar blood vessels.

    a. A rapid temperature swing in the airways after stopping exercise stimulates a reactive hyperemia, which causes airway narrowing.

      i. The time course of this "fits" pulmonary function data.

    b. However, this is unlikely to be a universal theory.

      i. It does not explain the bronchoconstriction reversal by β_2 agonists, or the prevention of EIB by mast cell stabilizing drugs.

    c. However, cold air should enhance airway dehydration such that the osmotic stimulus is more widespread.

Airway Cells Involved in EIB

A. Mast cells, T-lymphocytes, macrophages, neutrophils, and eosinophils have all been associated with EIB.

B. However, these cells may only be markers of chronic inflammation or result from exercise (e.g., elevated neutrophil counts) and have no direct relationship to acute EIB.

C. Some studies have shown high mast cell counts with normal neutrophil and eosinophil counts.

D. Others report elevated neutrophil and eosinophil counts with normal mast cell counts.

E. Exposure to chemical pollutants has been shown to cause elevated neutrophils and eosinophils.

F. Mast cells are probably important in EIB pathology since mediator release occurs in immunoglobulin (Ig)E-allergen-induced and in non-IgE-dependent stimulation (cold air). Important in non-atopic EIB.

G. Eosinophils are important in the pathogenesis of EIB in the asthmatic, but little evidence supports a role of eosinophil involvement in EIB in non-asthmatics.
  1. However, eosinophils are likely involved in chronic inflammation but do not contribute directly to the acute EIB exacerbation.
     a. The time course of eosinophilic inflammatory expression is several hours after a stimulus.

Mediators Involved in EIB

A. Evidence supports mast cell release of histamine, cysteinyl leukotrienes, and prostaglandins following exercise.
B. Histamine has been implicated as a marker of mast cell activation and EIB.
  1. Histamine H_1-receptor antagonists have shown 24–56% protection against EIB.
     a. Terfenadine decreased hyperreactivity by 24, 44, and 56% for exercise, hyperventilation, and hypertonic saline challenges, respectively.
     b. This suggests that the exercise response may be less histamine-dependent than surrogate challenges and implicates multiple mediator involvement in EIB.
C. Leukotriene (LT) involvement in EIB exacerbation has received much attention.
  1. LTs are formed via the 5-lipoxygenase pathway of arachidonic acid breakdown.
  2. LTs have been found to be 100 to 1000 times more potent than histamine.
  3. LT–receptor antagonists and 5-lipoxygenase inhibitors have been found to be 0–100% effective (median ~ 50%) in preventing EIB; again, suggestive of multiple mediators (Figure 2-6).
D. Products of arachidonic acid cyclooxygenation.
  1. PGD_2 and thromboxane $(Tx)A_2$ are potent bronchoconstrictors.
  2. Cyclooxygenase inhibition has been shown to be ~ 30% protective.
E. Current evidence supports multiple mediators in the pathogenesis of EIB.
  1. The inability of single antagonist therapy to completely inhibit EIB and the individual variability in single drug treatment response support this concept.

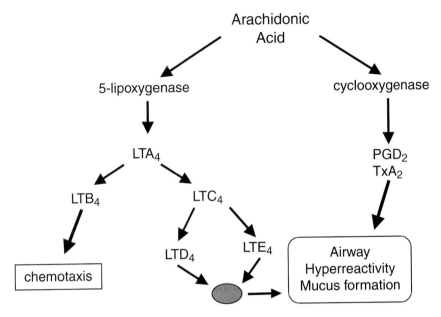

FIGURE 2-6 The breakdown of arachidonic acid forms leukotrienes and prostanoids involved in airway hyperreactivity. LTB_4 is a chemokine that may be involved in inflammatory cell infiltration to the airways. LTC_4, LTD_4, PGD_2, and TxA_2 are potent bronchoconstrictors.

DIAGNOSIS OF AIRWAY DYSFUNCTION IN COLD-WEATHER ATHLETES

Diagnosis should be based upon an objective measurement of reversible airflow obstruction with an appropriate EIB-provoking challenge.

Diagnosis Should Include Medical History

A. Detail symptoms.
  1. Observable clinical symptoms.
    a. Cough.
    b. Wheeze.
    c. Dyspnea.
    d. Excess mucus.
  2. Symptoms history should include instigating ambient conditions, exercise conditions, exercise mode, and frequency of EIB episodes.

   3. Performance-related symptoms.
      a. Climate- or seasonal-related symptoms and performance.
      b. Mismatch between performance and level of conditioning.
      c. Feeling of being out of shape or having "heavy legs."
   4. Symptoms-based diagnosis: See Symptoms-Based Diagnosis.
B. Individual and familial history of asthma or asthma-like symptoms.
C. Degree of exposure to environmental factors that might contribute to the severity of EIB or airway inflammation.
   1. Wax room exposure, internal combustion pollutants in the ice rink or urban environment, or mold or other allergens.
D. Sport patient participates in.
E. Exposure to tobacco smoke.

Diagnosis Should Include Physical Examination

A. Physical examination of an athlete with EIB often reveals a normal respiratory tract when the athlete is at rest.
B. However, with chronic inflammation the lower respiratory tract may show a prolonged expiratory phase and wheezing or coughing with inspiration.
C. Nasal passages should be thoroughly examined for inflammation, congestion, and nasal drainage to the pharynx.

Differential Diagnosis

A. Foreign bodies.
B. Respiratory infection.
C. Heart disease.
D. Paroxysmal atrial tachycardia (PAT).
E. Chronic obstructive pulmonary disease (COPD).
F. Gastroesophageal reflux disease (GERD).
G. Vocal cord dysfunction (VCD).
   1. Paradoxical closure of vocal cords especially during inspiration.
   2. Female preponderence (~10% female endurance athletes).
   3. Difficult to confirm diagnosis.
      a. May have flattened or truncated inspiratory loop during spirometry when symptomatic.
      b. May have post-exercise reduction in FVC when symptomatic.
   4. Often misdiagnosed as EIB.

    5. Symptoms include:
       a. A high-pitched inspiratory wheeze (stridor) during exercise.
       b. A feeling of throat tightness.
       c. Associated with psychologically stressful events such as hard workouts or competition.
       d. Highly variable and difficult to reproduce.
       e. Typically resolves within a couple of minutes after stopping the exercise bout.

Symptoms-Based Diagnosis

A. Symptoms are diverse and varied.
B. Some complain of symptoms (see Diagnosis Should Include Medical History.).
C. Others identify worsening problems with environmental exposure to allergens, pollutants, cold and/or dry air, and changes in weather.
D. Self-reported symptoms (Table 2-1) are unreliable: low sensitivity and specificity.
E. Be suspicious of a self-reported wheeze.
    1. Determine whether it occurs during exercise and whether it resolves quickly upon exercise cessation. If so, suspect VCD (see Differential Diagnosis, G).

Pulmonary Function Testing (PFT)

A. All pulmonary function maneuvers should follow this procedure:
    1. Three normal tidal volume breaths.

TABLE 2-1

Self-reported symptoms have been shown not to be of diagnostic value in and of themselves. Rundell et al. (2001) demonstrated that when compared to spirometry-based post-exercise fall in FEV$_1$, self-reported symptoms were not much better than a coin toss in making a diagnosis.

Symptom	Proportion of True Diagnosis	Sensitivity	Specificity
Cough	0.66	0.61	0.69
Wheeze	0.61	0.17	0.82
Chest tightness	0.63	0.20	0.83
Excess mucus	0.65	0.22	0.85

2. A maximal inhalation followed by a forced maximal exhalation lasting at least 6 seconds.
3. Concluding with a second maximal inhalation.
4. The best of three PFT maneuvers based on forced vital capacity and forced expiratory volume in 1 second (FEV_1) should be used as baseline (resting) values for analysis.
5. After baseline spirometry values are established, subjects then perform the designated provocation challenge, followed by PFT maneuvers at 5, 10, and 15 minutes post-exercise.

B. The following spirometric measures should be analyzed:
1. Forced vital capacity (FVC).
2. FEV_1.
3. Forced expiratory flow between 25% and 75% of FVC (FEF_{25-75}).
4. Forced expiratory flow at 50% of FVC (FEF_{50}).
5. Peak expiratory flow (PEF).
6. FEV_1/FVC.
7. FEF_{50}/FVC.

C. Postchallenge falls in pulmonary functions should be determined by subtracting each postchallenge PFT value from the best of three prechallenge baseline values and dividing by baseline values.
1. Falls $\geq$ 10% in FEV_1 at any point postchallenge should be considered EIB positive (EIB+).
2. Subjects who do not meet this cutoff are grouped as normal (EIB–).

D. Resting spirometry.
1. Abnormally low resting spirometry may reflect a state of chronic inflammation or airway remodeling (Table 2-2).
2. Chronic exposure to air pollutants may result in low resting baseline measurements.
   a. Especially mid-expiratory flow rates (e.g., FEF_{50}, FEF_{25-75}).

TABLE 2-2

Interpretation of resting spirometric measurements. Cutoff criteria presented as percent of predicted values.

	FVC	FEV_1	FEV_1/FVC	FEF_{25-75}
Normal	> 80	> 80	> 70	> 67
Mild obstruction	66–80	66–80	60–70	50–67
Marked obstruction	< 66	< 66	< 60	< 50

Protocols and Challenges for Provoking EIB

A. Four primary challenge categories: pharmacological, osmotic, hyperventilation, and exercise.

B. Pharmacological challenges.
1. Typically used to define the presence of asthma.
2. May not be sensitive or specific to EIB.
3. Increased doses, followed by PFTs until an upper-limit dose or cutoff criteria are met (e.g., 10% fall in FEV_1).
4. Histamine challenge.
   a. Causes airway obstruction by activation of bronchial smooth-muscle and mediator receptors.
5. Methacholine challenge.
   a. Functions by:
      i. Inducing bronchoconstriction.
      ii. Increasing airway inflation pressure.
      iii. Contracting of the trachealis muscle.
6. Bronchodilator test.
   a. A positive test is defined as a 12% or greater increase in FEV_1 calculated as a percent of the predicted FEV_1 (and exceeds 200 mL) after the administration of an inhaled β_2 agonist.

C. Osmotic challenges.
1. Osmotic challenges demonstrate sensitivity and specificity to exercise and are economical, stable, and easy to administer.
2. Inhaled mannitol powder challenge.
   a. Same general protocol as methacholine or histamine; e.g., increased doses of mannitol are administered followed by PFTs.
   b. The stimulating mechanism acts by changing airway surface liquid (ASL) osmolarity followed by inflammatory mediator release.
3. Inhaled AMP challenge.
   a. Follows same procedure as mannitol challenge and targets mast cell degranulation.
4. Hypertonic saline challenge.
   a. Involves inhalation of nebulized hypertonic saline that acts by altering ASL osmolarity with a similar response to the mannitol challenge.

D. Eucapnic voluntary hyperventilation (EVH).
1. Based on the premise that increased ventilation causes bronchoconstriction in susceptible individuals.
2. Dries ASL and alters osmolarity.
3. Involves breathing a dry air mixture containing 5% CO_2 to ensure eucapnia.

      a. This mixture protects against hyperventilation-induced hypocapnia.

  4. EVH breathing is done at a predetermined rate of 60–85% of maximal voluntary ventilation (MVV).

      a. With a high-level athlete, breathing should be a minimum of 85% MVV.

      b. Individual breathing rate can be determined by taking a percentage of $35 \times FEV_1$ (a calculated estimate of MVV; e.g., $30 \times FEV_1 \approx 85\%$ MVV).

      c. However, because of variability in estimated MVV, it is best to perform an MVV maneuver to determine actual MVV for intensity calculations prior to the EVH challenge.

      d. EVH is the International Olympic Committee Medical Commission (IOC-MC) recommended challenge for EIB identification among Olympic athletes. However, an appropriate field-based exercise challenge or a bronchodilator challenge is also accepted.

  5. Grades of severity.

      a. Mild: 10–19% fall in FEV_1 at a minute ventilation of $\geq 60\%$ of MVV.

      b. Moderate: 20–29% fall in FEV_1 at a minute ventilation of $\geq 60\%$ of MVV.

      c. Severe: $\geq 30\%$ fall in FEV_1 at any level of ventilation or a $\geq 10\%$ fall at a ventilation of $\leq 30\%$ of MVV.

E. Exercise challenge.

  1. Intuitively makes sense to test for exercise-induced broncospasm with an exercise challenge.

  2. Exercise intensity, duration, mode, and environmental conditions must all be considered when defining an appropriate EIB-provoking challenge.

      a. Intensity for high-level athletes must be greater than for a nonathletic population.

         i. For an athlete, exercise intensity must be 90% of HR max or greater; 85% for a nonathlete.

         ii. Competition intensity is best.

      b. Duration should be 6 to 8 minutes.

         i. However, shorter and longer durations of exercise have been found to be EIB-provoking.

         ii. Speed skaters have been evaluated at durations of 2 minutes of high intensity with success.

            • Mathematical modeling of airway drying has shown that 2 minutes of near-maximal ventilation is sufficient to cause significant water loss of the ASL.

   c. Exercise mode has received attention; some studies have suggested that some modes are more effective in triggering airway reactivity than others.

      i. The exercise environment and ventilation requirement appear to be most critical to the response.

   d. Environmental conditions are primary to the response to exercise.

      i. Cold/dry air is primary for most challenges.

         • Rundell et al. (2000) demonstrated that 78% of winter athletes who tested EIB+ with a cold/dry field challenge tested negative in a laboratory environment of 21°C, 50% RH (Figure 2-7).

      ii. Other conditions that trigger the response should be considered for special populations.

         • Ice rink air pollution for figure skaters, speed skaters, and hockey players (see EIB in the Ice Rink Athlete).

         • High chlorine levels in indoor pools may trigger the response in swimmers.

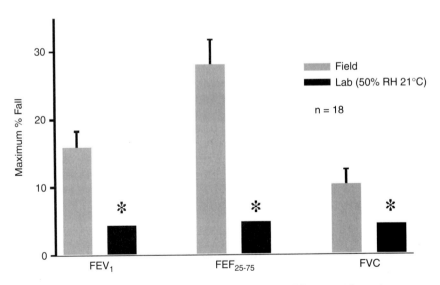

FIGURE 2-7 Eighteen of 23 cold-weather athletes with spirometry-defined EIB (>10% fall in FEV_1 after field-based exercise challenge) tested normal when retested in room temperature, 50% relative humidity. This study demonstrates the importance of appropriate temperature and humidity when evaluating for EIB. Figure redrawn from Rundell et al. (2000).

TREATMENT OF EIB

Long-Term Control: The Primary Objective

A. Limit EIB exacerbations and allow symptom-free competition and training.

B. Assessment and monitoring.
   1. The severity of the hyperreactive response must be defined.
      a. Mild, moderate, or severe.
   2. Efficacy of medication and the treatment regimen should be seasonally evaluated.

C. Pharmacological and nonpharmacological therapy.
   1. Initial treatment is to control exercise-related reactivity.
      a. Treat promptly with short-acting β_2 agonist.
      b. Prompt communication with physician.
   2. First line of treatment and/or prophylaxis is a short-acting β_2 agonist such as Salbutamol (albuterol).
      a. As prophylaxis, the $\beta2$ agonist should be administered 20–30 minutes prior to exercise.
      b. Maximal duration of action is 3–4 hours, but peak effect occurs within 1 hour.
      c. Frequent use (i.e., more than 2 times per week) may result in the development of a tolerance and other interventions should be considered.
      d. Relaxes smooth muscle, increasing air flow.
      e. Decreases vascular permeability.
      f. Moderately inhibits mediator release.
      g. Recently, the efficacy of β_2-agonist use in EIB management has been challenged.
         i. Wilber et al. (2001) found that a short-acting β_2 agonist did not improve airway function in EIB+ short-track speed skaters.
            • This study suggests that:
               – Underlying inflammation was not addressed by the β_2 agonist.
               – The skaters had become tachyphylactic.
               – The ice rink–related EIB may be pathologically different from the classic hyperreactive response.
   3. Long-acting β_2 agonists.
      a. Function similarly to short-acting β_2 agonists, but may provide protection for up to 12 hours.
      b. Studies have shown a synergy with corticosteroid use in controlling inflammation.

   c. Similar to the short-acting β_2 agonists, tachyphylaxis will also occur.
   d. There has been recent concern about a tachyphylactic effect of long-acting β_2 agonists on the short-acting β_2 agonists, those used as rescue medication.
4. Cromolyn sodium can be an effective prophylaxis when provided in high doses.
   a. May function by blocking chloride ion flux into the mast cells, epithelial cells, and neurons, thus preventing mediator release.
5. Leukotriene modifiers such as montelukast, zafirlukast, and zileuton have shown promise in protection against EIB.
   a. Demonstrated importance as treatment against EIB, although results have varied from 0% to 100% protection.
6. Inhaled corticosteroids may be necessary and may be underused.
   a. Because chronic inflammation is often present in EIB-symptomatic patients, inhaled corticosteroids can be effective and appropriate treatment of EIB.
   b. Inhaled corticosteroid use by mild asthmatics often controls EIB.
   c. Have been found effective in reducing inflammation, preventing inflammatory mediator release, and reducing airway eosinophil counts.
7. Refractory period.
   a. The initial EIB-provoking exercise will attenuate the bronchoconstricting response to a second exercise bout if the second bout is performed within 2 hours of the initial exercise.
      i. This means that the severity of the post-exercise bronchoconstriction can be reduced by a pre-exercise warm-up.
      ii. This may provide a nonpharmacological way to control EIB.
   b. Depletion of bronchoconstricting mediators has been suggested to be a responsible mechanism.
      i. If this is true, duration of the initial exercise and the time between the first and second exercise bouts should be important. However:
         • Studies demonstrating refractoriness have utilized exercise durations ranging from 8 × 30 seconds with 1.5-minute recovery to 30-minute steady-state exercise.
         • Others have utilized rest durations between exercise bouts from 2 minutes to 2 hours.

- The protection in these studies indicates that mediator depletion occurs early in the initial exercise and/or the rest duration between bouts has no impact on the degree of protection.
  c. This refractory period has given rise to the notion that an EIB-triggering warm-up can be used as prophylaxis to EIB.
  d. Studies in the laboratory setting using asthmatic subjects have demonstrated moderate protection for some.
  e. The efficacy of this warm-up prophylaxis for mild EIB-suffering athletes is not yet established.
      i. Rundell et al. (2003) found no significant refractoriness among elite cold-weather athletes who suffered from mild EIB.

EIB IN THE ICE RINK ATHLETE: A SPECIAL POPULATION WITH SPECIAL CONCERNS

Ice Resurfacing: What's in That Air?

A. Ice rink resurfacing involves cutting down the ice and laying a thin layer of water to refreeze a new surface.
B. Done hourly during daily rink activities.
C. Machines are typically propane- or gas-powered; however, electric-powered equipment is becoming more popular.
D. Carbon monoxide (CO) has been found at levels as high as 125 parts per million (ppm). Cutoff standards in some states have been set at 25–30 ppm.
E. Nitrogen dioxide (NO_2) has been found at levels greater than 3000 parts per billion (ppb). The World Health Organization 1-hour guideline value is 213 ppb NO_2 for indoor air.
F. Ultrafine and fine particulate matter (PM_1) has been shown to elevate to over 400,000 particles cm^{-3}. Outdoor air is typically 2000 to 5000 particles cm^{-3} (Figure 2-8).
G. Gas-powered resurfacers emit higher CO, and propane-powered resurfacers emit higher NO_2. Both emit equally high PM_1 (Figure 2-9).

Does Rink PM_1 Affect Airway Hyperreactivity?

A. Prevalence of EIB in figure skaters and hockey players is about 30% and exacerbations are worsened by rink air quality.
B. Peripheral airways appear to be affected more.

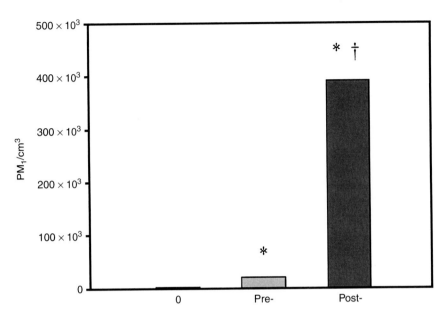

FIGURE 2-8 Ultrafine and fine particulate matter ($PM_1 \cdot cm^{-3}$) in an indoor ice rink before and after ice rink edging with a gas-fueled machine compared to outdoor $PM_1 \cdot cm^{-3}$ (0). Note the manyfold increase in particulate matter from edging.

Does Rink PM$_1$ Cause Airway Inflammation?

A. Women's Hockey Team: February 2001
  1. 0.7 of 22 (32%) were EIB+.
  2. 8 of 22 (36%) had low resting mid-expiratory flows (one was EIB+).
    a. 58% of a predicted normal value for athletes.
B. Current evidence suggests that PM_1 emitted from fossil-fueled ice resurfacers may be the cause of airway inflammation and hyper-reactivity.
  1. When evaluating skaters, this should be taken into consideration.

SUMMARY

Prevalence of EIB

EIB is prevalent among cold-weather athletes at a rate of 20–50% depending on specific athlete populations.

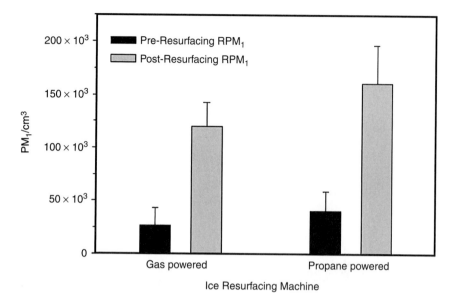

FIGURE 2-9 Pre- and post-ice resurfacing $PM_1 \cdot cm^{-3}$ from gas- or propane-powered resurfacing machines. Note that no difference in PM_1 concentration between the two fuel sources is apparent. Redrawn from Rundell (2003).

A. EIB in the cold-weather athlete may be pathologically different from frank asthma in many cases.
B. Are the repeated high ventilation rates of training cold-weather athletes the underlying cause of EIB, or are inhaled allergens and/or airborne pollutants critical to EIB etiology?

Typical EIB Response

The typical EIB response is normal bronchodilation during exercise followed by bronchoconstriction after exercise.
A. However, broncoconstriction can and does occur during exercise in a large percentage of EIB+ athletes.
    1. As such, EIB may affect athletic performance.

Characterization of EIB

EIB is characterized by:
A. +/− airway inflammation.
B. + airway hyperreacticity.

C. +/− symptoms such as cough, wheeze, dyspnea, chest tightness, and excess mucus.

D. Airway remodeling of the basement membrane may contribute to persistent symptoms.

Most Likely Triggers

EIB is most likely triggered by water loss of the ASL, osmolarity change in airway cells, and release of inflammatory mediators.

A. Pathogenesis supports multiple mediator involvement.
  1. Histamine.
  2. Leukotrienes.
  3. Prostanoids.

Diagnosis

Diagnosis of EIB should be based on objective measurements of variable, reversible airflow obstruction and/or the presence of chronic inflammation.

A. Spirometry coupled with an appropriate EIB-provoking challenge should be the foundation for diagnosis.

B. Symptoms-based diagnosis has been found to be unreliable.

Treatment

A. Treatment should be based on an objective diagnosis, not self-reported symptoms.

B. Key is symptom-free exercise.

C. If underlying inflammation is identified, inhaled corticosteroids should be considered.
  1. A reduction in inflammation typically reduces hyperreactivity.

D. Short-acting β_2 agonist is preferred pre-exercise prophylaxis, but use should be limited to 2–3 times per week.
  1. If prophylaxis is required on a daily basis, alternative treatment regimens should be explored.

E. Cromolyn sodium in high doses may provide protection from acute exacerbations.

F. Montelukast may be used as prophylaxis.

The Ice Rink

A. Poor air quality is often characteristic of the indoor ice rink environment.

B. High airway inflammation and hyperreactivity among ice rink athletes suggest a relationship between PM_1 exposure and airway dysfunction.

CONCLUSIONS

Airway dysfunction is high among cold-weather athletes and in many cases is different from classic asthma.

The precise pathophysiology of EIB is not yet defined, but is likely a physiological response to protect the airways.

Suggested Readings

Alderoth E, Morris MM, Hargreave FE, et al. Airway responsiveness to leukotrienes C_4 and D_4 and to methacholine in patients with asthma and normal controls. *N Eng J Med* 1986;315:480–4.

Alton EW, Norris AA. Chloride transport and the actions of nedocromil sodium and cromolyn sodium in asthma. *J Allergy Clin Immunol* 1996;98:S102–6.

American Thoracic Society. Lung function testing: Selection of reference values and interpretative strategies. *Am Rev Respir Dis* 1991;144:1202–18.

Anderson SD. Airway drying and exercise-induced asthma. In: McFadden ER Jr, ed. *Exercise-Induced Asthma*. New York: Marcel Dekker, Inc; 1999:77–114.

Anderson SD, Argyros GJ, Magnussen H, et al. Provocation by eucapnic voluntary hyperpnoea to identify exercise-induced bronchoconstriction. *Br J Sports Med* 2001;35:344–47.

Anderson SD, Brannan J, Spring J, et al. A new method for bronchial-provocation testing in asthmatic subjects using a dry powder of mannitol. *Am J Respir Crit Care Med* 1997;156:758–65.

Anderson SD, Connolly NM, Godfrey S. Comparison of bronchoconstriction induced by cycling and running. *Thorax* 1971;26:396–401.

Anderson SD, Daviskas E. Pathophysiology of exercise-induced asthma: The role of respiratory water loss. In: JM Weiler, ed. *Allergic and Respiratory Disease in Sports Medicine*. New York: Marcel Dekker, Inc, 1997;87–114.

Anderson SD, Daviskas E. The mechanism of exercise-induced asthma is…. *J Allergy Clin Immunol* 2000;106:453–59.

Anderson SD, Holzer K. Exercise-induced asthma: Is it the right diagnosis in elite athletes? *J Allergy Clin Immunol* 2000;106:419–28.

Anderson SD, Schoeffel RE. Respiratory heat and water loss during exercise in patients with asthma: Effect of repeated exercise challenge. *Eur J Respir Dis* 1982;63(5):472–80.

Anderson SD, Schoeffel RE, Follet R, et al. Sensitivity to heat and water loss at rest and during exercise in asthmatic patients. *Eur J Respir Dis* 1982;63(5):459–71.

Anderson SD, Seale JP, Ferris L, et al. An evaluation of pharmacotherapy for exercise-induced asthma. *J Allergy Clin Immunol* 1979;64:612–24.

Anderson SD, Smith CM, Rodwell LT, et al. The use of non-isotonic aerosols for evaluating bronchial heperresponsiveness. In: Spector S, ed. *Provocation Challenge Procedures*. New York: Marcel Dekker; 1995:249–78.

Backer V, Ulrik CS. Bronchial responsiveness to exercise in a random sample of 494 children and adolescents from Copenhagen. *Clin Exp Allergy* 1992;22(8):741–47.

Barnes NC, Marone G, Di Maria GU, Visser S, Utama I, Payne SL. A comparison of fluticasone propionate, 1 mg daily, with beclomethasone dipropionate, 2 mg daily, in the treatment of severe asthma. International Study Group. *Eur Respir J* 1993;6:877–85.

Bar-Yishay E, Godfrey S. Mechanisms of exercise-induced asthma. *Lung* 1984;162(4):195–204.

Beasley CR, Robinson C, Featherstone RL, et al. 9 alpha, 11 beta-prostaglandin F2, a novel metabolite of prostaglandin D2 is a potent contractile agonist of human and guinea pig airways. *J Clin Invest* 1987;79 (3):978–83.

Beck KC, Offord KP, Scanlon PD. Bronchoconstriction occurring during exercise in asthmatic subjects. *Am J Respir Crit Care Med* 1994;149:352–57.

Becker AB, Simons FE. Formoterol, a new long-acting selective beta-2 agonist, decreases airway responsiveness in children with asthma. *Lung* 1990;168 (suppl):99–102.

Belcher NG, Lee TH, Rees PJ. Airway resonses to hypertonic saline, exercise, and histamine challenges in bronchial asthma. *Eur Respir J* 1989;2:44–48.

Boulet LP, Becker A, Bérubé A, et al. Canadian asthma consensus report, 1999. *C Med Assoc J* 1999;161(suppl 11):S1–S62.

Brannan JD, Koskela H, Anderson SD, et al. Responsiveness to mannitol in asthmatic subjects with exercise- and hyperventilation-induced asthma. *Am J Respir Crit Care Med* 1998;158:1120–26.

Brauer M, Lee K, Spengler JD, et al. Nitrogen dioxide in indoor ice skating facilities: An international survey. *J Air Waste Manag Assoc* 1997; 47(10):1095–102.

Brauer M, Spengler JD. Nitrogen dioxide exposures inside ice skating rinks. *Am J Public Health* 1994 Mar;84(3):429–33.

Brugman SM, Simons SM. Vocal cord dysfunction. *Physician Sports Med* 1998;26:63–74.

Bye MR, Kerstein D, Barsh E. The importance of spirometry in the assessment of childhood asthma. *Am J Dis Child* 1992;146:977–78.

Charpin D, Vercloet D, Charpin J. Epidemiology of asthma in Western Europe. *Allergy* 1988;43:481–92.

Chen WY, Horton DJ. Heat and water loss from the airways and exercise-induced asthma. *Respiration* 1977;34:305–13.

Clough JB, Hutchinson SA, Williams JD, et al. Airway response to exercise and methacholine in children with respiratory symptoms. *Arch Dis Child* 1991; May;66(5):579–83.

Collaboration Investigators. *Arch Intern Med* 1999 Jun 14;159(11):1237–43.

Coreno A, Skowronski M, Kotaru C, et al. Comparative effects of long-acting β_2 agonists, leukotriene receptor antagonists, and 5-lipoxygenase inhibitor on exercise-induced asthma. *J Allergy Clin Immunol* 2000;106:500–6.

Costa DL, Dreher KL. Bioavailable transition metals in particulate matter mediate cardiopulmonary injury in healthy and compromised animal models. *Environ Health Perspect* 1997;105(suppl 5):1053–60.

Crapo RO. Pulmonary-function testing. *N Engl J Med* 1994;331:25–30.

Dahl R, Lundback B, Malo JL, et al. A dose-ranging study of fluticasone priopionate in adult patients with moderate asthma. International Study Group. *Chest* 1993;104:1352–58.

D'Alonzo GE, Nathan RA, Henochowicz S, et al. Salmeterol xinafoate as maintenance therapy compared with albuterol in patients with asthma. *J Am Med Assoc* 1994;271:1412–16.

Davis MS, Freed AN. Repeated hyperventilation causes peripheral airways inflammation, hyperreactivity, and impaired bronchodilation in dogs. *Am J Respir Crit Care Med* 2001 Sep 1;164(5):785–89.

Deal EC, McFadden ER Jr, Ingram RH, et al. Role of respiratory heat exchange in production of exercise-induced asthma. *J Appl Physiol* 1979;46(3): 467–75.

Deal EC, McFadden ER Jr, Ingram RH, et al. Hyperpnea and heat flux: Initial reaction sequence in exercise-induced asthma. *J Appl Physiol* 1979;46 (3):476–83.

Drazen JM, Austen KF. Leukotrienes and airway responses. *Am Rev Respir Dis* 1987;136:985–88.

Drazen JM, Israel E, O'Byrne PM. Treatment of asthma with drugs modifying the leukotriene pathway. *N Eng J Med* 1999;340:197–206.

Eady RP. The pharmacology of nedocromil sodium. *Eur J Respir Dis Suppl* 1986;147:112–19.

Eggleston PA, Rosenthal RR, Anderson SA, et al. Guidelines for the methodology of exercise challenge testing of asthmatics. *J Allergy Clin Immunol* 1979;64:642–45.

Eiser NM. Histamine antagonists and asthma. *Pharmacol Ther* 1982;17:239–50.

Fabbri L, Burge PS, Croonenborgh L, et al. Comparison of fluticasone propionate with beclomethasone dipropionate in moderate to severe asthma treated for one year. International Study Group. *Thorax* 1993;48:817–23.

Feinstein RA, LaRussa J, Want-Dohlman A, et al. Screening adolescent athletes for exercise-induced asthma. *Clin J Sport Med* 1996 Apr;6(2):119–23.

Finnerty JP, Holgate ST. Evidence of the role of histamine and prostaglandins as mediators in exercise-induced asthma: The inhibitory effect of terfenadine and flurbiprofen alone and in combination. *Eur Respir J* 1990;3:540–57.

Finnerty JP, Twentyman OP, Harris A, et al. Effect of GR 32191, a potent thromboxane receptor antagonist, on exercise-induced bronchoconstriction in asthma. *Thorax* 1991;46:190–92.

Finnerty JP, Wilmot C, Holgate ST. Inhibition of hypertonic saline-induced bronchoconstriction by terfendine and flurbiprofen: Evidence for the predominant role of histamine. *Am Rev Respir Dis* 1989;140:593–97.

Finnerty JP, Wood-Baker R, Thomson H, et al. Role of leukotrienes in exercise-induced asthma: Inhibitory effect of ICI 204219, a potent leukotriene D4 receptor antagonist. *Am Rev Respir Dis* 1992;145:746–49.

Fitch KD, Godfrey S. Asthma and athletic performance. *J Am Med Assoc* 1976 Jul 12;236(2):152–57.

Folinsbee LJ. Does No2 exposure increase airways responsiveness? *Toxicol Ind Health* 1992;8:273–83.

Fujitaka M, Kawaguchi H, Kato Y, et al. Significance of the eosinophil cationic protein/eosinophil count ratio in asthmatic patients: Its relationship to disease severity. *Ann Allergy Asthma Immunol* 2001;86(3):323–29.

Gaddy JN, Margolskee DJ, Bush RK, et al. Bronchodilation with a potent and selective leukotriene D4 (LTD4) receptor antagonist (MK-571) in patients with asthma. *Am Rev Respir Dis* 1992;146:358–63.

Ghosh SK, DeVos C, McIlory I, et al. Effect of cetirizine on exercise-induced asthma. *Thorax* 1991;46:242–44.

Godfrey S. Clinical and physiological features. In: McFadden ER, ed. *Exercise-Induced Asthma*. New York: Marcel Dekker, Inc; 1999:11–45.

Greening AP, Ind PW, Northfield M, et al. Added salmeterol versus higher-dose corticosteroid in asthma patients with symptoms on existing inhaled corticosteroid. Allen & Hanburys Limited UK Study Group. *Lancet* 1994; 344:219–24.

Griffen M, Weiss JW, Leitch AG, et al. Effects of leukotriene D on the airways in asthma. *N Eng J Med* 1983;308:436–39.

Haahtela T, Jarvinen M, Kava T, et al. Comparisons of a beta-2 agonist, terbutaline, with an inhaled corticosteroid, budesonide, in newly detected asthma. *N Engl J Med* 1991;325:388–92.

Haby MM, Anderson SD, Peat JK, et al. An exercise challenge protocol for epidemiological studies of asthma in children: Comparison with histamine challenge. *Eur Respir J* 1994;7:43–49.

Haby MM, Peat JK, Mellis CM, et al. An exercise challenge for epidemiological studies of childhood asthma: Validity and repeatability. *Eur Respir J* 1995;8:729–36.

Hartley JPR, Norgrady SG. Effect of inhaled antihistamine on exercise-induced asthma. *Thorax* 1980;35:675–79.

Hedberg K, Hedberg CW, Iber C, et al. An outbreak of nitrogen dioxide–induced respiratory illness among ice hockey players. *J Am Med Assoc* 1989 Dec 1;262(21):3014–17.

Heir T. Longitudinal variations in bronchial responsiveness in cross-country skiers and control subjects. *Scand J Med Sci Sports* 1994;4:134–39.

Heir T, Oseid S. Self-reported asthma and exercise-induced asthma symptoms in high-level competitive cross-country skiers. *Scand J Med Sci Sports* 1994;4:128–33.

Helenius I, Haahtela T. Allergy and asthma in elite summer sport athletes. *J Allergy Clin Immunol* 2000 Sep;106(3):444–52.

Helenius IJ, Tikkanan HO, Haahtela T. Exercise-induced bronchospasm at low temperature in elite runners. *Thorax* 1996 Jun;51(6):628–29.

Helenius IJ, Tikkanen HO, Haahtela T. Association between type of training and risk of asthma in elite athletes. *Thorax* 1997 Feb;52(2):157–60.

Helenius IJ, Tikkanan HO, Haahtela T. Occurrence of exercise-induced bronchospasm in elite runners: Dependence on atopy and exposure to cold air and pollen. *Brit J Sports Med* 1998;32:125–29.

Hoshino M, Fukushima Y. Effect of OKY-046 (thromboxane A_2 synthetase inhibitor) on exercise-induced asthma. *J Asthma* 1991;28:19–29.

Israel E, Cohn J, Dube L, et al. Effect of treatment with zileuton, a 5-lipoxygenase inhibitor, in patients with asthma: A randomized controlled trial. Zileuton Clinical Trial Group. *J Am Med Assoc* 1996;275:931–36.

Judelson DA, Williams SD, Rundell KW. Gender differences in pulmonary function of elite ice hockey players. *Med Sci Sports Exer* 2001;33(5).

Karjalainen EM, Laitinen A, Sue-Chu M, et al. Evidence of airway inflammation and remodeling in ski athlete with and without bronchial hyperresponsiveness to methacholine. *Am J Respir Crit Care Med* 2000;161(6): 2086–91.

Kumlin M, Dahlen B, Bjorck T, et al. Urinary excretion of leukotriene E4 and 11-dehydro-thromboxane in response to bronchial provocations with allergen, aspirin, leukotriene D4, and histamine in asthmatics. *Am Rev Respir Dis* 1992;146(1):96–103.

Kumlin M, Stensvad F, Larsson L, et al. Validation and application of a new simple strategy for measurements of urinary leukotriene E_4 in humans. *Clin Exp Allergy* 1995;25(5):467–79.

Laitinen LA, Laitinen A, Haatela T. Airway mucosal inflammation even in patients with newly diagnosed asthma. *Am Rev Respir Dis* 1993;147: 697–704.

Lal S, Dorow PD, Venho KK, et al. Nedocromil sodium is more effective than cromolyn sodium for the treatment of chronic reversible obstructive airway disease. *Chest* 1993;104:438–47.

Langdeau JB, Boulet LP. Is asthma over- or under-diagnosed in athletes? *Respir Med* 2003;97(2):109–14.

Larsson L, Hemmingsson P, Boethius G. Self-reported obstructive airway symptoms are common in young cross-country skiers. *Scand J Med Sci Sports* 1994;4:124–27.

Larsson K, Ohlsen P, Larsson L, et al. High prevalence of asthma in cross-country skiers. *BMJ* 1993 Nov 20;307(6915):1326–29.

Lee K, Yanagisawa Y, Spengler JD, et al. Carbon monoxide and nitrogen dioxide exposures in indoor ice skating rinks. *J Sports Sci* 1994 Jun;12(3): 279–83.

Levy JI, Lee K, Yanagisawa Y, et al. Determinants of nitrogen dioxide concentrations in indoor ice skating rinks. *Am J Public Health* 1998;88(12): 1781–86.

Li JT, O'Connell EJ. Clinical evaluation of asthma. *Ann Allergy Asthma Immunol* 1996;76:1–15.

Lin CC, Wu JL, Huang WC, et al. A bronchial response comparison of exercise and methacholine in asthmatic subjects. *J Asthma* 1991;28(1):31–40.

Mannix ET, Farber MO, Palange P, et al. Exercise-induced asthma in figure skaters. *Chest* 1996;109:312–15.

Mannix ET, Manfredi F, Farber MO. A comparison of two challenge tests for identifying exercise-induced bronchospasm in figure skaters. *Chest* 1999;155:649–53.

McFadden ER Jr, Gilbert IA. Exercise-induced asthma. *N Engl J Med* 1994 May 12;330(19):1362–67.

McFadden ER Jr, Lenner KAM, Strohl KP. Postexertional airway rewarming and thermally induced asthma: New insights into pathophysiology and possible pathogenesis. *J Clin Invest* 1986;78:18–25.

McFadden ER, Zawadski DK. Vocal cord dysfunction masquerading as exercise-induced asthma. *Am J Respir Crit Care Med* 1996;153:942–47.

McFarlane PI, Heaf DP. Selective histamine blockade in childhood asthma: The effect of terfenadine on resting bronchial tone and exercise-induced bronchoconstriction. *Thorax* 1991;46:190–92.

McKenzie DC, McLuckie SL, Stirling DR. The protective effects of continuous and interval exercise in athletes with exercise-induced asthma. *Med Sci Sports Exerc* 1994 Aug;26(8):951–56.

The Medical Letter. Drugs for asthma. *Med Lett Drugs Ther* 2000;42:19–24.

Meltzer EO, Weiler JM, Widlitz MD. Comparative outdoor study of the effi-cacy, onset, and duration of action, and safety of cetirizine, loratadine, and place-bo for seasonal allergic rhinitis. *J Allergy Clin Immunol* 1996; 65:46–50.

Morris JF. Spirometry in the evaluation of pulmonary function. Medical Progress, *West J Med* 1976;125:110–11.

Nagakura T, Obata T, Schihijo K, et al. GC/MS analysis of urinary excretion of 9alpha,11beta-PGF2 in acute and exercise-induced asthma in children. *Clin Exp Allergy* 1998;28(2):181–86.

National Heart, Lung, and Blood Institute. *Expert Panel Report 2: Guidelines for the Diagnosis and Management of Asthma.* 1st ed. Bethesda: NIH Publications, 1997:1–146.

Noviski N, Bar-Yishay E, Gur I, et al. Exercise intensity determines and cli-matic conditions modify the severity of exercise-induced asthma. *Am Rev Respir Dis* 1987 Sep;136(3):592–94.

Nystad W, Harris J, Borgen JS. Asthma and wheezing among Norwegian elite athletes. *Med Sci Sports Exerc* 2000;32(2):266–70.

Oberdorster G, Gelein RM, Juraj F, et al. Association of particulate air pollu-tion and acute mortality: Involvement of ultrafine particles? *Inhal Toxicol* 1995;7:111–24.

O'Donnell AE, Fling J. Exercise-induced airflow obstruction in a healthy mil-itary population. *Chest* 1993;103(3):742–44.

Ortega-Carr D, Bush RK. Asthma in adults and adolescents. In: Rakel RE, ed. *Conn's Current Therapy 1995.* Philadelphia: WB Saunders Co; 1995: 678–82.

O'Sullivan S. On the role of PGD2 metabolites as markers of mast cell activa-tion in asthma. *Acta Physiol Scand Suppl* 1999;644:1–74.

O'Sullivan S, Roquet A, Dahlen B, et al. Evidence for mast cell activation dur-ing exercise-induced bronchoconstriction. *Eur Respir J* 1998;12(2):345–50.

Patel KR. Terfenadine in exercise-induced asthma. *BMJ* 1987;288:1496–97.

Peters SP. Mechanism of mast-cell activation. In: Busse WW, Holgate ST, eds. *Asthma and Rhinitis.* Boston: Blackwell Scientific Publications; 1995.

Pohunek P, Kucera P, Sukova B, et al. Serum ECP taken in the acute episode of bronchial obstruction can predict the development of bronchial asthma in young children. *Allergy Asthma Proc* 2001;22(2):75–79.

Potts J. Factors associated with respiratory problems in swimmers. *Sports Med* 1996 Apr;21(4):256–61.

Provost-Craig MA, Arbour KS, Sestilli DC, et al. The incidence of exercise-induced bronchospasm in competitive figure skaters. *J Asthma* 1996; 33:67–71.

Rabone SJ, Phoon WO, Anderson SD, et al. Hypertonic saline challenge in an adult epidemiological survey. *Occup Med* 1996;46:177–85.

Reiff DB, Choudry NB, Pride NB, et al. The effect of prolonged submaximal warm-up exercise on exercise-induced asthma. *Am Rev Respir Dis* 1989 Feb;139(2):479–84.

Rice SG, Bierman CW, Shapiro GG, et al. Identification of exercise-induced asthma among intercollegiate athletes. *Ann Allergy Asthma Immunol* 1985;55:790–93.

Riedler J, Reade T, Dalton M, et al. Hypertonic saline challenge in an epidemiologic survey of asthma in children. *Am J Respir Crit Care Med* 1994;150:1632–39.

Roche WR. Fibroblasts and asthma. *Clin Exp Allergy* 1991;21(5):545–48.

Roquet A, Dahlen B, Kumlin M, et al. Combined antagonism of leukotrienes and histamine produces predominant inhibition of allergen-induced early and late phase airway obstruction in asthmatics. *Am J Respir Crit Care Med* 1997;155(6):1856–63.

Rundell KW. High levels of airborne ultrafine and fine particulate matter in indoor ice arenas. *Inhal Toxicol* 2003;15(3):237–50.

Rundell KW, Im J, Mayers LB, et al. Self-reported symptoms and exercise-induced asthma in the elite athlete. *Med Sci Sports Exerc* 2001;33:208–13.

Rundell KW, Im J, Wilber RL, et al. Mid-expiratory flow rates of cold-weather athletes with exercise-induced asthma. *Med Sci Sports Exerc* 2001;33 (suppl 5):S12.

Rundell KW, Jenkinson DM. Exercise-induced bronchoconstriction in elite athletes. *J Sports Med* 2002;32(9):583–600.

Rundell KW, Judelson DA, Williams SD. Diagnosis of exercise-induced asthma in the athlete. In: Rundell KW, Wilber RL, Lemanske R, eds. *Asthma and Exercise*. Champaign: Human Kinetics; 2001.

Rundell KW, Spiering BA. Inspiratory stridor in elite athletes. *Chest* 2003;123:468–74.

Rundell KW, Spiering BA, Judelson DA, Wilson MH. Bronchoconstriction during cross-country skiing: Is there really a refractory period? *Med Sci Sports Exerc* 2003;35(1):18–26.

Rundell KW, Wilber RL, Szmedra L, et al. Exercise-induced asthma screening of elite athletes: Field versus laboratory exercise challenge. *Med Sci Sports Exerc* 2000;32:309–16.

Rupp NT, Guill MF, Brudno DS. Unrecognized exercise-induced bronchospasm in adolescent athletes. *Am J Dis Child* 1992;146(8):941–44.

Ryu JH, Scanlon PD. Obstructive lung diseases: COPD, asthma, and many imitators. *Mayo Clin Proc* 2001;76(11):1144–53.

Schnall RP, Landau LI. Protective effects of repeated short sprints in exercise-induced asthma. *Thorax* 1980 Nov;35(11):828–32.

Schwartz HJ, Blumenthal M, Brady R, et al. A comparative study of the clinical efficacy of nedocromil sodium and placebo: How does cromolyn sodium compare as an active control treatment? *Chest* 1996;109:945–52.

Sears MR. Epidemiological trends in bronchial asthma. In: Kaliner MA, Barnes PJ, Persson CGA, eds. *Asthma, Its Pathology and Treatment.* New York: Marcel Dekker Inc; 1991.

Singh AK, Cydulka RK, Stahmer SA, et al. Sex differences among adults presenting to the emergency department with acute asthma. Multicenter Asthma Research Collaboration Investigators. *Arch Intern Med* 1999; 159(11):1237–43.

Smith CM, Anderson SD. Inhalation provocation tests using non-isotonic aerosols. *J Allergy Clin Immunol* 1989;84:781–90.

Smith LJ, Greenberger PA, Patterson R, et al. The effect of inhaled leukotriene D_4 in humans. *Am Rev Respir Dis* 1985;131:368–72.

Sporik R, Holgate ST, Platts-Mills TA, et al. Exposure to house-dust mite allergen (Der p I) and the development of asthma in childhood. *N Eng J Med* 1990;323(8):502–7.

Sterling GM. The mechanism of bronchoconstriction due to hypocapnia in man. *Clin Sci* 1968;34:277–78.

Storms WW. Exercise-induced asthma: Diagnosis and treatment for the recreational or elite athlete. *Med Sci Sports Exerc* 1999 Jan;31(suppl 1): S33–38.

Sue-Chu M, Larsson L, Moen T, et al. Bronchoscopy and bronchoalveolar lavage findings in cross-country skiers with and without "ski-asthma." *Eur Respir J* 1999;13(3):626–32.

Sue-Chu M, Karjalainen EM, Laitinen A, et al. Placebo-controlled study of inhaled budesonide on indices of airway inflammation in bronchoalveolar lavage fluid and brochial biopsies in cross-country skiers. *Respiration* 2000;67(4):417–25.

Suman OE, Beck KC, Babcock MA, et al. Airway obstruction during exercise and isocapnic hyperventilation in asthmatic subjects. *J Appl Physiol* 1999 Sep;87(3):1107–13.

Tan RA, Spector SL. Exercise-induced asthma. *Sports Med* 1998;25:1–6.

Togias AG, Naclerio RM, Proud D, et al. Nasal challenge with cold dry air results in release of inflammatory mediators. *J Clin Invest* 1985;76: 1375–81.

Togias AG, Proud D, Lichtenstein LM, et al. The osmalality of nasal secretions increases when inflammatory mediators are released in response to inhalation of cold, dry air. *Am Rev Respir Dis* 1988;157:625–29.

United States Olympic Committee, Division of Sports Medicine. *Asthma.* 1999.

Van Essen-Zandvliet EE, Hughes MD, Waalkens HJ, et al. Effects of 22 months of treatment with inhaled corticosteroids and/or beta-2 agonists on lung function, airway responsiveness, and symptoms in children with asthma. The Dutch Chronic Nonspecific Lung Disease Study Group. *Am Rev Respir Dis* 1992;146:547–54.

Von hertzen LC. The hygiene hypothesis in the development of atopy and asthma: Still a matter of controversy? *Q J Med* 1998;91:767–71.

Voy RO. The U.S. Olympic Committee experience with exercise-induced bronchospasm, 1984. *Med Sci Sports Exerc* 1984;18(3):328–30.

Wagner EM, Jacoby DB. Methacholine causes reflex bronchoconstriction. *J Appl Physiol* 1999;86:294–97.

Weiler JM, Layton T, Hunt M. Asthma in U.S. Olympic athletes who participated in the 1996 summer games. *J Allergy Clin Immunol* 1998;102: 722–26.

Weiler JM, Ryan EJ III. Asthma in U.S. Olympic athletes who participated in the 1998 Olympic winter games. *J Allergy Clin Immunol* 2000;106:267–71.

Weiss JW, Drazen JM, Coles N, et al. Bronchoconstrictor effects of leukotriene C in humans. *Science* 1982;216:196–98.

Westcott JY. The measurement of leukotrienes in human fluids. *Clin Rev Allergy Immunol* 1999;17(1–2):153–77.

Wilber RL, Rundell KW, Judelson DA. Efficacy of asthma medication regimen in elite athletes with exercise-induced asthma. *Med Sci Sports Exerc* 2001;33(suppl 5):S12.

Wilber RL, Rundell KW, Szmedra L, et al. Incidence of exercise-induced bronchospasm in Olympic winter sport athletes. *Med Sci Sports Exerc* 2000 Apr;32(4):732–37.

Williams PV, Shapiro GG. Asthma in children. In: Rakel RE, ed. *Conn's Current Therapy 1995*. Philadelphia: WB Saunders Co; 1995:682–91.

Williams SD, Judelson DA, Rundell KW. High levels of airborne particulate matter in indoor ice arenas. *Med Sci Sports Exerc* 2001;33(suppl 5):S12.

COLD INJURY

William O. Roberts

GENERAL

Injuries and Emergencies

The injuries and emergencies associated with physical activity in the cold include:
A. Chilblains.
B. Frostbite.
C. Hypothermia.

Recognition of Cold Injury

A. Suspect in cold exercise settings.
    1. Hypothermia can occur with ambient temperatures in the 60–70°F range especially when the athlete's energy levels are depleted.
B. Environment reflects greatest risk of cold injury.
    1. Nordic skiing limits race starts to –20°C (–4°F) and warmer.
    2. Windchill cooling effects increase risk of cold injury.
    3. Duration of exposure.
        a. Short duration exposure in extreme cold can lead to injury.
        b. Longer duration exposure required in moderate temperatures.

Prognosis

A. Rapid onset and rapid correction result in better outcome.

PHYSIOLOGY OF COLD EXPOSURE

Normal Range of Core Temperature

A. 37°C (98.6°F) considered normal body temperature.
  1. 1°C normal diurnal variation.
  2. 36.5–38.5°C (97–100.6°F) considered normal in clinical medicine.
  3. 36.5–40°C (97–104°F) is the physiologic range during activity.

Definition

Hypothermia is defined as core temperature < 36.5°C (97°F).

Effects of Cell Cooling on Cells

A. Decreased cell metabolism with lower cell temperature.
B. Cold promotes cell preservation until cell contents freeze.
C. Cardiac tissue cooling causes tissue instability.
  1. Can lead to cardiac arrhythmias.
  2. Rewarming the victim is an important component of treating an unstable cardiac rhythm.
D. Transfer, then treat.
  1. "Second freeze damage" occurs when a victim is rewarmed and then is immediately reexposed to the cold environment.
  2. Rewarming complications may occur, so it is best to rewarm at a facility in which complications can be addressed.

Heat Balance

A. Heat exchange mechanisms.
  1. Conduction.
    a. Direct contact heat exchange.
    b. Ground and air in contact with the body.
  2. Convection.
    a. Fluid flow across an object exchanges heat energy.
    b. Air and water are common fluids.
    c. Windchill temperature is convective heat loss.
  3. Radiation.
    a. Radiation is the transfer of energy between two objects (radiant heat).
      i. Warmer, high-energy object gives off heat to the cooler, lower-energy object.
    b. Body transfers heat to surroundings in cold conditions.

   4. Evaporation.
      a. Removes 0.58 kcal of heat per mL of sweat vaporized.
      b. Body produces sweat during activity in the cold.
         i. Inuits say "sweat kills."
      c. Respiratory heat losses are through evaporation.
B. Body heat production and loss.
   1. Heat production.
      a. Muscle work is 25% energy-efficient.
      b. Remainder of muscle work creates waste heat.
         i. Keeps athletes warm during exercise.
         ii. Active heat removal is necessary to keep core from overheating, even in cold environments.
      c. Prolonged exercise can deplete energy store.
         i. Depleted energy store is a risk factor for cold injury.
         ii. Core body temperature cannot be maintained.
   2. Heat loss in the cold during exercise.
      a. Sweat evaporation.
      b. Wet clothing or skin surface augments convective and conductive losses.
      c. Body heat radiation to surroundings.
C. Temperature regulation.
   1. Thermoregulatory system.
      a. Central control in preoptic hypothalamus.
      b. Peripheral control from temperature-sensitive receptors in the skin.
   2. Cold conditions.
      a. Heat conservation system activated.
         i. Increases insulation by vasoconstriction of blood flow to skin and subcutaneous tissues.
         ii. Causes relative hypervolemia and diuresis.
      b. Heat energy removal still necessary when exercising to prevent hyperthermia.

TEMPERATURE MEASUREMENT

Thermometer

Low-temperature thermometer is essential, should read to < 70°F.

Temperature Gradient

Core–shell temperature gradient may be 20°C in the cold.

A. Core temperature measurements accessible from:
  1. Rectum.
     a. Diagnostic and treatment criteria are based on rectal temperature.
     b. Reliable in the field.
     c. Lags behind esophageal and actual core temperatures.
  2. Esophagus.
  3. Urine.
     a. Supply-dependent.
     b. Tends to follow rectal temperature.
B. Shell temperature equals skin surface temperature.
  1. Natural openings may be influenced by the shell temperature.
     a. Mouth.
     b. Nasopharynx.
     c. Aural canal.
     d. Tympanic membrane.
  2. Cooled by environment.
  3. Poor accuracy and precision in field conditions.

CHILBLAINS AND FROSTBITE/FROSTNIP

Chilblains

A. Chronic vasculitis of dermis.
B. Caused by chronic exposure to cold conditions above freezing.
C. Affected areas.
  1. Face.
  2. Anterior tibia.
  3. Dorsum of hands and feet.
D. Prevention.
  1. Keep feet dry and warm.
  2. Aluminum chlorhydrate solution to prevent sweating.
  3. Change into dry socks 2 to 3 times per day for chronic exposures.

Frostbite and Frostnip

A. Definition.
  1. Freezing of tissue including intracellular contents.
     a. Occurs at 28–31°F.
     b. Eutectic point of saline solution.
B. Frostnip is present when superficial skin layers freeze; injury is considered frostbite when deeper tissue layers become involved.
  1. Risk is greatest in appendages and vascular watershed areas.
     a. Fingers and toes.

        b. Ears.

        c. Nose.

        d. Cheeks.

        e. Feet and hands.

        f. Genitalia.

            i. "Testicular nip."

C. Clinical picture.

    1. White, cold, firm or hard tissue.

    2. Vascular changes and inflammation occur with rewarming.

        a. Free radical oxidative stress damages tissue.

        b. Blood clots form in the microvasculature.

D. Classification based on initial exam.

    1. Superficial.

        a. Mobile subcutaneous tissue.

    2. Deep.

        a. Deep tissue is hard.

        b. Tissue remains cool and insensitive post-thawing.

E. Severity rating is determined several days after freeze injury.

    1. First degree.

        a. Numbness.

        b. Erythema.

        c. Edema.

    2. Second degree.

        a. Clear, fluid-filled blisters.

        b. Erythema.

        c. Edema.

    3. Third degree.

        a. Hemorrhagic blisters.

    4. Fourth degree.

        a. Injury to bone and muscle.

        b. Tissue mottled and lifeless.

F. Treatment of frostbite.

    1. Protect and insulate the frozen tissue until rewarmed.

    2. Do not rewarm frozen tissue until there is no chance of refreezing.

    3. Rapid rewarming in a water bath at 40–42°C (104–108°F).

    4. Pharmacologic interventions can be instituted to improve healing of tissue.

        a. Topical aloe vera (70% aqueous extract) qid.

            i. Dermaide™ aloe cream.

        b. Oral ibuprofen.

            i. 400 mg bid.

        c. Prophylactic antibiotic use is controversial.

    5. Observe for demarcation of viable tissue.

6. Surgical debridement or amputation of nonviable tissue is required.
7. Anticipate complicating conditions and possible long-term tissue changes.

G. Lewis-Hunting reaction to prevent frostbite.
1. Local vasodilatation due to paralysis of precapillary sphincter produces local rewarming.
2. Vasoconstriction response recurs as capillary sphincters warm and become functional.
3. Oscillation between threshold temperatures protects skin and subcutaneous tissue from freezing.
4. Most prominent in digits, ears, and face for frostbite protection.

HYPOTHERMIA IN ATHLETES AND ACTIVE PEOPLE

Lack of Studies

There are few centers with high-casualty incidence to launch prospective studies.

A. Greatest knowledge gains have been from high-risk areas and activities.
1. High-altitude medical stations.
   a. Mount Everest.
   b. Denali National Park.
2. Antarctica medical stations.
3. Cold-weather races.

The Condition

Hypothermia is a multisystem disease with lower survival rates at lower initial core temperatures.

A. Lowest surviving accidental hypothermia victim had a core temperature of 15.2°C.
1. Induced surgical hypothermia low core temperature is 6°C.
B. Below 30°C core temperature, the body is poikilothermic, which means that the body's temperature will drift toward the temperature of the surrounding environment.
C. Victims are not considered clinically dead until warm and dead.
1. Warm = 32–35°C core or rectal temperature.

Definitions and Classification

A. 36.5–38.5°C (97–100.6°F) considered normal body temperature in clinical medicine.

B. Core body temperature < 36.5°C (97°F) considered hypothermic.
1. Mild: 34–36°C (93–97°F).
2. Moderate: 30–34°C (86–93°F).
3. Severe: < 30°C (< 86°F).

Etiology of Hypothermia in Athletes

A. Accidental.
1. Rapid.
   a. Cold water immersion.
   b. Severe exposure to extreme cold.
2. Slow.
   a. Exposure to cool and/or wet weather.
   b. Hiker's hypothermia.

Morbidity and Mortality

A. Mild casualties.
1. General recovery with endogenous heat production.
2. Morbidity and mortality low.
B. Moderate casualties.
1. General recovery with active rewarming.
2. Morbidity and mortality slightly higher than mild casualties, but overall still low.
C. Severe casualties.
1. 30–80% mortality reported in the literature.
   a. More recent data shows 30% mortality.
   b. In the mid-1980s, 55–100% mortality was reported for severe accidental hypothermia.
2. Pulse present at initial exam indicates better survival prognosis.
3. Longer duration of hypothermia associated with increased morbidity.

Pathophysiology of Cold Exposure

A. Intense vasoconstriction.
1. Constriction of peripheral vasculature.
   a. Shunts blood to the core.
   b. Increases the risk of frostbite in the periphery.
2. Progressive contraction of core vasculature occurs to protect vital organs; this increases body insulation by a factor of 6.
3. Produces relative increase in blood volume.
   a. Cold exposure alone augments urine flow.
   b. Results in diuresis (see below) and volume depletion.
B. Tissue cooling causes a decrease in metabolic rate of ~ 6% for each 1°C.

C. Diving reflex occurs with face immersed in cold water.
   1. Decreased metabolic rate in response to sudden cold immersion.
   2. Decrease in heart rate and respiratory rate.
   3. May be present in children.
   4. Probably lost in adults.
D. Diuresis.
   1. Kidney sees increased volume due to peripheral (and later core) vasoconstriction.
   2. Kidney attempts to reestablish normal volume with increased urine production.
   3. Results in dehydration.
   4. Not as severe in rapid-onset immersion hypothermia with early intervention.
E. Hyperglycemia.
   1. Cold exposure leads to inhibited sympathetic insulin secretion.
   2. Direct cooling of insulin-secreting cells inhibits their function.
   3. Elevated blood sugar levels can contribute to diuresis and volume contraction.
F. Blood chemistry changes do occur but are of limited diagnostic value.
   1. Elevated enzyme markers of cell injury are typically noted.
   2. Combined respiratory and metabolic acidosis is commonly seen.

Cardiac Effects of Decreased Core Temperature

A. Cardiac contractility usually remains normal even to profoundly cold temperatures.
B. Heart rate slows with decreasing core temperature.
   1. < 3 beats/min at 10°C below normal.
C. Atrial fibrillation commonly encountered below 30°C.
D. Heart muscle becomes irritable at 28°C.
   1. Ventricular fibrillation.
      a. Greatest risk 20–24°C.
      b. Difficult to treat if core temperature remains below 28°C.
   2. Alcohol may lower arrhythmia threshold by 2–5°C.
E. Asystole is common below 20°C.
F. Poor cardiac tissue response to treatment when core temperature measures below 30°C.
   1. Defibrillation.
   2. Antiarrhythmic drugs.
   3. Cardioactive drugs.
   4. Pacemaker.
G. J-wave noted on EKG tracing.

1. Extra deflection at QRS-ST junction.
2. Was once considered pathognomonic of hypothermia.
   a. Also found in sepsis and CNS lesions.
   b. Presence not obligatory for hypothermia.
      i. Found in 80% of hypothermic victims.

Clinical Presentation of Hypothermia

A. Mental status changes.
   1. Impaired judgment.
      a. Paradoxical undressing in moderate range.
   2. Confusion.
   3. Apathy.
   4. Decreased level of consciousness.
      a. Loss of consciousness common between 30–32°C.
   5. Coma.
B. Shivering: the body's heating system to counter core cooling.
   1. Decreases at core temperatures below 33°C, possibly to preserve energy stores.
   2. Can occur at body temperatures as low as 24°C.
C. Muscle stiffness: increases as cell temperatures drop.
D. Decreased pulse.
E. Decreased respiratory rate.
   1. Response to decreased O_2 demands.
   2. Decreased metabolic rate.

Rewarming treatment

A. Rewarming physiology
   1. Peripheral rewarming.
      a. Vasodilatation of extremities can cause shock.
      b. Reducing vasoconstriction can override compensation for hypovolemia.
   2. Increased O_2 demand in warmed tissues.
   3. Afterdrop during rewarming.
      a. Drop in core temperature after cooling stimulus is removed and warming has started.
         i. 2–3°C adults.
         ii. 5°C children.
      b. Mechanism of afterdrop is heat exchange cooling of the blood circulating through cold peripheral tissues.
         i. Initially thought to be recirculation of cold blood from the extremities.
   4. Cardiac catheterization may not be as risky as once believed.

B. Passive rewarming methods utilize endogenous heat production.
  1. 1°C increases in temperature per hour at basal metabolic rate.
  2. 2°C per hour if shivering.
  3. Exercise for rewarming initiated only for temperature > 35°C.
C. Active external (surface) rewarming methods use exogenous energy.
  1. Warm water immersion.
      a. Water temperature = 40–45°C.
      b. Keep the victim's extremities out of water.
      c. Body temperature can increase by 5°C+ per hour.
      d. Problems.
          i. Difficult to perform CPR if needed.
          ii. Evaporative heat loss when taken from tub.
  2. Heating blankets.
      a. Increase body temperature by 0.5°C–3°C per hour.
      b. Burn risk exists.
  3. Warmed air "blankets."
      a. Bair Hugger™.
      b. Heater air ducts into blankets.
  4. Plumbed garments.
      a. Bare Hugger™.
  5. Heated objects or containers.
      a. Blankets warmed in a dryer or microwave.
  6. Radiant heat.
      a. Radiant heaters.
      b. Heat lamps.
      c. Open fires.
      d. Other animal bodies (field technique).
D. Internal (core) rewarming techniques.
  1. Extracorporeal cardiopulmonary bypass.
      a. Increases body temperature by 3–10°C per hour.
          i. 1–2°C every 3–5 minutes.
      b. Bleeding risk from heparin.
      c. Method of choice in cardiac arrest.
  2. Continuous thoracostomy (pleural) lavage.
      a. Two-chest-tube method.
      b. Rewarming of up to 8°C per hour.
  3. Peritoneal irrigation (peritoneal dialysis).
      a. Increases body temperature by 4–6°C per hour.
      b. Simple procedure.
      c. Two bladder catheters.
      d. Ringer's lactate or saline warmed to 40°C in a blood warmer.
          i. Lavage rate: 10–12 L/hr.
  4. Mediastinal lavage.
      a. Increases body temperature by 2–3°C per hour.

  5. Extracorporeal hemodialysis.
  6. Airway inhalation.
      a. Can be utilized in the field.
      b. Better methods available in hospital.
  7. Warmed IV fluids.
  8. Gastric irrigation.
      a. Increases body temperature by 1–1.3°C per hour.
      b. Augments other methods.
  9. Rectal irrigation.
      a. Not well described.
      b. Augments other methods.
  10. Bladder irrigation.

Field Treatment and Initial First Aid for Hypothermia

A. Handle the injured tissue gently (handle the patient gently in general).
B. Stop the core temperature drop.
  1. Remove from cold environment.
  2. Remove wet clothing.
  3. Dry the skin.
  4. Insulate with prewarmed blankets.
      a. Prewarm.
      b. Clothes dryer.
C. Use O_2 if available.
D. Consider intravenous dextrose 50% in water.
E. EKG monitoring if available.
  1. Electrodes may not stick.
  2. Puncture skin with needle through electrode pad.
  3. Maximum amplification.
F. CPR.
  1. Initiate if victim is:
      a. Pulseless.
          i. Not for bradycardia.
          ii. May need to monitor for prolonged period of time to detect a pulse.
      b. Apneic.
  2. Initiate only if CPR can be continued to the hospital.
  3. Cardiac monitor.
      a. Pierce skin and electrode with needle if electrodes will not stick to cold skin.
      b. Do not use needle-piercing technique for cardioversion.
G. Rewarming in the field can be attempted in mild to moderate cases as long as the victim is conscious and refreezing can be avoided.

1. Walk to generate intrinsic heat.
2. Warm packs in neck, axilla, and groin for mild to moderate cases.
   a. Hot-water bottles.
   b. Warmed IV bags.
3. Insulate with warmed blankets.
4. Breathe warmed, humidified air.
   a. 42–46°C.
   b. Bennett respirator.
   c. Bird respirator.
5. Blanket with circulation tubes for warmed air or fluid.
   a. Bare Hugger™.
   b. Bair Hugger™.
H. Field disposition.
   1. Mild casualties can be released if victim becomes normothermic and stable.
   2. Moderate to severe cases will need hospital evaluation.

Hospital Treatment of Hypothermia

A. Rewarming for mild, conscious victim.
   1. Passive techniques.
   2. Active external techniques.
B. Rewarming for moderate victims.
   1. Passive and active external techniques.
   2. Use caution with active external rewarming in unconscious victims due to skin burn risk.
C. Rapid internal techniques are utilized for severe hypothermia.
   1. Extracorporeal rewarming is method of choice.
      a. Extracorporeal bypass.
      b. Extracorporeal hemodialysis.
   2. Peritoneal dialysis or two-chest-tube irrigation.
   3. Centrally administered warmed IV fluids at 43°C.
   4. Heated, humidified O_2.
D. Monitor temperature at 5- to 10-minute intervals.
E. End point for rewarming.
   1. Stop rewarming at 32–34°C.
   2. Stopped at this level to avoid hyperthermia and increased cell metabolism.
F. System support.
   1. Support hypovolemia with fluid resuscitation.
      a. Saline.
      b. No lactated Ringer's.
         i. Cold liver cannot metabolize lactate.

   2. If victim has altered mental status:
      a. D50%W, 50 mL IV.
      b. Thiamine, 100 mg IV.
      c. Naloxone, 0.8 mg IV.
   3. O_2 administration.
   4. Monitor laboratory values.
      a. Glucose.
      b. Electrolytes.
      c. Chemistries.
   5. CPR.
   6. Antibiotics.
G. Cardioversion of arrhythmias.
   1. The victim typically needs to be rewarmed for defibrillation to be successful.
      a. Can attempt at low core temperature but do not give up.
      b. Defibrillation trial up to 3 shocks for temperature < 30°C.
   2. Cardiac arrhythmia prophylaxis with bretylium (5 mg/kg).
      a. For core temperature < 28°C.

Complications of Hypothermia

A. Pneumonia.
B. Pulmonary edema.
C. Cardiac arrhythmia.
D. Myoglobinuria.
E. Disseminated intravascular coagulation (DIC).
F. Seizures.
G. Compartment syndromes.

PREVENTION

General Precautions

Hypothermia is a preventable illness in athletic settings.
A. Preventing emergencies during athletic competition in cold conditions.
   1. Define environmental conditions that pose a threat to the athletes' safety (Table 3-1).
   2. Have contingency plans in case of hazardous conditions.
      a. Cancel the event.
      b. Postpone the event.
      c. Modify the event.

TABLE 3-1

Wet bulb globe temperature and ambient temperature cascades.

Temperature (°C/°F)	Flag	ACSM Road Race	MSHSL Heat & Cold Guide (based on ASCM & FIMS recommendations)
< −29/−20 Ambient	—		Recommended lower limit for practice
< −20/−4 Ambient	Blue		Cancel Nordic races and events > 1 min duration
< 10/50 WBGT	White	Increased hypothermia risk	Hypothermia risk
10/50 to 18/65 WBGT	Green	Low risk hyperthermia and hypothermia	Normal activity

3. Administrative actions in cold conditions are the most powerful form of prevention.
   a. Stop activities in high-risk settings.
   b. Provide appropriate shelters.
   c. Provide warming devices.
      i. Blankets.
      ii. Heaters.
   d. Create an emergency plan in case of moderate to severe cold injury, including evacuation plan.
B. Preventing cold-related injuries and illness.
   1. Athlete education.
      a. Hydration.
      b. Nutrition.
      c. Proper clothing.
   2. Buddy system with athletes watching each other.
   3. Coach education.
      a. Signs and symptoms.
      b. Risk conditions and modifications.

Adaptations to Environmental Cold Stress

A. Behavioral adaptation.
   1. Move indoors.
   2. Increase layers of clothing.
   3. Seek shelter outdoors.

   4. Find an external heat source.
   5. Psychologic.
   a. Mental adaptations to cold conditions can increase late-season risk.
   b. Conditions "feel" warm, but heat loss risk is still present.
   6. Normal behavioral responses in athletic competition may not take place.
   a. "Removed" from the athlete.
   b. The athlete feels that:
     i. The safety of the competitive arena is left to the event administration.
     ii. Coaches and event administrators will not send them out in hazardous conditions.
B. Physiologic adaptations to cold stress.
   1. Limited capacity for physiologic adaptation in humans.
   2. Increased peripheral vasoconstriction.
   a. Noted in Australian aborigines.
   3. Increased fat layer.
   a. Increased skinfold thickness in men in Antarctica has been reported.
   4. Increased metabolic heat production.
   a. Seen in deep-water pearl divers.

Frostbite Prevention

A. Risk factors for athletes.
   1. Outdoor activity in ambient temperatures $< 31°C$.
   2. Previous frostbite increases risk twofold.
   3. Altered mental status.
   a. Hypothermia.
   b. Exercise exhaustion.
   4. Tobacco use.
   5. Black race.
   6. Petroleum product spills.
   a. Liquid petroleum products cool to temperatures well below tissue freezing levels.
   b. Rapid evaporation adds to heat loss.
B. Prevention strategies.
   1. Education of athletes regarding:
   a. Protective clothing for genitals, hands, feet, and ears.
     i. Avoid tight and constricting clothing.
     ii. Carry extra equipment and clothing.
   b. Signs and symptoms of impending cold injury.
   c. First aid.

2. Remove metal jewelry.
   a. Especially circumferential and pierced.
3. Eye protection to prevent corneal freeze and blindness.
4. Buddy system reasons and importance.
5. Event planners need to take appropriate precautions.
   a. Assess risk of cold injury on day of event.

Hypothermia Prevention

A. Risk factors.
   1. Environment.
      a. Temperature < 18°C (64°F).
      b. Wind speed and windchill factor (Table 3-2).
         i. 40°F with 15 mph wind speed = 32°F windchill.

TABLE 3-2

Wind chill chart (National Weather Service, 2001).

Temperature (°F)

	Calm	40	30	20	10	0	−10	−20	−30	−40
Wind (mph)	5	36	25	13	1	−11	−22	−34	−46	−57
	10	34	21	9	−4	−16	−28	−41	−53	−66
	15	32	19	6	−7	−19	−32	−45	−58	−71
	20	30	17	4	−9	−22	−35	−48	−61	−74
	25	29	16	3	−11	−24	−37	−51	−64	−78
	30	28	15	1	−12	−26	−39	−53	−67	−80
	35	28	14	0	−14	−27	−41	−55	−69	−82
	40	27	13	−1	−15	−29	−43	−57	−71	−84
	45	26	12	−2	−16	−30	−44	−58	−72	−86
	50	26	12	−3	−17	−31	−45	−60	−74	−88
	55	25	11	−3	−18	−32	−46	−61	−75	−89
	60	25	10	−4	−19	−33	−48	−62	−76	−91

Frostbite Times

	30 minutes
	10 minutes
	5 minutes

Wind Chill (°F) = 35.74 + 0.6215T − 35.75 (V$^{0.16}$) + 0.4275T (V$^{0.16}$)

Where, T = Air Temperature (°F)

V = Wind Speed (mph)

    c. Extreme cold.

    d. Wet conditions.

       i. Sweating.

       ii. Raining or sleeting.

       iii. Cold water immersion.

          • Thermal conductivity 32 times greater than air.

2. Age.

    a. Older athletes have a decreased metabolic rate.

    b. Younger athletes have larger body surface to mass ratio, which leads to greater surface heat loss.

3. Alcohol.

    a. Behavior changes are the greatest risk associated with alcohol consumption.

    b. Vasodilatation may contribute to mild hypothermia.

       i. Significant vasodilatation does not occur until sublethal blood alcohol levels are reached.

4. Pharmacologic.

    a. Barbiturates, halothane, phenothiazines, and ether.

       i. Direct effect on temperature regulation center.

       ii. Reduce thermogenic shivering.

       iii. Induce cutaneous vasodilatation.

       iv. Lower the basal metabolic rate.

5. Hypoglycemia.

    a. Depleted glycogen stores.

       i. Prolonged shivering.

       ii. Physical exertion.

    b. Diabetes mellitus.

6. Medical conditions that lead to hypothermia or increase risk.

    a. Head injury.

       i. Decreases body temperature through central mechanisms.

       ii. Loss of shivering thermogenesis.

       iii. More commonly a cause of slow-onset hypothermia.

    b. Hypothyroidism.

       i. Decreased metabolic rate.

    c. Hypopituitarism.

    d. Hypoadrenalism.

    e. Sepsis.

       i. Decreases body temperature through central mechanisms.

B. Prevention strategies.

    1. Take environment precautions during activity.

    2. Education.

    a. Hydration before and during activity to maintain blood flow.

    b. Appropriate nutrition maintains energy stores during activity and prevents "hiker's hypothermia."

    c. Proper clothing.

        i. Avoid cotton to keep dry layer next to skin.

        ii. Use layers and vented clothing to regulate temperature and avoid excessive sweating.

SUMMARY

Cold injury and illness of moderate to severe degree are best treated in the hospital rather than in the field.

    Severe cold injury and illness are not common in athletes.

A. Can occur quickly in a cold outdoor setting in an injured athlete who cannot move to shelter quickly.

B. Evacuation protocols established in advance of an event are critical for remote activities.

Athletes involved in prolonged activity are at greater risk for hypothermia if energy sources and fluids are not replaced throughout the activity.

    Wet environments increase risk of hypothermia at "warmer" temperatures.

    Prevention is critical to athlete safety and cold-injury reduction.

Suggested Readings

American College of Sports Medicine. Position statement on exercise and fluid replacement. *Med Sci Sports Exerc* 1996;28(1):i–vii.

American College of Sports Medicine. Position statement on heat and cold illnesses during distance running. *Med Sci Sports Exerc* 1996; 28(12):i–vii.

Armstrong LE, CM Maresh, AE Crago, R Adams, WO Roberts. Interpretation of aural temperatures during exercise, hyperthermia, and cooling therapy. *Med Exerc Nutr Health* 1994;3(1):9–16.

Bracher MD. Environment and thermal injury. *Clin Sports Med* 1992;11(2):419–36.

Brengelman GL. The dilemma of body temperature measurement. In: Shiraki K, Yousef MK, eds. *Man in Stressful Environments: Thermal and Work Physiology*. Springfield: Thomas; 1987.

Channa AB, MA Seraj, AA Saddique, GH Kadiwal, MH Shaikh, AH Samarkandi. Is dantrolene effective in heat stroke patients? *Crit Care Med* 1990;18(3):290–92.

Coyle EF, SJ Montain. Benefits of fluid replacement with carbohydrate during exercise. *Med Sci Sports Exerc* 1992;24(suppl 9):S324–S330.

Finley JB, AF Hartman, RC Weir. Post-swim orthostatic intolerance in a marathon swimmer. *Med Sci Sports Exerc* 1995;27(9):1231–37.

Hayward JS, M Collis, JD Eckerson. Thermographic evaluation of relative heat loss areas of man during cold water immersion. *Aerospace Med* 1973; 44(7)708–11.

Heggers JP, MC Robson, et al. Experimental and clinical observations on frostbite. *Ann Emerg Med* 1987;16(9):1056–62.

Lazar HL. The treatment of hypothermia (editorial). *N Eng J Med* 1997; 337(21):1545–47.

McCann DJ, WC Adams. Wet bulb globe temperature index and performance in competitive distance runners. *Med Sci Sports Exerc* 1997;29(7):955–61.

McCauley RL, JP Heggers, MC Robson. Frostbite: Methods to minimize tissue loss. *Post Grad Med* 1990;88(8):67–77.

Mills WJ. Field care of the hypothermic patient. *Int J Sports Med* 1992; 13(suppl 1):199–202.

Roberts WO. Assessing core temperature in collapsed athletes. *Phys Sportsmed* 1994;22(8):49–55.

Roberts WO. Environmental concerns. In: Kibler WB, ed. *ACSM's Handbook for the Team Physician*. Baltimore: Williams & Wilkins; 1996.

Roberts WO. Exercise-associated collapse in endurance events: A classification system. *Phys Sportsmed* 1989;17(5):49–55.

Walpoth BH, BN Walpoth-Aslan, HP Mattle, et al. Outcome of survivors of accidental deep hypothermia and circulatory arrest treated with extracorporeal blood warming. *N Eng J Med* 1997;337(21):1500–05.

Weinberg AD. Hypothermia. *Ann Emerg Med* 1993;22(2 pt2):370–77.

DOPING

Sami F. Rifat
James L. Moeller

OVERVIEW

Definition

Doping is the administration to or the use by a competing athlete of any substance foreign to the body or any physiologic substance taken in abnormal quantity with the sole intention of increasing in an artificial and unfair manner his/her performance.

Historical Perspective

A. The ancient Greeks used stimulants and hallucinogenic mushrooms to improve their athletic performance in the first Olympic games.
B. In 1889 French physiologist Charles Edward Brown-Séquard claimed to reverse the aging process after he self-injected testicular extracts.
C. Testosterone was first synthesized in 1935.
D. In the 1940s athletes began using anabolic steroids to increase muscle mass.
E. In the 1950s amphetamines began to be extensively used by athletes.
F. The International Olympic Committee (IOC) banned the use of anabolic steroids and amphetamines in the early sixties.
G. Drug testing began at the 1968 Olympic games.
H. The World Anti-Doping Agency (WADA) was formed in 1999.

1. An international cooperative effort between governments and sporting federations.
2. Mission is to fight against doping of any kind in all sports.

ANABOLIC STEROIDS

General Considerations

A. Anabolic steroids are testosterone and testosterone-like substances that result in anabolic and androgenic effects.
B. History.
   1. Anabolic steroids were developed in the 1930s in Germany.
   2. The Germans gave them to their own soldiers to make them more aggressive.
   3. They were first introduced into athletics in the 1950s.
   4. Athletes quickly realized the benefits in strength and endurance.
C. Prevalence.
   1. In 1999 a federal study found that 2.7% of all eighth and tenth graders and 2.9% of all twelfth graders had tried anabolic steroids at least once.
   2. This trend seems to be rising.
   3. The prevalence among elite athletes is not well known.
      a. Difficult to study.

Mechanisms of Action

A. Induce protein synthesis in muscle cells.
B. Stimulate the release of endogenous growth hormone.
C. Reverse the effects of cortisol.

Administration

A. Anabolic steroids may be administered orally or parenterally.
   1. Oral forms are less hepatotoxic.
   2. Oral anabolic steroids are detectable via drug testing for a longer period of time.
B. Athletes often use 10 to 40 times greater than the normal therapeutic dose.
C. Stacking is the process of combining anabolic steroids.
D. Anabolic steroids are often taken in cycles of 6- to 12-week duration.
E. Pyramiding refers to the practice of increasing the dose of steroid throughout the cycle with the hope of maximizing beneficial effects while minimizing the harmful ones.

Uses

A. Accepted clinical uses:
1. Treatment of hypogonadism.
2. Treatment of impotence.
3. Reversal of wasting secondary to burns or chronic debilitating illness.

B. Use in athletics.
1. Proven effects.
   a. Increased lean body mass.
   b. Increased strength.
2. Strong anecdotal evidence.
   a. Increased speed.
   b. Decreased recovery time.
   c. Increased endurance.

Adverse Effects

A. Liver carcinoma.
B. Male reproductive system.
1. Impotence, usually reversible.
2. Testicular atrophy.

C. Virilization in females.
1. Deepening of voice.
2. Male pattern baldness, usually irreversible.

D. Musculoskeletal.
1. Tendon rupture.
2. Osteonecrosis of the hip.

E. Skin.
1. Acne.
2. Gynecomastia in males, usually irreversible.
3. Alopecia.

F. Cardiovascular.
1. Myocardial infarction.
2. Stroke.
3. Cardiomyopathy.
4. Increased blood pressure.
5. Increased risk of thromboembolism.

G. Psychological.
1. Psychosis.
2. Aggressiveness.
3. Mood swings.
4. Depression.

Testing

A. The ratio of testosterone to epitestosterone (T:E) has been used to identify the use of exogenous steroids.
  1. Epitestosterone is an isomer of testosterone.
  2. The normal T:E ratio is 1:1.
  3. When exogenous testosterone is taken, the serum testosterone is elevated and out of proportion to epitestosterone.
  4. A ratio of 6:1 or greater is considered to be a positive test.
  5. Some athletes take epitestosterone to maintain a "normal" ratio.
B. Recently a test to differentiate naturally occurring testosterone from chemically manufactured testosterone has been developed.
C. Masking agents.
  1. Substances used to hide the presence of anabolic steroids during drug testing.
  2. Probenecid.
    a. A renal tubular blocking agent.
    b. Masks the presence of steroid in the urine by blocking the excretion of the drug.
    c. Probenecid itself is a banned substance.
  3. Diuretics.
    a. Dilute the concentration of the steroid in the urine.
    b. Most drug tests use a minimum specific gravity to counteract the use of diuretics as masking agents.
  4. Human chorionic gonadotropin (hCG).
    a. Naturally occurring hormone produced by the placenta.
    b. In women it is used to induce ovulation in order to get pregnant.
    c. In men it stimulates the production of androgens.
    d. When used with anabolic steroids it helps to reduce the T:E ratio.

HUMAN GROWTH HORMONE (hGH)

General Considerations

A. Growth hormone is a naturally occurring polypeptide hormone found in the anterior pituitary gland.
B. History.
  1. In the 1930s animal breeders discovered that animals fed pituitary glands developed increased muscle mass and increased lean body mass.
  2. In the 1950s it was found that hGH stimulated growth.
  3. In 1985 the first synthetic hGH was sold in the United States.
C. Prevalence of use in athletes is unknown due to difficulty in detection.

Mechanism of Action

A. In hGH-deficient children the administration of exogenous growth hormone results in a positive nitrogen balance and stimulation of skeletal and soft tissue growth.
B. Other effects.
    1. Anti-insulin effect by inhibiting the cellular uptake of glucose.
    2. Stimulates the mobilization of lipids from adipose tissue.

Administration

A. Therapeutic dose in deficient individuals is approximately 0.2 mg/kg/wk divided daily or three times a week.
B. Little is known about dosing in athletes though it is believed that some athletes use 20 times the normal therapeutic dose.
C. It is extremely expensive and its use may be cost-prohibitive for many athletes.

Uses

A. Acceptable clinical uses.
    1. Treatment of short stature.
    2. Turner syndrome.
    3. Chronic renal failure.
B. Use in athletics.
    1. Perceived benefits.
        a. Increased muscle mass.
        b. Increased strength.
    2. Documented benefits.
        a. No published evidence of an effect on muscle strength in trained power athletes.
        b. No change in body composition in healthy, lean, trained athletes.
        c. Possible flaws of the published studies.
            i. Doses studied are less than abusing athlete uses.
            ii. Low sample size.

Adverse Effects

A. Fluid retention.
B. Arthralgia.
C. Insulin resistance and impaired glucose tolerance.
D. Type 2 diabetes.
E. Hypertension.

F. Dyslipidemia.
G. Acromegaloid features.
H. Malignancies of the gastrointestinal tract.
I. Carpal tunnel syndrome.
J. Transient peripheral edema in children.
K. Pseudotumor cerebri due to transient peripheral edema.

Testing

A. hGH is banned by the IOC.
B. Blood and blood/urine tests for hGH have recently been reported.
C. The validity of these tests has not been definitively determined.

CREATINE

General Considerations

A. Creatine is an amino acid naturally occurring in the body.
  1. Primarily found in skeletal muscle.
  2. 60% is stored as creatine phosphate.
B. Produced in the liver, kidneys, and pancreas at a rate of 2 g/day.
C. Not currently banned by the International Olympic Committee.

Mechanism of Action

A. Plays a critical role in skeletal muscle energy metabolism.
B. Maintains high cellular ATP/ADP ratios.
C. Physiologic buffer to ATP use.
D. Energy transport.
  1. Facilitates energy translocation from mitochondria to sites of ATP utilization.
  2. Secures energy availability for work of all kinds.

Administration

A. Loading dose 15–25 g per day for 5 days.
B. Maintenance dose 2–5 g per day.

Uses

A. Accepted clinical uses: none.
B. Use in athletics.
  1. Perceived benefits.
     a. Increased strength.
     b. Increased size.

    c. Increased speed.
    d. Decreased fatigue and quicker recovery.
    e. More intense workouts.
  2. Documented benefits with moderate to long-term use along with an appropriate training program.
    a. Increased repeated sprint performance.
    b. Decreased decay in jumping ability on repeated testing.
    c. Increased lower-body maximal strength.
    d. Increased lower- and upper-body power.
    e. No documented effects in endurance activities.

Adverse Effects

A. Documented effects.
  1. Weight gain.
  2. Increased urinary creatinine.
    a. No evidence of renal impairment in the healthy kidney.
    b. Probably should not be used by those with renal dysfunction or the potential for renal dysfunction (e.g., diabetes).
B. Anecdotal effects.
  1. Muscle cramping.
  2. Muscle strain.
  3. Tendon injury.
    a. Tendonitis.
    b. Tendon rupture.
  4. GI upset and diarrhea.
  5. Dehydration.
C. To date there have been no long-term outcome studies demonstrating serious adverse effects from creatine use.

ANDROSTENEDIONE

General Considerations

A. Androstenedione is a dietary supplement and a direct precursor of testosterone.
  1. Converted in the liver to testosterone.
  2. Converted by 17-beta hydroxysteroid dehydrogenase.
B. Used since the 1970s.

Mechanism of Action

A. Androstenedione is considered a prohormone.
B. Its action is derived from its conversion to testosterone.

C. The conversion of exogenously administered androstenedione to testosterone has not yet been proven in the scientific literature.
   1. Some studies have shown that androstenedione consumption does not lead to a predictable increase in testosterone level.
   2. Other studies have shown no increase in testosterone at all.
   3. Leder et al. (2000) demonstrated increased testosterone when 300 mg/day was ingested.
D. Androstenedione supplementation has been found to increase estrogen and estrogen derivatives.

Administration

A. Androstenedione is widely available.
B. It typically is taken orally, although nasal sprays and transdermal forms are also available.
C. The usual dose is 100–300 mg/day.

Uses

A. Perceived benefits.
   1. Increased strength.
   2. Increased size.
   3. Increased power.
B. Proven benefits.
   1. Studies have not consistently demonstrated positive functional benefits, such as changes in body composition or exercise performance.

Adverse Effects

Adverse effects are not well documented but are believed to be similar to those seen in exogenous testosterone administration.

Testing

A. Androstenedione use is banned by the IOC, NCAA, and various other organizations, though currently no test is available for the detection of androstenedione use.
B. Studies of over-the-counter supplements containing androstenedione have shown mislabeling to be prevalent.
   1. Actual amount of androstenedione present is typically inaccurate.
   2. Testosterone has been found in some formulations, enough to lead to a positive drug test.

DHEA

General Considerations

A. Dehydroepiandrosterone (DHEA) is a steroid hormone and precursor to testosterone and estrogen.

B. In its natural form it is made from cholesterol by the adrenal glands.

Mechanism of Action

A. Believed to increase serum testosterone levels although this effect has not been scientifically documented.

B. Increased levels of serum androstenedione have been documented; however, neither serum testosterone nor estrogen appear to increase with oral administration.

Uses

A. No proven clinical benefits.

B. Perceived benefits.
   1. Increased muscle mass.
   2. Increased strength.
   3. Greater sense of well-being.

BLOOD DOPING

General Considerations

A. Blood doping refers to the banking and reinfusion of red blood cells.

B. This practice increases oxygen-carrying capacity of the blood.

C. History.
   1. In 1947 fresh blood was transfused into military personnel and a 34% increase in endurance over control subjects was demonstrated.
   2. In 1984 seven U.S. cyclists were found to be doping at the 1984 Olympic games.
   3. In 1990 a study of 1018 Italian athletes found that 7% had tried blood doping.

Mechanism

A. Transfusion increases oxygen delivery to muscle tissue.

B. Red blood cell mass and Vo_2 max are well correlated.

C. Increased hemoglobin concentration.
D. Increased exercise tolerance.

Uses

A. Accepted clinical uses.
    1. Transfusion for symptomatic anemia.
B. Use in athletics.
    1. Improved oxygen-carrying capacity of the blood.
    2. Improved performance in endurance athletes.

Administration

A. 2000 mL homologous blood.
B. 900 to 1800 mL frozen autologous blood.

Adverse Effects

A. Transfusion reactions in improperly matched blood can be fatal.
B. Allergic reactions.
C. Bacterial contamination.
D. Disease transmission.
E. Immune sensitization.
F. Polycythemia.
    1. Ischemia.
    2. Thromboembolic events.

Testing

Though banned by WADA, the reinfusion of red blood cells is difficult to detect.

ERYTHROPOIETIN

Definition

Recombinant human erythropoietin (rEPO) is a synthetic hormone that enhances erythropoiesis by stimulating the formation of pro-erythroblasts and release of reticulocytes from bone marrow.

General Considerations

A. rEPO is a synthetic version of naturally occurring erythropoietin.
B. Has largely replaced blood doping.
C. Regulates erythropoiesis in the bone marrow.

Historical Perspective

A. Erythropoietin was discovered in 1953.
B. In 1957 the kidney was found to be the source of erythropoietin.
C. Recombinant human erythropoietin was first synthesized in 1987.
D. Banned by the IOC since 1990.

Prevalence

A. 7.6% of college athletes using anabolic steroids also admitted to using rEPO.
B. The unexplained deaths of 18 Dutch and Belgian cyclists in the early 1990s raised the suspicion of widespread rEPO abuse.

Use

A. Accepted clinical uses.
   1. Anemia.
     a. Chronic renal failure.
     b. Chemotherapy.
     c. In HIV-infected individuals.
   2. To reduced the need for allogenic blood transfusion in anemic patients prior to surgery.
B. Use in athletics is identical to blood doping.

Adverse Effects

A. Hyperviscosity of blood.
   1. May lead to ischemia.
   2. May lead to thromboembolic events.
B. Hypertension.
C. Flu-like symptoms.
D. Hyperkalemia.

Testing

A. Recently a reliable test for rEPO was developed.
B. It was first utilized on a large scale at the 2002 Salt Lake City Winter Olympic games.

AMPHETAMINES

General Considerations

A. Amphetamines are synthetic central nervous system stimulants.
B. Amphetamines are commonly referred to as speed.

C. History.
 1. First synthesized in 1887.
 2. They were first used in the 1930s to treat congestion, obesity, and narcolepsy.
 3. In the 1950s the effect on human performance was studied.
 4. Danish cyclist Kurt Jensen died of an amphetamine overdose during the 1960 Olympic games.

Administration

A. Amphetamines are usually administered orally.
B. They come in long- and short-acting forms with varying dosages.

Uses

A. Accepted clinical uses.
 1. Attention deficit disorder.
 2. Narcolepsy.
A. Use in athletics.
 1. Perceived benefits.
  a. Increased performance.
 2. Documented benefits.
  a. No clear evidence of improved athletic performance, though a few studies have shown modest gains in performance.

Adverse Effects

A. Nervous system.
 1. Restlessness.
 2. Insomnia.
 3. Tremor.
 4. Dizziness.
 5. Cerebral hemorrhage.
B. Psychiatric.
 1. Addiction.
 2. Psychosis.
 3. Anxiety.
C. Cardiovascular.
 1. Arrhythmias.
 2. Aggravation of angina.

Testing

A. Amphetamines are banned by the IOC and NCAA.
B. Amphetamines are easily detected in the urine.

β_2 AGONISTS

General Considerations

A. β_2 agonists are considered to be anabolic agents and stimulants.
B. The exact mechanism of the β_2 agonists' anabolic effects has not been determined.

Administration

A. The β_2 agonists can be administered by inhalation, orally, or intravenously.
B. The inhaled β_2 agonists have no significant anabolic effects.

Uses

A. Accepted clinical uses.
   1. Asthma.
   2. Chronic obstructive pulmonary disease.
B. Use in athletics.
   1. Increased muscle size.
   2. Decreased body fat.
   3. Stimulant effect.

Adverse Effects

A. Palpitations.
B. Headache.
C. Nausea.
D. Sweating.
E. Muscle cramps.
F. Dizziness.

Testing

A. The IOC bans all oral and injectable β_2 agonists.
B. The inhaled forms of albuterol (Salbutamol), salmeterol, terbutaline, and formoterol are allowed.
   1. Clinical and laboratory proof that the athlete needs the medication is required.
C. The presence of β_2 agonists can be detected in the urine.

OTHER NUTRITIONAL SUPPLEMENTS

TABLE 4-1

Miscellaneous nutritional supplements.

Supplement	Purported Benefits	Proven Benefits
B-Complex vitamins	Enhanced physical power Enhanced energy Anxiolytic	None
Caffeine	Increased mental awareness Increased metabolic rate Reduced perception of fatigue	Increased time to exhaustion in prolonged exercise Improves end-of-run sprint performance, though not sprinting in general No apparent effect on untrained people
Calcium	Increased physical power Enhanced ATP use Decreased lactic acid production	Useful in those with inadequate dietary calcium intake Increased bone mineral density in amenorheic women
Chromium	Increases lean body mass Improves glucose metabolism	None
Ephedrine	Improved athletic performance Improved concentration Promotes loss of body fat	None
Ginseng	Increased resistance to catabolic effect of exercise Increased cortisol response to strenuous exercise Protection of the immune system Enhanced muscle glycogen synthesis after exercise	None

TABLE 4-1 (*Continued*)

Miscellaneous nutritional supplements.

Supplement	Purported Benefits	Proven Benefits
Magnesium	Increased physical power Increased muscle mass	None
Pseudoephedrine	Increased muscle strength	None
Vitamin C	Improved physical power Improved aerobic capacity Enhanced immunity	None
Vitamin E	Reduced delayed-onset muscle soreness	None
Zinc	Increased muscle contraction strength Increased muscle power Increased muscle endurance	None

Suggested Readings

Bouchard R, Weber AR, Geiger J. Informed decision making on sympathomimetic use in sport and health. *Clin J Sport Med* 2002;12:209–24.

Leder BZ, Longcope C, Catlin DH, Ahrens B, Schoenfeld DA, Finkelstein JS. Oral androstenedione administration and serum testosterone concentrations in young men. *JAMA* 2000;283(6):779–82.

Pipe A, Ayotte C. Nutritional supplements and doping. *Clin J Sport Med* 2002; 12:245–49.

Schwenk TL, Costley CD. When food becomes a drug: Nonanabolic nutritional supplement use in athletes. *Am J Sports Med* 2002; 30(6):907–16.

Silver MD. Use of ergoneic aids by athletes. *J Am Acad Ortho Surg* 2001; 9(1):61–70.

www.wada-ama.org

5

ALPINE SKIING

Sami F. Rifat

GENERAL CONSIDERATIONS

History

A. The use of implements to slide across the snow dates back as far as 5000 years ago.

B. Early hunters and fisherman in northern Europe used animal tusks to transport themselves across the snow and over frozen bodies of water.

C. Precursors of modern skis dating back to 2000 BC have been found in Scandinavia and Siberia.

D. The first written record describing skiing was found in China and dates back to 600 AD.

E. In the sixth century the Finns used rudimentary skis to increase their mobility on the snow and gain military advantage over their enemies.

Competitive Skiing

A. Started in Norway in the late 1700s and by the 1800s it was firmly entrenched.

B. In the mid-1800s, skiing was introduced into the mining camps of the western United States but did not gain popularity until the Lake Placid Olympics in 1932.

C. Today it is estimated that there are approximately 15 million skiers in the U.S. and 200 million worldwide.

D. Alpine events.
  1. There are ten Olympic Alpine skiing events: five for men and five for women.
      a. The courses for men and women differ, but the rules are the same.
      b. All events are run against the clock and time is measured down to one-hundredth of a second. In each event, the fastest time or combined time wins.
  2. Downhill:
      a. The downhill is the longest course and features the highest speeds.
      b. Each competitor makes a single run down a single course.
  3. Super-G:
      a. Combines the speed of the downhill with the turns of the slalom.
          i. The course is shorter than the downhill.
          ii. Fewer turns to navigate than slalom.
          iii. The skier makes a single run down a single course.
  4. Giant Slalom (GS):
      a. Similar to the slalom; however, it has fewer and wider turns.
      b. The skier makes two runs down two different courses on the same slope and the times are totaled.
  5. Slalom:
      a. The shortest course with the quickest turns.
      b. Each skier makes two runs down two different courses on the same slope.
  6. Combined:
      a. "Combines" one downhill with two slalom runs.
      b. The combined courses are shorter than those used for the regular downhill and slalom events.

Injury Statistics

A. The most recent data indicates 2 to 3 skier injuries per 1000 skier days.
  1. Injury rates have declined steadily over the past 50 years.
      a. Prior to 1970, injury rates were 5 to 8 injuries per 1000 skier days.
      b. The majority of this reduction can be attributed to improvements in ski equipment, especially boots and bindings.
  2. Although rates have been declining, it is believed that the current rates underestimate injury due to underreporting.

    3. Women and children appear to be at slightly greater risk of skiing-related injury compared to men.

        a. Women have an overall greater risk of knee injury.

           i. The increased risk of ACL injuries observed in many sports does not appear to apply to skiing.

           ii. The greater incidence of knee injuries has been attributed to the increased incidence of less severe collateral ligament injury.

        b. In children, the increased risk of injury is a reflection of a significantly higher incidence of tibial fractures compared to adults.

B. The anatomical distribution of injury has changed over the years.

    1. In 1982 the ratio of lower extremity to upper extremity injury was 4:1. By 1993 that ratio declined to 2:1.

        a. This decline is believed to be due to a decrease in lower extremity injuries as opposed to an increase in upper extremity injury.

    2. Over the same period there was a significant decline in the rate of ankle injuries and tibial fractures with a corresponding rise in ACL tears.

        a. The rate of ACL injury in skiers is now comparable to that of a collegiate football player.

MEDICAL ISSUES

Abdominal Injuries

A. General considerations.

    1. Though more common in contact or collision sports, abdominal injury has been reported in skiing.

    2. Abdominal trauma is the second most common cause of death in skiing, behind head injury.

    3. Skiers can suffer injury to the abdominal wall or viscera.

    4. Diagnosis is a challenge because the initial signs of many severe abdominal injuries are often quite subtle.

B. Abdominal wall contusion.

    1. Mechanism of injury.

        a. Direct injury: A direct blow caused by collision with another skier or piece of equipment can cause contusion and hematoma.

        b. Indirect injury: A sudden, violent contraction of the abdominal musculature can cause indirect injury of the muscle tissue.

2. Diagnosis.
   a. Typically the patient complains of pain with trunk flexion or rotation.
   b. Examination usually reveals local tenderness and ecchymosis.
3. Additional tests are not necessary to make the diagnosis.
4. Treatment.
   a. These injuries are usually self-limited and may be treated with relative rest, ice, and analgesics.
   b. More significant abdominal wall muscle contusions may be treated with rehabilitation in order to regain motion, strength, and endurance.

C. Rectus sheath hematoma.
   1. General considerations.
      a. The rectus abdominis muscles are particularly vulnerable because of the risk of injury to the epigastric or large intramuscular vessels.
      b. Injury to the muscle can cause hemorrhage with formation of a large hematoma within the rectus sheath.
   2. History.
      a. Individuals usually complain of sudden abdominal pain with rapid swelling.
      b. Nausea and vomiting may be present.
   3. Physical examination.
      a. Rectus sheath hematoma can mimic an acute abdomen with guarding and rigidity of the abdomen.
      b. The individual is most comfortable with the trunk in the supported flexed position.
      c. A tender palpable mass may be noted, most often below the umbilicus.
      d. Active flexion of the trunk produces pain.
   4. Diagnostic tests.
      a. Ultrasound is a good screening tool.
      b. The presence of a hematoma is confirmed by CT scan.
   5. Treatment.
      a. Ice, relative rest, and analgesics.
      b. Avoidance of activities that require flexion or rotation of the trunk.
      c. Stretching of the abdominal musculature.
      d. Large hematomas may require surgical evacuation and ligation of the epigastric artery, if torn.
      e. After the acute period, the athlete should begin rehabilitation with emphasis on regaining flexibility, strength, and endurance.

    f. Generally patients may return to activity as symptoms allow and when they have regained normal function.

D. Liver injury.

  1. General considerations.

    a. The liver is the most frequently injured abdominal organ.

    b. Two mechanisms of liver injury:

      i. Deceleration: As the body stops motion, the liver continues to move and lacerates its relatively thin capsule and underlying attached parenchyma.

      ii. Direct blow: Direct blows typically cause crush injury to the liver that often results in subcapsular or interparenchymal hematoma.

    c. The severity of liver injury ranges from minor capsular tear without parenchymal injury to extensive disruption of both lobes.

  2. History.

    a. Right upper-quadrant pain that may radiate to the right shoulder or neck.

    b. Nausea and vomiting may be reported.

    c. Some athletes complain of dizziness or light-headedness.

  3. Physical examination.

    a. Overlying ribs may be tender.

    b. Patients are typically tender in the right upper quadrant and sometimes demonstrate abdominal guarding.

    c. Flank bruising (Grey-Turner sign) may be present.

    d. Be sure to evaluate and document blood pressure and pulse.

  4. Diagnostic tests.

    a. Imaging is critical to the successful management of liver injury.

    b. CT scan is the "gold standard" (Figure 5-1); however, ultrasound is sometimes used for rapid screening.

    c. Diagnostic peritoneal lavage (DPL) is used if the patient is unconscious.

    d. Laboratory tests.

      i. Complete blood count.

      ii. Liver enzymes.

  5. Treatment:

    a. Depends on the level of consciousness and hemodynamic status of the athlete.

      i. Conscious athlete, hemodynamically unstable with peritoneal signs: immediate laparotomy.

      ii. Conscious athlete, hemodynamically stable: CT scan should be performed to determine the extent of the injury to the liver and optimize treatment.

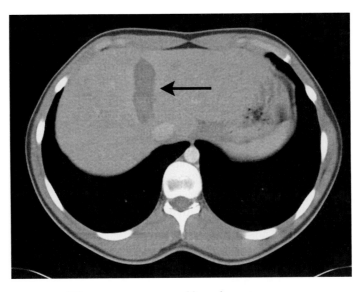

FIGURE 5-1　CT scan appearance of liver hematoma.

       iii. Unconscious athlete or physical signs are equivocal: DPL is generally recommended.
- An exploratory laparotomy is performed if the DPL is positive.

  b. A great deal of the management of liver injury is predicated on the fact that 50–80% of all liver injuries stop bleeding spontaneously.
      i. This fact has led to the trend toward nonoperative management of the hemodynamically stable patient with a success rate of up to 94%.

  c. Nonoperative management involves:
      i. Rest.
      ii. Careful observation.
      iii. Fluid support.
      iv. Though CT documentation of improvement and resolution was once the standard of care, follow-up CT scan is no longer recommended unless clinically indicated.

  d. Despite the current trend toward nonoperative treatment, a significant number of patients require laparotomy to control bleeding, as well as to repair or resect the liver, depending on the extent of the injury.

    e. Return to play criteria after liver injury have not been inves-
tigated and are not known.
      i. The basic principles of return to play should be used to
guide the team physician.
      ii. In general, the athlete should not be returned to play
until anatomic and functional healing have occurred.
        • In this setting, normalization of liver enzymes may be
a useful indicator of functional healing.

E. Splenic injury.
  1. General considerations.
    a. Spleen injury is the most common cause of death due to
abdominal trauma in sports.
    b. Injury to the spleen usually occurs as a result of direct trau-
ma to the left lower chest wall or left upper quadrant of the
abdomen.
    c. Because the splenic capsule can contain bleeding, the signs
of splenic injury are often delayed.
  2. History.
    a. Initially the pain of splenic injury is sharp, followed by a
continued dull left-sided ache.
      i. Pain may radiate to the left or right shoulder secondary
to free intraperitoneal blood irritating the diaphragm.
    b. Nausea and vomiting may be reported.
    c. Some athletes complain of dizziness or light-headedness.
  3. Physical examination.
    a. The abdomen may be distended.
    b Generalized abdominal tenderness.
      i. Rebound tenderness and abdominal guarding may also
be present.
    c. There may also be tenderness over the left 10th, 11th, and
12th ribs.
    d. Be sure to evaluate and document blood pressure and pulse.
  4. Any athlete with suspicion of spleen injury should be transported to the hospital for further evaluation.
  5. Diagnostic tests.
    a. Plain abdominal X-rays may show fading of the splenic out-
line and a growing splenic shadow.
    b. Ultrasonography may be helpful in screening splenic
injury.
    c. CT scan is the current diagnostic imaging standard of
care. CT staging of splenic injury does not predict the need
for laparotomy and does not correlate with clinical outcome.

> **d.** DPL classically is positive if any significant bleeding has occurred from injury to the spleen or other abdominal organ.
> **e.** A complete blood count should be obtained.
>> **i.** Hemoglobin and hematocrit can indicate the extent of any blood loss, though reduction in these levels may be delayed.
>> **ii.** An elevated white blood count may be present if a sub-scapular hematoma has developed.

6. Treatment.
> **a.** Splenic preservation is preferred over splenectomy.
>> **i.** Currently, nonoperative management of hemodynamically stable patients is the preferred method of treatment, especially in the pediatric population.
>> **ii.** This approach requires meticulous attention and has become possible because of the emergence of sophisticated and accurate imaging techniques.
> **b.** Exploratory laparotomy is indicated if the individual is hemodynamically unstable.
> **c.** Splenectomy is performed if the injury is extensive or the hemorrhage is otherwise uncontrollable.

7. Delayed rupture.
> **a.** More common in the spleen than in the liver.
> **b.** The clinician should maintain a high index of suspicion in anyone with a history of splenic trauma; however, currently available data does not support the use of routine follow-up imaging of children following blunt splenic injury.

8. Return to play.
> **a.** Controversy exists over the length of activity restriction after nonoperative management of blunt splenic injury.
>> **i.** Most authors recommend a three-month period of activity restriction with the first three weeks after hospital discharge spent in "quiet" activity at home.
>> **ii.** Ironically, athletes who undergo splenectomy often return to activity before their nonsurgical counterparts.
> **b.** Post-splenectomy patients may return to full activity when their surgical incisions have healed and they are feeling up to the rigors of competition.

F. Injury to other abdominal organs.
> **1.** General considerations.
>> **a.** Injuries to the stomach, intestine, and pancreas have been reported in sport.
>> **b.** These injuries occur from direct blows to the abdomen.
>> **c.** These injuries are rare in alpine skiing.

2. History.
   a. Usually present with persistent abdominal pain with signs of chemical or bacterial peritonitis:
      i. Fever.
      ii. Nausea and vomiting.
   b. Referred pain to the shoulder may occur from diaphragmatic irritation.
3. Physical examination.
   a. Pain may be localized.
      i. Guarding and rebound tenderness may be present.
   b. Rigid abdomen may be noted.
   c. Loss of normal bowel sounds.
4. As is the case with injury to the solid organs of the abdomen, sideline suspicion of these injuries with prompt transportation to the hospital is paramount.
5. Diagnostic tests.
   a. Plain radiographs of the abdomen may be rapidly performed and may reveal free air under the diaphragm or abdominal wall.
      i. Unfortunately, free air is not always initially apparent on plain radiographs.
   b. CT scanning should be considered in hemodynamically stable athletes.
      i. May detect the majority of bowel and pancreas injuries; however, the diagnostic findings are often subtle and require meticulous attention.
      ii. At the very least, CT scanning is useful to rule out the presence of liver or spleen injury.
   c. DPL and laparotomy are indicated in hemodynamically unstable patients suspected of injury to the stomach, intestine, or pancreas.
   d. Nasogastric tube placement may be helpful to check for blood in the stomach.
   e. Laboratory tests.
      i. CBC.
      ii. Liver enzymes.
      iii. Amylase, lipase.
      iv. Urinalysis.
6. Treatment.
   a. Laparotomy is often required to make an accurate diagnosis and definitively treat individuals with injury to the stomach, intestine, and pancreas.

HEAD AND SPINE INJURY

Head Injury

A. General considerations.
1. Head injuries account for 12–20% of all skiing injuries and half of all deaths. Incidence is 0.25 per 1000 skier days.
2. Traumatic brain injuries (TBIs) including concussion, cerebral contusion, subdural hematoma, intracerebral hematoma, and epidural hematoma represent about half of all reported head injuries.
3. Demographics.
    a. Head injuries in skiing are seen predominantly in young males with a mean age of 23 to 31.
    b. Males account for 50–75% of all head injuries and generally suffer more severe injuries.
    c. Older skiers are less likely to suffer from concussion compared to younger skiers, but are more likely to experience other head injuries.
4. Mechanism of injury.
    a. Simple falls are the most common mechanism causing head injury in skiers.
        i. Simple falls are responsible for causing approximately two-thirds of all head injuries.
        ii. The majority of these injures are concussions.
    b. More severe or fatal head injury is more likely to occur from a collision with a stationary object.
B. Prevention.
1. The most important factor in injury prevention is responsibility.
    a. Skiers should ski within their limits.
    b. Maintain good control at all times.
2. Helmets.
    a. It is believed that helmets may reduce the incidence of head injury since most head injuries involve an impact mechanism.
        i. It is estimated that helmet use would address approximately half of all ski-related head injuries.
        ii. Unfortunately, little data regarding the efficacy of helmet use exists.
    b. From what is known, the head injury rate in skiers not wearing a helmet is twice that of those wearing a helmet.
    c. Helmets should conform to safety standards, such as Snell RS98 and EN1077.

        i. The Snell standard is the more stringent of the two, but both are believed to be adequate.

        ii. Helmets should be replaced every five years or after any large impact.

    d. Some individuals have argued against the use of helmets, stating that their use may increase the risk of spine injury; however, there is no current evidence that helmet use increases the risk of spine injury in alpine skiers.

C. Concussion.

    1. Concussion is the most common head injury in skiers.

    2. The majority occur from simple falls.

    3. The diagnosis and management of concussion in skiers are not unlike that of other winter sports. For a complete discussion of the diagnosis and management of concussion, see Chapter 11, Ice Hockey.

Spine Injury

A. Introduction.

    1. Spine injuries are not common in skiing. Incidence is 0.01 per 1000 skier days.

        a. When they do occur, the effects are potentially devastating and may result in permanent disability.

        b. Spine injuries rank as the third most common cause of death and disability in skiing, behind head and abdominal injury.

        c. The current spine injury rate in skiing is about one-fourth that of snowboarding; however, the gap is narrowing.

            i. Spine injury is usually the result of jumps, falls, or collisions.

            ii. The recent proliferation of jumps and terrain parks will likely increase the number of spine injuries in skiing.

B. Demographics.

    1. Spine injuries in skiers tend to occur predominantly in young males.

    2. Spine injuries in males outnumber those in females 3 or 4:1.

C. Types of injury.

    1. The anatomic distribution of spine injury is fairly even overall, with 30% cervical, 32% thoracic, 32% lumbar, and 6% sacral.

        a. Males have a very even distribution of injury.

        b. Females have far more thoracic (39%) and lumbar (37%) injuries and fewer cervical injuries (16%).

    2. The mean age of skiers suffering cervical injury is generally higher than that of skiers suffering thoracic or lumbar injury.

3. Neurological deficits occur in 17–36% of spine injuries, with cervical injuries accounting for the majority of cases.
   a. Among skiers with cervical spinal injury, 26% suffered incomplete deficits and 12% suffered complete spinal cord injury.
   b. In those with thoracic level injury, 6% suffered incomplete deficits and 15% suffered complete injury.
   c. Of those with injuries in the lumbar spine, only 10% suffer incomplete injury and complete injury usually does not occur.
D. Mechanism of injury.
   1. Spine injury in skiing results most often from falls.
      a. Simple falls account for the majority of all spine injury.
      b. Collision into a tree accounts for 29% of spine injury.
      c. Approximately 10% occur from falls after jumps.
      d. Skier versus skier collision is rare and accounts for less than 5% of all spine injuries.
   2. Falls after jumps account for the greatest number of thoracolumbar injuries.
      a. Compression fractures comprise the majority of these injuries.
      b. Low occurrence of neurological deficit.
   3. Skier versus skier collision results in the greatest incidence of cervical spine injury with subsequent neurological deficit.
   4. Most skiers tend to fall forward, as opposed to snowboarders, who tend to fall backward. This disparity probably helps to explain the increased incidence of cervical injuries in skiers.
E. Specific injuries.
   1. Cervical spine injury: The diagnosis and management of cervical spine injury are discussed in Chapter 11, Ice Hockey.
   2. Thoracolumbar compression fracture.
      a. General considerations.
         i. Describes a compression injury of the vertebral body.
         ii. Typically occurs as a result of a fall causing an axial load on the vertebrae.
         iii. Most commonly occurs at the thoracolumbar junction.
      b. History.
         i. Acute onset of pain after fall or trauma.
            • The pain is usually midline, without radiation.
         ii. The patient often complains of stiffness in the back.
         iii. Sitting or standing often exacerbates the symptoms.
         iv. Symptoms may worsen over a few hours after the injury.
      c. Physical examination.
         i. Loss of normal lordotic curvature.
         ii. Limited range of motion.

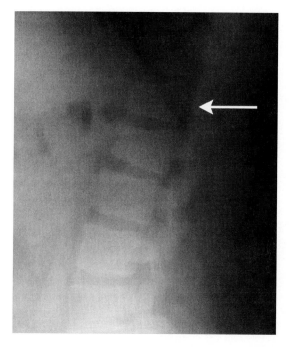

FIGURE 5-2 Lateral view of the spine showing thoracolumbar compression fracture.

  iii. Midline tenderness to palpation.
  iv. Neurological examination is usually normal.
 d. Diagnostic tests.
  i. X-rays should be obtained in all cases.
   • AP and lateral (Figure 5-2) radiographs are adequate for diagnosis.
  ii. CT scan may be necessary if any of the following are present:
   • Significant loss of vertebral height.
   • Associated neurological symptoms.
   • Lateral widening of the vertebral body on AP radiographs suggesting a burst fracture (Figure 5-3).
 e. Treatment.
  i. On the hill.
   • The downed skier should not be moved until the spine is palpated and the neurological function is assessed.
   • If spinal cord injury is suspected, the skier should be protected and immediately transported to the hospital.

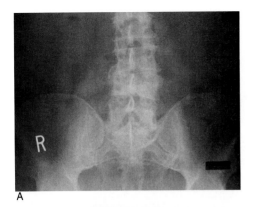

A

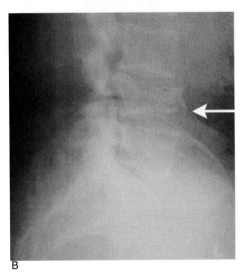

B

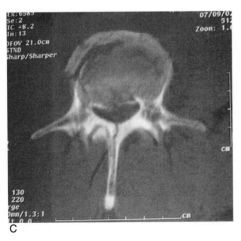

C

FIGURE 5-3   L4 burst fracture: a) AP radiograph shows vertebral body shortening and widening at L4, b) lateral radiograph shows anterior vertebral body wedging and fragmentation, c) CT scan of same injury shows the full extent of the injury including spinal canal narrowing.

    ii. "Simple" compression fracture with no significant loss of vertebral height and no neurological symptoms.
- Rest.
- Analgesics/NSAIDs.
- Calcitonin nasal spray for relief of bone pain.
- Thoracolumbosacral orthosis (TSLO).
- Strengthening program to prevent weakness and atrophy.

    iii. Burst fractures have a high risk of nerve root and/or spinal cord injury and should be referred to a surgical specialist.

UPPER EXTREMITY INJURIES

Ulnar Collateral Ligament Injury of the Thumb (Skier's Thumb)

A. General considerations.
1. Injury to the ulnar collateral ligament (UCL) is the most common upper extremity injury in skiers.
2. It accounts for one-third of all upper extremity injuries and about 8% of all injuries in skiers.
3. Injury to the UCL is the most common ski injury in the adolescent population.
4. Mechanism of injury.
   - **a.** The most common mechanism is a fall onto an outstretched hand with the ski pole in the palm of the hand.
   - **b.** The pole acts as a lever, placing a radial deviation stress on the UCL.

B. History.
1. In most cases the skier reports history of a fall onto an outstretched hand.
2. Swelling is present, and sometimes bruising.
3. The individual complains of pain at the base of the thumb and difficulty gripping objects.

C. Physical examination.
1. Edema and ecchymosis are sometimes seen.
2. Range of motion is often decreased secondary to pain.
3. There is typically local tenderness along the UCL.
4. Gentle valgus stress testing reproduces pain and, with complete tears, valgus opening with no demonstrable end point.

D. Diagnostic tests.
1. X-rays should be obtained to look for associated fracture.

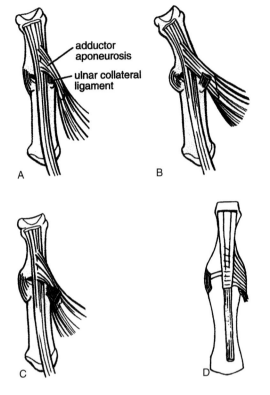

adductor
aponeurosis

ulnar collateral
ligament

A   B

C   D

FIGURE 5-4 Mechanism of formation of a Stener lesion of the thumb: a) Torn ulnar collateral ligament of the MCP joint of the thumb, b) valgus stress opens up the joint, c) the adductor aponeurosis slips past the proximal portion of the ruptured ulnar collateral ligament, and d) as alignment returns to normal, the adductor aponeurosis pushes the ulnar collateral ligament proximally to form the Stener lesion. Reprinted with permission from Brukner P, Khan K. *Clinical Sports Medicine*, rev. 2nd ed. New York: McGraw-Hill; 2002, p. 316.

E. Treatment.
1. Incomplete tears of the UCL may be treated with cast immobilization for approximately three weeks.
2. Because of the higher incidence of Stener lesions with complete UCL injury, surgical repair is often needed (Figure 5-4).
    a. Some authors recommend surgical exploration and repair in all patients because of the high incidence of Stener lesions in the skiing population.

Shoulder Injuries

A. General considerations.
1. Shoulder injuries account for 4–11% of all alpine skiing injuries and 22–41% of upper extremity injuries.
2. The rate of shoulder injury is 0.2 to 0.5 injuries per 1000 skier days.
3. Falls are the most common mechanism of shoulder injury.
    a. Direct blow.

      b. Axial load from landing on an outstretched arm.

      c. Eccentric muscle contraction associated with resisted abduction by the slope.

B. Rotator cuff contusion.

  1. Direct blow to the shoulder and/or axial load can contuse the rotator cuff musculature as well as the deltoid and trapezius muscles.

  2. History.

      a. Acute pain in the shoulder immediately after a fall (less commonly after a collision).

      b. Loss of motion.

  3. Physical examination.

      a. Edema and ecchymosis may be present.

      b. Local tenderness to palpation.

      c. Motion generally restricted because of pain.

      d. Rotator cuff weakness and tenderness on manual muscle testing.

      e. Impingement testing is often positive.

  4. Radiographs should be obtained and are typically negative.

  5. Treatment.

      a. Relative rest.

      b. Ice.

      c. Analgesics or NSAIDs.

      d Gentle range of motion exercises.

      e. Physical therapy may be necessary.

      f. Important to remember that the differential diagnosis includes rotator cuff tear.

  6. Athletes may return to activity when they have regained full range of motion and strength is nearly normal.

C. Rotator cuff tear.

  1. Up to 11% of all ski injuries involve the shoulder, with injury to the rotator cuff being the most common (nearly 25%).

  2. Mechanism of injury.

      a. A fall onto an outstretched arm producing an axial load to the shoulder is the most common mechanism of rotator cuff injury in skiers.

      b. A direct blow to the shoulder caused by a fall or collision can also cause injury.

      c. Both of these mechanisms can lead to complete or partial disruption of the rotator cuff tendon(s).

         i. The supraspinatus tendon is most frequently injured, usually at its insertion on the greater tuberosity of the humerus.

3. History.
   a. Pain in the shoulder.
      i. Typically referred to the anterolateral shoulder.
      ii. Increased with overhead or rotational activity.
      iii. Night pain is common.
   b. Motion loss may be noted.
4. Physical examination.
   a. Painful range of motion arc.
   b. Range of motion decreased.
   c. Positive impingement signs.
   d. Manual muscle testing reveals marked weakness.
   e. Atrophy may be present.
   f. Tenderness to palpation.
5. Diagnostic tests.
   a. Lidocaine injection may improve impingement signs and may indicate a tear if function or strength does not improve.
   b. Imaging.
      i. Plain radiographs including AP, axillary, and outlet views should be obtained.
         • Large rotator cuff tears may allow proximal migration of humeral head on AP view.
         • Spurring under the AC joint may be present.
         • Glenohumeral degenerative changes may be present.
         • Acromion morphology.
            – Type II or III acromion may predispose the individual to RC injury.
      ii. MRI.
         • Preferred imaging modality for rotator cuff injury.
         • Not necessary for initial management.
         • Consider contrast enhancement.
6. Treatment.
   a. Initial treatment is conservative and is similar to the treatment of rotator cuff tendinopathy.
      i. Relative rest.
      ii. Ice.
      iii. Analgesics or NSAIDs.
      iv. Physical therapy.
      v. Corticosteroid injection can be considered. (See Appendix.)
      vi. Surgery is considered if conservative treatment fails.
D. Anterior glenohumoral instability.
   1. Anterior glenohumoral dislocations and subluxations account for approximately 22% of all shoulder injuries in skiers.

2. Mechanism of injury.
  a. The typical mechanism for anterior dislocation is one in which the arm is forced into abduction, extension, and external rotation.
  b. Subluxation can occur from repeated overuse or as a result of previous dislocation.
3. The diagnosis and management of this injury are discussed in Chpater 6, Snowboarding.
E. Acromioclavicular (AC) sprains.
  1. Account for ~ 20% of all shoulder injuries in skiers.
  2. AC sprains typically occur from a direct blow to the shoulder.
    a. Usually due to a fall in which the tip of the shoulder impacts against packed snow.
  3. The diagnosis and management of this injury are discussed in Chapter 11, Ice Hockey.
F. Clavicle fractures occur in skiers and typically occur as a result of a fall onto the shoulder. This injury is discussed in Chapter 11, Ice Hockey.

LOWER EXTREMITY INJURIES

Tibial Shaft Fracture

A. General considerations.
  1. Tibial shaft fractures occur below the tibial plateau and above the malleoli.
  2. Most commonly occurs at the junction of the distal and middle thirds of the tibia.
  3. The incidence of tibial shaft fracture has decreased approximately 80% since the 1970s.
    a. This reduction is due to improvements in technology.
      i. Higher, stiffer boots.
      ii. Multimode (plane) binding release.
B. History.
  1. Sudden, severe pain after trauma.
    a. Often accompanied by a "crack."
  2. Unable to bear weight.
C. Physical examination.
  1. Gross deformity may be present in severe fractures.
  2. Edema and ecchymosis may be present.
  3. Focal bone tenderness.
  4. Crepitance may be present.

D. Special concerns.
   1. Be careful to determine if the fracture is open.
   2. Always note the neurovascular status of the leg.
E. Management on the hill.
   1. Splint to stabilize the leg.
   2. Transport for further treatment.
F. Radiographs are necessary and usually demonstrate the full extent of the injury clearly.
G. Treatment.
   1. Stable fractures with less than 5° of varus/valgus angulation:
      a. Long leg cast with partial weight bearing for 2 to 4 weeks.
      b. Fracture brace (allows knee and ankle motion) for 4 to 6 additional weeks.
   2. Stable fracture with more than 5° varus/valgus angulation:
      a. Reduction is necessary.
      b. Treatment as above.
   3. Unstable fractures require intramedullary nailing.
   4. Open fractures require irrigation, debridement, and antibiotics.

Knee Injuries

A. General considerations.
   1. Knee sprains are the most common injuries in alpine skiers.
   2. They account for approximately 30% of all injuries in adults.
B. Anterior cruciate ligament (ACL) sprains.
   1. General considerations.
      a. Partial or complete disruption of the ligament bundles.
      b. There are two bundles.
         i. Posterolateral.
         ii. Anteromedial.
      c. Ligament tears may occur at a number of locations:
         i. Femoral origin.
         ii. Tibial origin.
         iii. Midportion.
         iv. May be associated with avulsion of tibial spine in the young athlete.
   2. There are three common mechanisms of injury in skiers.
      a. Valgus-external rotation (Figure 5-5a).
         i. The skier falls forward while catching the inside edge of one of the skis.
         ii. The leg is abducted and externally rotated, leading to primary MCL injury.
         iii. May involve the ACL in 20% of cases.

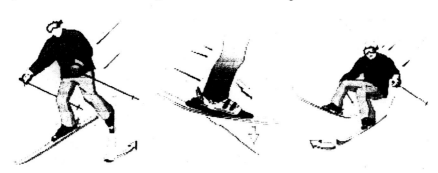

FIGURE 5-5 The common mechanisms of ACL injury in skiing: a) valgus external rotation, b) boot-induced anterior drawer, and c) phantom foot. Reprinted with permission from Koehle MS, Lloyd-Smith R, Taunton JE. Alpine ski injuries and their prevention. *Sports Med* 2002;32(12):785-93.

    b. Boot-induced anterior drawer (Figure 5-5b).
        i. Occurs when the skier lands from a jump with the knees extended.
        ii. The rear of the ski contacts the snow first, acting as a lever on the boot-binding complex and forcing the tibia anteriorly in relation to the femur.
        iii. This injury is more common among freestyle skiers but unusual in recreational skiers.
    c. Flexion-internal rotation (phantom foot) (Figure 5-5c).
        i. The skier loses balance and falls backward between the skis.
        ii. This causes weight to be distributed to the inside edge of the downhill ski.
        iii. As this edge catches, it results in a sudden internal rotation of the hyperflexed knee.
  3. History.
    a. Usually the patient complains of a loud "pop" at the time of injury.
    b. The feeling of instability or giving way is often described.
    c. Occasionally the acute event is accompanied by an autonomic response including nausea, dizziness, sweating, and light-headedness.
    d. Significant swelling is often noted within a few hours of the injury.
  4. Physical examination.

    a. In the acute setting, a large effusion/hemarthrosis is present.

    b. Positive Lachman test.

    c. Positive anterior drawer may be present; however, this test is typically not reliable.

    d. Positive pivot shift test may be present but is often difficult to perform acutely in the clinical setting.

5. Diagnostic tests.

    a. X-rays should be preformed routinely.

        i. Lateral capsular sign refers to an avulsion of the mid-portion of the lateral capsular ligament with a small fragment of the proximal lateral tibia visualized.

           • This finding is associated with a high incidence of ACL injury and anterolateral instability.

        ii. Tibial spine avulsion may be visualized.

        iii. Tibial plateau fracture should be ruled out.

    b. MRI (Figure 5-6).

        i. Accuracy rates of 85–95% in detecting ACL tears.

        ii. Not always required.

           • The clinical exam is usually more accurate and MRI adds no further information if the clinical exam is unequivocal.

        iii. MRI is especially helpful if clinical picture is not clear or other pathologies need to be ruled out.

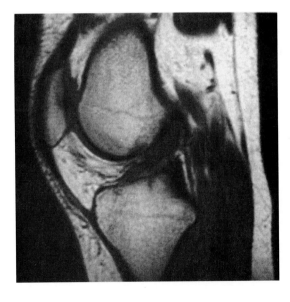

FIGURE 5·6 MRI showing ACL tear. Courtesy of I.F. Anderson. Reprinted with permission from Brukner P, Khan K. *Clinical Sports Medicine*, rev. 2nd ed. New York: McGraw-Hill; 2002, p. 451.

6. Treatment.
  a. Acute setting.
    i. Symptom control with crutches, ice, and analgesics.
    ii. Reduction of effusion.
      • Consider arthrocentesis if tense hemarthrosis is present.
      • Compression.
    iii. Establish normal range of motion.
    iv. Maintain quadriceps muscle tone.
    v. Consideration of reconstructive surgery.
  b. Individuals with chronic ACL injury may attempt functional stabilization through rehabilitation and lifestyle modification.
    i. Bracing.
      • Usually ineffective for individuals with complete ACL injury.
      • May be of some benefit in those with partial injury and good endpoint on Lachman.
  c. Surgery.
    i. Surgical reconstruction is indicated in those individuals with knee laxity who regularly engage in sports involving cutting and frequent change of direction.
    ii. Reconstruction is usually delayed at least three weeks to allow swelling to recede and establish normal range of motion.
    iii. Multiple techniques and graft types are available for reconstruction procedeures.
    iv. ACL reconstruction does not prevent future arthritis.
C. Posterior cruciate ligament (PCL) sprains.
  1. General considerations.
    a. Rare in skiing.
    b Usually caused by a valgus/varus stress in full extension.
    c. May also be caused by a direct blow to the anterior proximal tibia such as in a collision with a tree or other skier.
  2. History.
    a. Immediate onset of knee pain.
    b. Swelling is common and may come up within 24 hours.
    c. Feeling of instability.
  3. Physical examination.
    a. Effusion may be present.
    b. Positive posterior drawer sign.
    c. Positive gravity test or "sag" sign.

    4. Treatment.
        a. Mild injury usually responds to conservative treatment.
            i. Relative rest.
            ii. Ice.
            iii. Analgesics or NSAIDs.
            iv. Functional rehabilitation.
            v. Consideration of bracing.
        b. Surgical reconstruction is considered in certain cases:
            i. Severe laxity.
            ii. Failure of conservative treatment.
            iii. Chronic symptomatic injury.
D. Collateral ligament sprains.
    1. Injury to the medial collateral ligament (MCL) accounts for 18% of all injuries in skiers.
    2. Mechanism of injury.
        a. MCL sprains occur as a result of valgus stress.
        b. This usually occurs when a skier "catches a tip" and the ski is rapidly forced in a valgus direction.
    3. History.
        a. Acute onset of medial knee pain sometimes accompanied by a popping or tearing sensation.
        b. Usually no or minimal joint effusion, but may have local soft tissue swelling.
        c. Feeling of instability with lateral movement.
    4. Physical examination.
        a. Pain along the MCL or one of its attachment sites.
        b. Pain with valgus stress of the knee.
        c. Instability of the MCL with valgus stress testing depending on severity of injury.
            i. Valgus stress testing should be performed at full extension and 30° flexion positions.
              • Examination in full extension tests of the MCL and the central (ACL/PCL) ligaments.
              • Valgus stress testing with the knee in partial flexion is more specific for the MCL.
            ii. Grade I injury: no laxity but pain with valgus stress.
            iii. Grade II: partial ligament injury with mild (< 2 mm) laxity.
            iv. Grade III: complete ligament disruption, wide excursion without appreciable endpoint.
    5. Diagnostic tests.
        a. X-rays should be obtained routinely.

       i. Abduction stress films may be obtained in the skeletally immature to distinguish between MCL injury and growth plate injury.

   b. MRI is generally not necessary to make the diagnosis of MCL sprain.

 6. Treatment.

   a. Grade I and II sprains.

     i. Relative rest, crutches.

     ii. Analgesics or NSAIDs.

     iii. Ice.

     iv. Hinged knee brace.

     v. Functional rehabilitation.

     vi. May return to activity as function allows.

- The brace should be worn with activity for the first 1 to 2 months to protect the ligament until completely healed.

   b. Grade III injuries (isolated).

     i. Brace/immobilization.

- Immobilization should be considered with significant instability.
- The authors prefer a range of motion knee brace that can be locked initially, with motion introduced as healing progresses.

     ii. Function rehabilitation as symptoms allow.

     iii. Surgery may be considered if instability persists or if the MCL injury is associated with concomitant injury.

E. Meniscus injury.

 1. General considerations.

   a. Disruption of the meniscus cartilage may occur as a result of a single traumatic event, a degenerative process, or a combination of both.

   b. Meniscus tears can occur peripherally (more vascular) or centrally (less vascular).

     i. The location of the injury may impact surgical intervention decisions since healing is more likely to occur in the vascular zone.

   c. Tears take many forms, including bucket handle, radial, longitudinal, horizontal, or complex.

 2. Mechanism of injury.

   a. Meniscus injury usually occurs with a twisting or squatting mechanism.

    b. Often the skier will cross skis during a fall, causing a twisting and flexion injury.

3. History.

    a. The skier complains of joint-line pain.

    b. Mild to moderate swelling.

    c. Possible loss of motion or locking.

        i. A locked knee suggests a bucket handle meniscus tear.

4. Physical examination.

    a. Mild to moderate effusion.

    b. Joint-line tenderness to palpation.

    c. Positive McMurray's test.

        i. A palpable or audible joint-line "clunk" with flexion/circumduction of the joint.

        ii. Locking with the maneuver is also considered a positive test.

    d. Joint-line pain with flexion/circumduction.

        i. This is not the same as a positive McMurray's test.

        ii. This finding raises suspicion of a meniscus tear but is not diagnostic.

    e. Positive Appley's test.

        i. With the patient in a prone position, the knee is flexed to 90°.

        ii. Axial load is applied to the lower leg along with internal and external rotation.

        iii. If the above causes pain for the patient, the lower leg is distracted from the thigh and internal/external forces are again applied.

           • In the case of a meniscus tear, knee pain should be reduced with this distraction test.

5. Diagnostic tests.

    a. X-rays should be routinely obtained.

        i. Usually negative.

        ii. Weight-bearing views may reveal joint space narrowing and should be obtained if a degenerative process is suspected.

    b. MRI.

        i. Often identifies meniscus injury.

        ii. Most useful in determining whether to continue with conservative treatment or to proceed with surgery.

6. Treatment.

    a. A suspected meniscus injury with no ligamentous instability may initially be managed conservatively with symptomatic treatment and functional rehabilitation.

      i. Relative rest.
      ii. Crutches or other assistive device.
      iii. Analgesics or NSAIDs.
      iv. Ice.
      v. Range of motion exercises.
      vi. Physical therapy.

   b. If there is no improvement with conservative treatment, diagnostic and surgical arthroscopy may be required.

      i. Diagnostic arthroscopy is the most certain way to establish the diagnosis.
      ii. Tears located in the peripheral, vascular zone may be amenable to repair.
      iii. If repair is not possible, partial meniscectomy is performed.

Suggested Readings

Finch CF, Kelsall HL. The effectiveness of ski bindings and their professional adjustment for preventing alpine skiing injuries. *Sports Med* 1998;25(6):407–16.

Hunter RE. Skiing injuries. *Am J of Sports Med* 1999;27(3):381–89.

Kocher MS, Dupre MM, Feagin JA. Shoulder injuries from alpine skiing and snowboarding. *Sports Med* 1998;25(3):201–11.

Koehle MS, Lloyd-Smith R, Taunton JE. Alpine ski injuries and their prevention. *Sports Med* 2002;32(12):785–93.

Laskowski ER. Snow skiing. *Phys Med Rehab Clin North Amer* 1999;10(1): 189–211.

Levy AS, Smith RH. Neurologic injuries in skiers and snowboarders. *Sem Neurol* 2000:20(2): 233–45

Lyritis GP, Paspati I, Karachalios T, et al. Pain relief from nasal calcitonin in osteoporotic vertebral crush fractures: A double blind, placebo-controlled clinical study. *Acta Orthop Scand Suppl* 1997 Oct;275:112–14.

Natri A, Beynnon BD, Ettlinger CF, et al. Alpine ski bindings and injuries. *Sports Med* 1999;28(1):35–48.

6

SNOWBOARDING

Scott M. Koehler
James L. Moeller

INTRODUCTION

General

A. Snowboarding has emerged in the last twenty years as an exciting and increasingly popular winter sport at both the recreational and competitive levels.

B. The growing participation in snowboarding now includes millions worldwide and as many as 20–40% of the lift ticket holders at ski and snowboarding areas.

C. The overall injury rate appears to be approximately 4 to 6 injuries per 1000 snowboarder days. This rate is slightly higher than that seen in skiers.

D. Injuries are an accepted risk of snowboarding, and close attention has been given in recent years to the unique patterns of injuries in snowboarders.

  1. With the increase in participation, the injury patterns have become more completely defined.

  2. It is also helpful to review the biomechanics and injury mechanisms to help design and implement preventive measures.

History of Snowboarding

A. The origins of snowboarding are linked to sledding, skiing, and surfing.

  1. Attempts to go down a mountain or hill of snow standing on a sled or toboggan "surfer style" have occurred for years.

    2. Surfers and skiers have long referenced combining their sports to surf down a powder-covered slope.

B. Snowboard equipment.

    1. Evolution of the board.

        a. The "Snurfer" arose in the 1960s as an early snowboard design similar to two skis fixed together with the rider sailing down a sledding hill or ski slope.

            i. The feet were not fixed to the board.

            ii. The rider held a short tether to help with balance.

        b. The "Winterstick" was developed in the early 1970s.

            i. Designed like a long, narrow surfboard.

            ii. A tail fin was present in some variations and used for carving turns in deep powder.

        c. Tom Simms and Jake Burton Carpenter led development in the 1970s and 1980s of a more refined snowboard by combining these styles into a board design with fixed feet for more controlled riding.

        d. Boards were developed with metal edges to allow carving turns in packed snow.

    2. Boot style.

        a. A soft or pack style boot is the most commonly worn footwear, used by 70–90% of snowboarders.

            i. These boots usually have a mild amount of stiffness, but are much easier to hike in.

            ii. They are either strapped into fixed bindings, or snapped into step-in bindings (Figure 6-1).

        b. The hybrid snowboarding boot is similar to the soft boot with added stiffness. Some of these boots have a partial hard shell and soft upper boot, while others have added stiffness in the inner boot.

        c. The hard-shelled boots that are frequently worn by racers provide more ankle support. These boots are similar to ski boots but allow more freedom of ankle motion (Figure 6-2).

        d. The fixed boots and bindings in snowboarding allow for more torque and axial forces on the foot and ankle than in skiing.

            i. Releasable bindings have been developed for snowboarding, but have not become widely available yet.

C. Modern progression.

    1. 1977: Ski resort liability insurers agreed to cover snowboarders on the ski runs, and resorts slowly began to allow snowboarders on their slopes.

        a. Snowboarding on existing runs quickly became common, and in the 1980s snowboarding steadily grew in popularity.

        b. Most resorts now allow snowboarders.

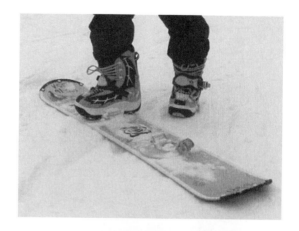

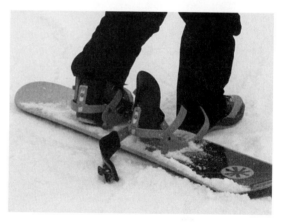

FIGURE 6·1 The common soft boot with (top) fixed step-in bindings and (bottom) fixed strap-in bindings. Photos courtesy of Scott M. Koehler, MD.

    2. Early snowboard competition included slalom and downhill.
    3. Half-pipe competition was added later, with competitors judged on style and tricks.
    4. In 1998, snowboarding was introduced as a medal sport to the Olympic Games (Nagano, Japan).

Epidemiology

A. Demographics.
    1. Snowboarding caught on initially with teenage and young adult winter sports enthusiasts and has grown to include all age groups, from toddlers to seniors. Because of its popularity with younger age groups and the relative newness of the sport, there is a significant predominance of younger age groups in snowboarding.

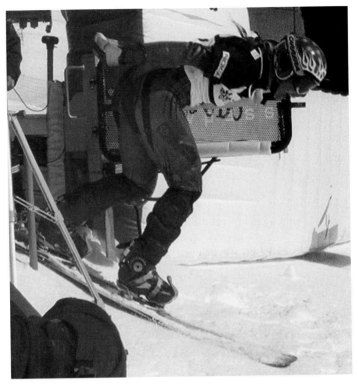

FIGURE 6-2   A slalom rider with hard-shelled boot. Photo courtesy of Scott M. Koehler, MD.

    2. There are two to three times more male than female snowboarders. The interest is increasing in girls and women, and their proportion is increasing.

    3. There is a higher proportion of beginners in snowboarding when compared to skiing, which likely accounts for the higher injury rate. This will probably change as the growth of snowboarding plateaus in future decades.

B. Injury data.

    1. Many studies of injury in snowboarders compare them to skiers.

      a. The main difference includes a higher proportion of upper extremity injuries and a lower proportion of lower extremity injuries in the snowboarders.

        i. This can be linked directly to the differences in technique and injury mechanics between the sports.

    2. Beginners.

      a. First-time snowboarders and skiers each suffer injuries at a rate of approximately 4% during their first outing.

  b. A significantly higher number of snowboarders need imme-
    diate medical attention due to the severity of the injury.
  c. Higher number of fractures, often of the wrist, when com-
    pared to alpine skiing.
  d. 53% of injuries are to the upper extremity and 15% are head
    injuries (mostly concussions).
 3. No significant difference has been identified thus far in the
   injury patterns between male and female snowboarders, except
   for groin injuries (see discussion of vulvar injuries below and
   in Chapter 11, Ice Hockey).
  a. Males are more likely to do aerial maneuvers that increase
    the risk of certain injuries.
  b. No significant difference in injury severity between men
    and women.
 4. Injuries that occur due to collisions are of interest, especially
   related to mixing skiers and snowboarders on the same slopes.
  a. There has not been a significant change in the amount or
    severity of collision injuries when skiers and snowboarders
    are mixed.
C. The vast majority of injuries from snowboarding that require
  treatment are acute/traumatic in nature.
 1. The more common injuries are discussed in detail below.
 2. Overuse injuries requiring medical attention are uncommon
   but do occur.
  a. These injuries are typically mild and rarely prevent the
    snowboarder from continuing.
   i. Wrist tendonitis may occur, especially in beginners, due
     to repetitively landing on the wrist and pushing off from
     the ground.
   ii. Prepatellar and olecranon bursitis may develop from
     repetitive minor trauma.
   iii. Knee tendonitis, especially of the pes anserine group and
     the patellar tendon, as well as patellofemoral arthralgia,
     is occasionally seen.
     • These seem to occur from overuse with the foot posi-
       tion fixed with too much external rotation.
     • Usually, foot position adjustment is required, in addi-
       tion to the usual treatments.
   iv. Achilles, peroneal, and posterior tibialis tendonitis have been
     seen in snowboarders. Planar fasciitis may also develop.
     • These seem to develop due to hiking in the snow-
       boarding boots.
       – E.g., the boarder who spends many days at the
         half-pipe, hiking up the pipe for each run.

TABLE 6-1

Approximate injury site in snowboarders (compiled from multiple sources).

Wrist	16–32%
Elbow	2–5%
Shoulder	8–16%
Foot	1–3%
Ankle	12–28%
Knee	12–20%
Spine	2–7%
Head	10–18%
Chest	1–3%
Abdomen	6%
Other	< 2% (hand, face, muscle, hip, pelvis)

- Treatment involves the usual local treatment plus footbed or boot modifications.
    b. There will be no further discussion of overuse injuries in this chapter.
D. Injuries related to anatomic area.
    1. A review of more than twenty studies related to injury epidemiology has been summarized in Table 6-1.
    2. The upper extremities are the most common areas to be injured in snowboarders.
        a. Studies show that up to 50% of snowboarding injuries are to the upper extremities.
        b. Snowboarders have nearly double the number of upper extremity injuries that skiers do.
            i. The snowboarder is seven to ten times more likely to injure the wrist.
        c. A series of 3645 upper extremity injuries (among 7430 total injuries) in snowboarders detailed the emerging trends in these injuries.
            i. 21.6% of all injuries occurred in the wrist.
            ii. 16.2% occurred in the shoulder.
            iii. 4.1% in the hand.
            iv. 3.8% in the elbow.
            v. 2.7% in the forearm region.
        d. Wrist and upper extremity injuries are more common in beginners than in the advanced boarders.

      i. Advanced snowboarders are more likely to have complex and severe wrist fractures, including more scaphoid fractures, and more hand, elbow, and shoulder injuries.

  3. Lower extremity injuries are common.

    a. Location.

      i. Ankle: 12–28% of all injuries.

      ii. Knee: 13–23%.

      iii. Foot: 1–3%.

    b. Most lower extremity injuries occur to the lead leg.

      i. Injury types are no different between lead and trail legs.

    c. Kirkpatrick et al. (1998) tabulated 3213 snowboarding injuries presenting for medical care, and detailed 549 injuries to the foot and ankle region.

      i. 15.3% (492/3213) were ankle injuries.

        • 52% of the ankle injuries were sprains.

        • 44% were fractures.

          – Many of the fractures occurred at the lateral process of the talus (LPT), which is a frequently missed, high-risk fracture.

      ii. 1.8% (57/3213) of the injuries were foot injuries defined as occurring distal to the talus.

        • 57% were fractures.

          – Most foot fractures occurred in the metatarsals.

        • 28% sprains.

        • 15% contusions, abrasions, and other soft-tissue injuries.

    d. The effect of boot style on injury type varies, but there appears to be a lower incidence of ankle sprains in hybrid boots and a higher incidence of LPT fractures in hard-shelled boots.

Special Concerns and Unique Aspects of Snowboarding

A. Catching an edge.

  1. One of the major causes of injury in snowboarders is from the abrupt fall that occurs when the downhill edge of the board catches the snow, stopping the board quickly (Figure 6-3). Typically this slams the snowboarder to the ground with great force.

    a. Toe edge falls (forward falls) put the upper extremities at risk.

    b. Heel edge falls.

      i. The wrists and upper extremities can be injured if the snowboarder reaches back to break his/her fall.

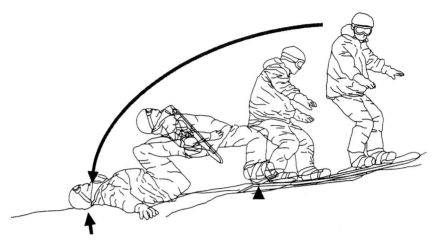

FIGURE 6-3 Drawing of the mechanism of the snowboarder catching the heel edge. These falls commonly lead to wrist injury if the athlete reaches back to break the fall, or to spine and head injury. Reprinted with permission from H. Nakaguchi and K. Tsutsumi, "Mechanisms of snowboarding-related severe head injury." *J. Neurosurg* 2002;97:542–548.

      ii. The spine and head are also at risk.

      iii. This mechanism, which has also been termed the "opposite edge phenomenon," actually occurs more easily in the flats or on a gentle slope because the opposite edge is closer to the snow and can get caught with a slight loss of balance.

B. Terrain variables.

    1. Open areas are common at ski and snowboarding resorts.

      a. On powdered runs, the snowboarder maneuvers much like a surfer, leaning the board and shifting weight to float through the snow.

      b. On groomed or packed trails, the snowboarder uses the edge of the board more exclusively to carve turns.

    2. Wooded areas are frequently enjoyed due to the challenge of riding "slalom style" through the obstacles.

      a. Resorts may thin out the trees from forested areas to create glades of spaced trees to vary the terrain.

      b. There is an increased risk of collision injuries if the rider loses control in wooded areas.

    3. The half-pipe.

      a. The half-pipe is a half-tube of snow created with steep edges to allow a run of steady banked turns or aerial tricks. (Figure 6-4).

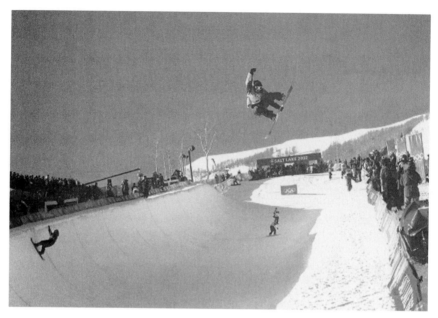

FIGURE 6-4 Half-pipe with aerial maneuvers. Photo courtesy of Scott M. Koehler, MD.

      i. The half-pipe can be created in any size, including the super-pipe of professional and Olympic competition that is 200 feet long, 15 to 18 feet deep, and 50 feet across at the lip.

   b. Aerial maneuvers have been shown to have a higher risk of injury to the head, spine, and abdomen.

  4. The terrain park: The creation of terrain parks to attract more snowboarders has been successful.

   a. A run or runs are modified by setting up fixed objects such as rails, table-tops, half-pipes, and jumps for the enjoyment and challenge of snowboarders and skiers.

   b. The area is often informally referred to as the "trauma park" by local medical providers due to the steady supply of injuries.

C. Ski lifts: Ski lifts are a challenge for snowboarders, especially while learning.

  1. Loading and unloading from the lift requires unhooking one foot from the snowboard, which decreases control of balance and steering.

  2. Up to 8% of snowboarding injuries occur while loading and unloading from lifts, especially on the steep slope at the top end of lifts.

Racing

Various racing formats are used by snowboarders.

A. The slalom is occasionally run in snowboarding with tightly spaced gates, but more commonly a giant slalom format is used, in which the gates are more widely spaced.

B. The parallel giant slalom is the current racing format at the World Cup and Olympic levels.
   1. Two competitors race on side-by-side courses, and then switch sides to race a second time.
   2. The winner has the fastest total time for the two runs.

C. Downhill races have the gates widely spaced apart, and the riders descend the mountain at high speeds.

D. The "snowboard cross" is an event in which two to six riders simultaneously board race down a course of varied terrain. The course is typically made up of banked turns, jumps, and flats in an all-out race to the finish.

Snowboard Event Coverage

A. Snowboarding event coverage should be coordinated with the ski patrol at the area.
   1. A minimum of dedicated ski patrol staff at the site is important for any organized event.
   2. Ski patrol personnel are trained and experienced first responders, and will help injury management go smoothly.
   3. For competitions, it is ideal to also have experienced certified athletic trainer and physician coverage.

B. For large events, local access to radiographs and splinting materials is helpful. Be sure to have injury documentation capabilities on-site.

C. To prepare for life-threatening emergencies, ambulance pickup sites and helicopter landing zones must be predetermined.

EXERCISE PHYSIOLOGY

Cardiac Demands

A. Snowboarding is characterized as a high static, low dynamic activity. Most of the athlete's energy is used to maintain balance and muscular tone to control the activity.

B. When a significant amount of hiking is involved, such as backcountry snowboarding or hiking to the top of each run, the activity demands more of the cardiovascular system.

Biomechanics of Snowboarding

A. There are some unique aspects of snowboarding that affect the injury patterns and make them distinctly different from patterns found in skiing.
   1. Riders stand sideways on the board.
      a. Both legs are fixed with no independent motion to widen the stance to break a fall.
         i. Because of this, the arms are commonly used to absorb the force of a fall.
         ii. As a result, the snowboarder is much more likely to injure the upper extremity.
      b. Roughly two-thirds of snowboarders use a left leg forward regular stance, while right foot forward riding is termed the "goofy" stance.
   2. Most bindings are nonreleasing and the forces on the board are transmitted directly to the lower extremities.

MEDICAL ISSUES

Frostbite and Hypothermia

A. For a full discussion, see Chapter 3, Cold Injury.

High-Altitude Illness

B. Acute mountain sickness (AMS) is the most common form of high-altitude illness.
   1. Epidemiology.
      a. Noted in up to 25% of people at moderate (1920–2957 m) altitudes.
      b. More common at altitudes > 2500 m.
      c. Children and adults appear to be at similar risk.
      d. Athletes and nonathletes appear to be at similar risk, although exercise may exacerbate symptoms.
   2. Risk factors.
      a. Rate of ascent.
      b. Altitude reached, particularly sleeping altitude.
      c. Individual susceptibility.
         i. Previous episode of AMS.
         ii. Permanent residence < 900 m.
   3. History: Complaints are vague and usually appear 6 to 12 hours after arriving at altitude.

       a. Headache.
       b. Anorexia.
       c. Nausea and vomiting.
       d. Fatigue.
       e. Dizziness.
       f. Sleep disturbance.
    4. Physical examination is typically normal.
B. High-altitude cerebral edema (HACE).
    1. Felt to be the end stage of AMS.
    2. Pathophysiology.
       a. Not fully understood.
       b. Theorized that hypoxemia causes neurohumoral and hemo-dynamic responses that eventually lead to:
          i. Increased cerebral blood flow.
          ii. Altered permeability of the blood–brain barrier.
          iii. Cerebral edema.
    3. History.
       a. Progression of AMS symptoms.
       b. Confusion.
       c. Exhaustion.
    4. Physical examination.
       a. Ataxia.
       b. Altered level of consciousness.
          i. May progress rapidly to coma and death.
       c. Ocular changes.
          i. Retinal hemorrhage.
          ii. Papilledema.
       d. Focal neurological deficits sometimes noted.
    5. Treatment.
       a. Descent from altitude.
       b. Supplemental oxygen.
          i. Hyperbaric O_2 also effective.
       c. Corticosteroid administration.
       d. Acetazolamide or other diuretic.
C. High-altitude pulmonary edema (HAPE).
    1. Typically occurs 2 to 4 days after arrival at altitude (> 2500 m).
       a. Risk factors are the same as those noted for AMS and HACE.
    2. Pathophysiology.
       a. Noncardiogenic pulmonary edema.
       b. Exaggerated pulmonary hypertension leads to overperfu-sion and vascular leakage.
    3. History.

     a. Different from HACE in that AMS symptoms do not precede HAPE in all cases.

     b. Dyspnea.

       i. Initially present on exertion.

       ii. Eventually may be present at rest.

     c. Decreased exercise tolerance.

     d. Cough.

       i. Starts as dry, annoying.

       ii. Advances to productive cough with blood-tinged sputum.

  4. Physical examination.

     a. Findings may be subtle at onset.

       i. Tachypnea at rest.

       ii. Tachycardia at rest.

     b. Later in disease course.

       i. Low-grade fever is common.

       ii. Crackles on auscultation.

  5. Diagnostic tests.

     a. Chest X-ray may be nonspecific.

     b. EKG may show right ventricular strain.

  6. Treatment.

     a. Descent from altitude.

     b. Supplemental oxygen.

       i. Hyperbaric O_2 also effective.

       ii. Continuous positive airway pressure may be helpful.

     c. Diuretic.

     d. Nifedipine 10 mg followed by 20–30 mg slow release every 12 to 24 hours can be considered as well.

D. Prevention of altitude sickness.

  1. Ascend gradually.

  2. Descend for rest/sleep.

  3. Acetazolamide may be useful for prophylaxis in at-risk individuals.

Snow Immersion Injury and Death

A. Due to the fixed nature of the feet in snowboarding, it can be difficult to get out from deep snow after a fall.

B. A number of deaths have occurred of snowboarders who were buried upside-down in the deep, soft powder of a tree-well because of inability to get out.

C. Snowboarders should always ride the deep powder and forested areas in pairs.

D. Back-country snowboarders should take full avalanche precautions.

Head Injuries in Snowboarders

A. Head injuries in snowboarding continue to be a problem despite the increased frequency of helmet use in the sport. There is a growing body of evidence showing that helmets decrease the incidence and severity of head injuries in snowboarders.

1. The cause of head injuries in snowboarders can be broken down into falls (40–50%), errors while jumping (30%), and collisions (18–20%).

2. The most common site of contact is to the occiput, as most of the injuries occur from catching the heel edge and falling backward.

   a. The arms are less able to protect from a head injury in these falls.

3. Head injuries include contusions, abrasions, lacerations, concussions, fractures, and intracranial injuries.

   a. There are a concerning number of subdural hematomas among snowboarders.

4. Although head injuries only account for 3–15% of the overall injuries in snowboarders, they are estimated to total 50–88% of the fatalities in snowboarding.

B. Detailed studies of head injuries in snowboarders have been presented in the medical literature.

1. Fukuda et al. (2001) analyzed 634 head injuries requiring emergency department evaluation in snowboarders from an estimated 6.95 million snowboarder visits to resorts in a Japanese area serviced by only one hospital.

   a. Head injury incidence was 6.3 per 100,000 snowboarder visits (versus 1.03 per 100,000 skier visits).

      i. Other studies show the rate in skiers as high as 3 to 4 per 100,000 visits.

   b. None of the injured snowboarders were wearing helmets.

      i. The U.S. Consumer Product Safety Commission summarized in its 1999 report that the use of helmets "will reduce the risk of head injury associated with skiing and snowboarding."

2. Nakaguchi et al. (1999) did a separate review of snowboarders with 143 head injuries that occurred in a catchment area including 2.2 million snowboarder visits over two ski seasons.

   a. This study reported a head injury rate of 6.5 per 100,000 snowboarder visits.

   b. Snowboarders had a five times greater incidence of major head injuries (defined as a positive CT scan) when compared to skiers.

3. These and other studies show that snowboarders have a significantly higher proportion of beginners with head injuries.
4. Compared to skiers, snowboarders suffer more:
   a. Head injuries from falls while jumping.
   b. Head injuries from occipital impact.
   c. Major head injuries (positive CT scan).
      i. Superficial hematomas.
      ii. Subdural hematomas.
         • Present in 46% of positive CT scans.
      iii. Skull fractures.
         • Present in 41% of positive CT scans.
      iv. Subarachnoid and cortical bleeds.
C. Subdural hematomas.
   1. Many develop distant to the site of impact.
      a. Coup injury: brain injury directly below the area of impact.
      b. Countercoup injury: brain injury directly opposite the area of impact.
   2. Many seem to occur from rotational and shear forces that tear the subdural bridging veins perpendicular to the force of the blow.
      a. A pattern of temporal and parietal subdural hematomas from occipital impact has been suggested.
D. Head injury evaluation.
   1. Detailed history of the injury including the mechanism, and immediate and delayed symptoms.
   2. A mental status examination including assessment of level of consciousness, orientation, memory, and concentration along with a complete neurological exam should be documented.
      a. Glasgow Coma Scale is the most commonly utilized tool to assess level of consciousness after severe head injury.
         i. Scores based on best patient response in three areas (Table 6-2).
            • Eye opening.
            • Verbal response.
            • Motor response.
         ii. Scores can range from 3 to 15.
   3. Head and neck musculoskeletal exam along with examinations of sites of other potential associated injury is undertaken.
      a. Injuries at other sites may be masked by the symptoms of a head injury.
      b. Treat the injured athlete as if there is an associated neck injury if there is any decreased level of consciousness.
   4. A period of observation for evolution of symptoms can help further define the injury.

TABLE 6-2

The Glasgow Coma Scale.

Eye Opening	Verbal Response	Motor Response
4 Spontaneous	5 Alert and oriented	6 Follows commands
3 To speech	4 Disoriented conversation	5 Localizes pain
2 To pain	3 Nonsensical speech	4 Withdrawal from pain
1 No response	2 Unintelligible sounds	3 Decorticate flexion
	1 No response	2 Decerebrate extension
		1 No response

    a. Due to the possible delayed development of symptoms, such as following a lucid period from a slowly growing subdural hemorrhage, close follow-up and discharge instructions that include observation by a responsible adult are vital.

    5. Emergent imaging with a CT scan is often necessary due to significant or progressive symptoms or exam findings.

    6. Any athlete with symptoms of a head injury should not be allowed to continue to snowboard, and typical concussion guidelines should be followed.

E. Treatment.

    1. Emergent neurosurgery consultation is necessary for athletes with acute intracranial injury.

F. Concussion: For full discussion of concussion, see Chapter 11, Ice Hockey.

Pregnancy

A. It is unwise to learn snowboarding while pregnant due to the increased risk of injury.

B. Accomplished snowboarders must take care while boarding when pregnant due to the increased risk of abdominal trauma, especially after the first trimester. The risk may outweigh participation for all but a few skilled riders.

TRAUMATIC INJURIES

Distal Radius Fractures

A. A statistically significant increase in the risk of wrist fracture is present in each of the following groups:

      1. Those not wearing wrist guards.

        a. Wrist guards have been shown to decrease incidence and severity of wrist injuries in randomized, controlled trials.

        b. The braces seem to provide protection by absorbing and dispersing the force of a fall on the outstretched hand.

        c. Wrist brace use should be especially encouraged for beginners, during lessons, and when learning new tricks.

      2. Younger snowboarders.

      3. Those with less experience.

B. Mechanism of injury.

      1. Typically occurs when the outstretched hand is used in an attempt to break a fall.

        a. More likely to occur when falling backward (toward the heel edge).

C. History.

      1. Pain in the wrist, usually present immediately after a fall.

        a. Pain increased with attempted motion.

        b. The snowboarder often supports the injured wrist with the opposite hand to relieve discomfort.

      2. Deformity may or may not be present.

      3. Paresthesias may or may not be present.

D. Physical examination.

      1. Observe.

        a. Gross deformity.

        b. Edema.

        c. Skin changes.

        d. Spontaneous motion.

      2. Palpate.

        a. May wish to obtain radiographs first.

        b. Try to pinpoint area of maximal tenderness.

          i. Distal radius versus anatomical snuff box.

          ii. Palpate the entire wrist, not just the radial side.

      3. Test and document neurovascular status.

E. Radiographs should be obtained in all cases of traumatic wrist pain in a snowboarder.

      1. Standard, properly aligned, three-view radiographs of the wrist should be obtained.

        a. Understanding the normal radiocarpal relationship is important in determining if the alignment is acceptable.

          i. The normal position of the distal radius should reflect an anterioposterior view radial inclination of 20–25° and a lateral view volar inclination of 10–12° (Figure 6-5).

      2. A coned-in scaphoid view can be added if there is suspicion of scaphoid injury.

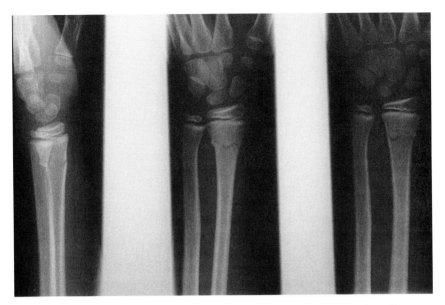

FIGURE 6-5 Lateral, oblique, and AP X-rays of a distal radius fracture display reversal of the normal volar inclination and subtle loss of radial inclination. Images courtesy of Scott M. Koehler, MD.

      3. Description of the fracture should include:
        a. Position.
          i. Many of these fractures are displaced.
        b. Alignment.
        c. Involvement of the distal radioulnar or radiocarpal joint.
        d. Degree of comminution.
          i. Many of these fractures are comminuted.
  F. Treatment is guided by the type of fracture.
      1. Nondisplaced fracture or minimally angulated buckle fracture.
        a. Splint for 5 to 7 days.
        b. Repeat the examination and radiographs at that time prior to definitive casting.
        c. Short arm cast is typically adequate.
          i. Healing time is 4 to 6 weeks.
          ii. Repeat radiograph at intervals of every 2 to 3 weeks.
      2. Extraarticular, angulated fracture.
        a. Initial treatment.
          i. Closed reduction with hematoma block.
          ii. Place in a double sugar tong splint until follow-up (if postreduction alignment is acceptable in the splint).

    b. Follow-up in 3 to 4 days with a provider who is comfortable treating these injuries.
      i. High chance of displacement or angulation of fracture fragments even when appropriately splinted/casted.
      ii. Typically treated by an orthopedic surgeon.
  3. Comminuted or displaced interarticular fractures.
    a. Usually require closed reduction with percutaneous pinning or open reduction internal fixation (ORIF) to maintain position and articular surface integrity.
    b. Immediate orthopedic surgery referral recommended.
  4. Significantly comminuted or shortened fractures may need external fixation to preserve the length of the radius.
    a. Immediate orthopedic surgery referral recommended.

Scapholunate Dissociation

A. Mechanism of injury.
  1. Fall on outstretched hand.
B. History.
  1. Pain in dorsal aspect of wrist.
  2. Worsened with weight-bearing activities, such as pushing the ground to get back onto board after a fall.
  3. May describe a click or snap with activities.
C. Physical examination.
  1. No gross deformities noted in most cases.
  2. Neurovascular status intact.
  3. Tender in region of scapholunate joint on dorsal palpation of wrist.
  4. Positive Watson test.
    a. Stabilize scaphoid tubercle with wrist in ulnar deviation/extension position.
    b. Maintain scaphoid stabilization while passively moving wrist into radial deviation/flexion position.
    c. If scapholunate ligament intact, scaphoid will flex despite being stabilized by examiner.
    d. If scapholunate disrupted, scaphoid will not flex and forces will therefore be transmitted to the scapholunate joint.
      i. Typically causes pain.
      ii. Subluxation of the scaphoid noted as a "clunk."
D. Radiographic evaluation.
  1. X-rays are necessary when scapholunate dissociation is suspected.

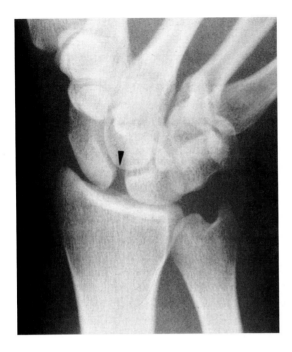

FIGURE 6·6 Scapholunate dissociation. Image courtesy of I.F. Anderson. Reprinted with permission from Brukner P, Khan K. *Clinical Sports Medicine,* rev. 2nd ed. New York: McGraw-Hill; 2002, p. 301.

    a. AP view in neutral and clenched-fist positions.
        i. Assess the width of the scapholunate joint.
           • Gap of > 3 mm considered positive (Figure 6-6).
             – "Terry Thomas" sign.
           • Comparison views of contralateral wrist may be helpful.
    b. Lateral view.
        i. Assess alignment of carpal bones.
           • The radius, lunate, capitate, and third metacarpal should be collinear.
           • A collapsing pattern may be noted in the unstable wrist.
  2. MRI is not needed if physical exam and X-rays are positive.
E. Treatment.
  1. Referral to an orthopedic or hand surgeon is advised for consideration of surgical stabilization of the joint.

Shoulder Dislocation

A. Shoulder injuries, in general, account for 8–16% of snowboarding injuries and occur at nearly twice the rate of these injuries in skiers.

1. These injuries occur more commonly from falling forward, or toward the toe edge.
2. Common shoulder injuries in snowboarding include rotator cuff strains, glenohumeral subluxations and dislocations, acromioclavicular separations, and clavicle fractures.
    a. Other sprains, strains, and fractures also occur.
3. Shoulder and clavicle injuries are more common in advanced snowboarders compared to beginners.

B. Anterior glenohumeral stability issues.
1. General considerations.
    a. Dislocation is a complete separation of the articular surfaces and can be either anterior or posterior.
    b. Subluxation is an abnormal translation of the humeral head on glenoid without complete separation of the articular surfaces.
2. Mechanism of injury.
    a. The typical mechanism for anterior dislocation is one in which the arm is forced into abduction, extension, and external rotation.
    b. Subluxation can occur from repeated overuse or as a result of previous dislocation.
3. Anterior shoulder dislocation.
    a. History.
        i. Acute onset of pain in the shoulder after a fall.
        ii. Reduced shoulder ROM. Some athletes are unable to move the shoulder at all.
        iii. Paresthesias in the upper arm may be reported.
    b. Physical examination.
        i. Observation.
            • Patients with acute anterior dislocation present in pain, holding the arm in slight abduction with external rotation.
            • A void in the posterior aspect of the shoulder and abnormal contour to the joint may be apparent.
        ii. The patient is unable to internally rotate or abduct the shoulder.
        iii. Neurovascular status should be documented.
            • Axillary nerve involvement is very common.
            • Be sure to reassess neurovascular status after reduction.
        iv. Apprehension with anterior stability testing.
            • If the shoulder is already reduced, relocation test relieves discomfort and apprehension.

   c. Diagnostic testing.
      i. X-rays including AP, axillary lateral, and transcapular views should be obtained.
- Often obtained prior to attempted reduction in order to rule out fracture.
- Axillary lateral view is important.
  – Verifies the direction of the dislocation.
  – More easily shows Hill-Sachs lesions.

      ii. MRI may be considered in those over the age of 40 who do not regain normal strength within three weeks of the dislocation injury, due to the higher incidence of rotator cuff injury in older individuals.

   d. Treatment.
      i. Prompt reduction of the dislocation.
- This may be performed at the venue by a physician competent in the procedure if fracture is not suspected.
  – Reduction close to the time of injury is usually easier to perform because muscle spasm has not yet set in.
  – Intravenous sedation may be necessary if the shoulder has been dislocated for a while and muscle spasm has set in.
- Multiple techniques may be employed to achieve reduction of the joint.

      ii. Post-reduction treatment.
- Obtain post-reduction X-rays.
- Sling is used for comfort and usually may be discontinued in about one week.
- Protected ROM (90° abduction and forward flexion).
- Analgesic medications.
- Ice.
- Rotator cuff strengthening program can commence when acute pain resolves.

   e. Return to play.
      i. Considered when:
- Range of motion is full.
- Strength is full.
- There is no pain or apprehension on stability testing.

      ii. The risk of redislocation is high, particularly if the initial dislocation occurs at a young age. This should be reviewed with the athlete.

f. Surgical intervention.
 i. Appropriate in the treatment of recurrent dislocation.
 ii. There is a great deal of debate surrounding the topic of surgical intervention after first dislocation in young athletes.

Elbow Dislocation

A. General information.
 1. Elbow injuries account for 2–5% of snowboarding injuries.
  a. Common elbow injuries include contusions, sprains, strains, fractures, and dislocations.
  b. These injuries are more common in snowboarders than skiers.
 2. A fall on the snowboard puts the elbow at increased risk, especially of hyperextension and longitudinal forces along the radius and ulna.
 3. The elbow is the second most commonly dislocated joint (following the shoulder) in the snowboarder.
  a. The majority of the dislocations are posterior (the ulna dislocating posteriorly in relationship to the humerus).
   i. This puts the coronoid process and the proximal radius at risk, especially due to the combined longitudinal force along the radius.
    • Fractures at these two sites are most commonly involved in fracture dislocations.
B. Mechanism of injury.
 1. Fall onto outstretched arm.
  a. Elbow is partially flexed in most cases.
  b. Axial load to joint.
  c. Rotational forces commonly take place at the time of injury as well.
C. History.
 1. Immediate pain throughout elbow.
 2. Gross deformity.
 3. Inability to move elbow.
 4. Numbness/tingling may be present.
D. Physical examination.
 1. On-field.
  a. Document neurovascular status.
   i. If neurovascular compromise present, on-field attempt at reduction may be necessary.
   ii. If neurovascular status intact, reduction is urgent but does not have to be attempted in the field.

      b. Stabilize extremity and transport to appropriate area/facility.

        i. Allows for more thorough evaluation.

        ii. Removes injured athlete from cold-weather environment.

  2. In medical facility.

      a. Expose the extremity and observe.

        i. Gross deformity.

          • Olecranon in a posterior location.

          • Angular deformities should raise suspicion of concurrent fracture.

        ii. Skin color changes.

        iii. Associated injuries.

      b. Document neurovascular status.

        i. May change from initial (on-field) exam.

      c. Presence of dislocation is usually plainly evident.

E. Radiographic evaluation.

  1. X-rays must be obtained in all cases of elbow dislocation (Figure 6-7).

      a. Most recommend obtaining X-rays prior to attempted reduction.

        i. Rule out fracture.

        ii. More fully evaluate the orientation of the dislocation.

      b. Must obtain at least an AP and lateral view.

        i. It is important to remember to evaluate the lateral elbow radiograph carefully for subtle signs of hemarthosis, which suggests an occult fracture in an otherwise normal radiograph series.

        ii. In skeletally immature snowboarders, it is critical to be sure the anterior humeral cortical line bisects the capitellum to rule out an occult growth plate fracture.

          • Comparison views of the contralateral elbow are advised particularly if there is uncertainty of physeal injury or position.

  2. Additional diagnostic studies not typically needed prior to reduction.

F. Treatment.

  1. Reduce the dislocated joint (the following describes treatment of posterior dislocation).

      a. Reduction often requires two people.

      b. Distract the ulna from the humerus with axial traction.

      c. Once distracted, flex the elbow.

        i. Click often felt/heard as the olecranon engages the articular surface of the humerus.

        ii. Gently pushing the olecranon may assist the reduction.

      d. Pain decreases significantly upon reduction of the joint.

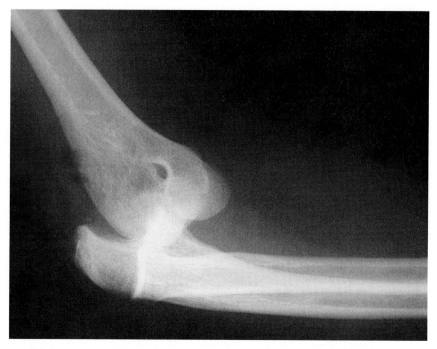

FIGURE 6-7   Posterior elbow dislocation. Image courtesy of Scott M. Koehler, MD.

2. After reduction accomplished.
   a. Reassess neurovascular status.
   b. Obtain post-reduction X-rays.
   c. Move elbow through range of motion passively to ensure stability.
   d. Place elbow in a splint with at least 90° flexion and the forearm slightly supinated.
3. Further management.
   a. Reevaluate the patient in 24 to 48 hours for signs of vascular compromise.
   b. Try to initiate motion exercises as early as possible.
      i. Can often be started in 3 to 5 days post-injury.
      ii. Greater periods of immobilization post-injury are associated with:
          • A greater likelihood of long-term flexion contracture.
          • More severe pain symptoms at follow-up.
      iii. ROM brace is a helpful tool to provide protection while allowing graduated return to full motion.

Forearm Injuries

A. Uncommonly, the force of a fall in snowboarding can cause a fracture to one or both bones of the forearm.
   1. A diaphyseal fracture of one forearm bone with dislocation of the other may occur.
B. Monteggia fracture/dislocation.
   1. Fracture of the proximal ulna with associated dislocation of the proximal radius.
      a. Type I (frequency: 60%).
         i. Anterior dislocation of the radial head.
         ii. Anterior angulation of the diaphyseal ulna fracture.
      b. Type II (frequency: 15%).
         i. Posterior or posterolateral dislocation of the radial head.
         ii. Posterior angulation of the diaphyseal ulna fracture.
      c. Type III (frequency: 20%).
         i. Lateral or posterolateral dislocation of the radial head.
         ii. Fracture of ulnar metaphysis.
      d. Type IV (frequency: 5%).
         i. Anterior dislocation of the radial head.
         ii. Fracture at proximal one-third of radius.
         iii. Fracture of ulna at same level.
   2. Treatment.
      a. Prompt orthopedic surgery referral for treatment is appropriate.
      b. Closed treatment is appropriate in most cases in children.
         i. Closed reduction performed under general anesthesia.
         ii. Types I, III, and IV injuries are immobilized in long arm cast at 100–110° elbow flexion for 4 to 6 weeks.
         iii. Type II injuries are immobilized in long arm cast at 90° elbow flexion for 4 to 6 weeks.
      c. In adults, ORIF of the ulna fracture along with reduction of the dislocated radius.
         i. Immobilization for six weeks after surgery.
            • Types I, III, and IV.
               – 110° elbow flexion best position to maintain reduction of radius.
               – Supination (not forced).
            • Type II.
               – 70° elbow flexion.
C. Galeazzi fracture/dislocation.
   1. Fracture of the radius at the junction of the mid and distal one-thirds associated with dislocation of the distal radioulnar joint.
   2. Internal fixation is recommended in all cases to assure adequate outcome.

    a. High risk of malunion and continued radioulnar joint dislo-
    cation if closed reduction attempted.

    b. Surgery is followed by six weeks of splint immobilization of
    the elbow.

Fractures of the Lateral Process of the Talus (LPT)

A. General information.
1. Understanding this "snowboarder's fracture" is critical in the treatment of snowboarders.
2. This once-rare injury has become common with the growth of snowboarding.
    a. LPT fractures represent ~15% of ankle injuries in snow-boarders.
3. Outside of snowboarding this injury is present in <1% of ankle injuries.
    a. This fracture is often misdiagnosed.

B. Mechanism of injury.
1. Axial loading of the ankle in an inverted and dorsiflexed position.
    a. Research models of this injury suggest that external rotation of the ankle may also be involved.
    b. Typically occurs when landing hard from a jump with body weight too far over the toe edge of the board.
2. An eversion ankle injury mechanism has recently been demonstrated.

C. History.
1. Presents similar to an inversion ankle sprain.
    a. Pain in the lateral ankle.
        i. Increased with weight bearing.
    b. Lateral ankle swelling.
    c. Lateral ankle and dependent foot bruising.

D. Physical examination.
1. Lateral ankle edema.
2. Ecchymosis.
3. Point-tender to palpation of the lateral ankle.
    a. Often difficult to distinguish bony tenderness from ligamentous tenderness.
        i. LPT lies between and beneath the anterior talofibular and the calcaneofibular ligaments.
4. Ligamentous testing.
    a. Anterior drawer test.
        i. Ankle held in slight plantar flexion.
        ii. The foot (talus) is translated anteriorly within the ankle mortise.

    iii. Increased excursion compared to the uninjured side is indicative of ligamentous injury.
- This will likely be painful in the case of LPT fracture as well as an acute sprain.
- Athletes with a history of previous ankle sprain may have residual laxity, making the anterior drawer test more difficult to interpret.

  b. Talar tilt test.
    i. Ankle held in neutral (90°) position.
    ii. The talus is tilted into inversion.
    iii. As noted with the anterior drawer test, this will likely be painful in both the fracture and sprain situations.
- Increased excursion is more suggestive of a ligamentous injury.

E. Diagnostic studies.
  1. X-ray.
    a. Because of the relatively high incidence of LPT fractures, radiographs should be obtained in cases of acute ankle injury in a snowboarder.
    b. Radiographs are not always necessary in cases of acute ankle injury in other sports.
    c. X-ray series should include AP, lateral, and mortise projections.
    d. The fracture is often difficult to see (Figure 6-8a) and may not be visible in 20–40% of cases.
  2. CT scan.
    a. Often needed to recognize or fully define these subtle fractures (Figure 6-8b,c).
    b. If X-rays appear negative, consider CT scan in the snowboarder with lateral point tenderness and inability to bear weight if symptoms don't improve over the first 5 to 7 days.

F. Treatment.
  1. Treatment depends on fragment size, displacement, and involvement of the articular surfaces.
    a. Fracture morphology is defined by CT scan in all but the simplest cases.
  2. Large LPT fractures.
    a. High risk of disability due to potential involvement of both the talocrural and subtalar joints.
    i. Perfect anatomic alignment is important as in some cases degenerative subtalar changes have been described within 6 to 24 months of this fracture.

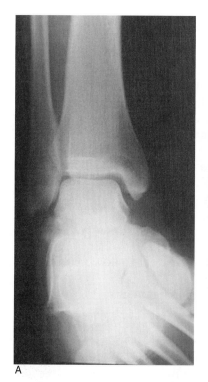

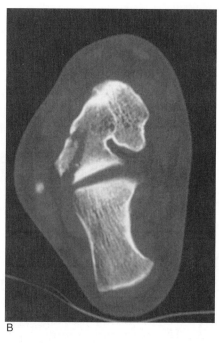

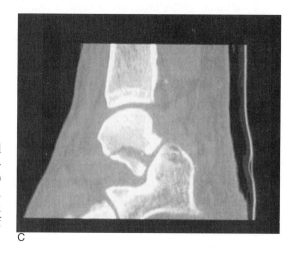

FIGURE 6-8 Lateral process of the talus fracture: a) AP radiograph, b) coronal CT scan image, and c) sagittal CT scan image. Images courtesy of Keith A. Stuessi, MD.

    b. ORIF to stabilize the fragment and preserve the articular surfaces.

        i. Followed by six weeks in a non-weight-bearing (NWB) cast.

  3. Small, nondisplaced fractures of the tip of the process.

    a. Four weeks in NWB cast followed by two weeks of gradual weight bearing in a walking cast.

    b. Progressive ankle rehabilitation begins when immobilization complete.

  4. Comminution and/or extension into the body of the talus typically requires ORIF, possibly with excision of small fragments.

Lateral Ankle Sprains

A. Roughly half of all injuries to the ankle in snowboarding are sprains.

  1. Most sprains are of the lateral ankle ligaments.

    a. Anterior talofibular ligament.

    b. Calcaneofibular ligament.

  2. The injury more commonly occurs to the lead foot.

B. Mechanism of injury, history, and physical examination findings are similar to what is seen with LPT fractures (see Traumatic Injuries, Fractures of the Lateral Process of the Talus (LPT), page 151.

  1. Differentiating between lateral ankle sprain and LPT fractures clinically is very difficult.

  2. Subtle differences in the physical examination findings may include:

    a. More tenderness over the anterior talofibular or calcaneofibular ligament than the LPT.

        i. Due to the anatomical location of the LPT in relationship to the ligaments, palpation is not reliable.

    b. Increased excursion on ligamentous testing.

        i. Usually indicates acute ligamentous injury.

        ii. If the snowboarder has suffered a previous lateral ankle sprain, some residual laxity can be present.

C. Diagnostic testing.

  1. Although X-rays are not always necessary in cases of lateral ankle injury in many sports, a standard three-view ankle series should be obtained in all snowboarders with an acute lateral ankle injury.

  2. The Ottawa Ankle Rules outline situations in which ankle X-rays should be obtained in the acute injury setting.

    a. Patient unable to walk four consecutive steps.

    b. Tenderness on palpation of the posterior half of the medial malleolus.

    c. Tenderness on palpation of the posterior half of the lateral malleolus.

D. Treatment.

    1. In the past, immobilization was a mainstay of ankle sprain treatment. Early, active rehabilitation is now recommended for most athletes.

        a. Allows for faster recovery and return to play.

        b. May be more uncomfortable than immobilization in the early stages of treatment.

    2. Treatment can be divided into five basic stages.

        a. Control of pain and swelling: PRICE.

            i. Protection.

                • External ankle brace.

                    – May be very helpful to reduce risk of recurrent injury upon return to sport.

                • ROM walking boot.

            ii. Rest.

                • Crutches may be needed early on.

            iii. Ice.

                • Reduces blood flow and swelling to the area.

                • Reduces early inflammation.

                • Reduces pain.

            iv. Compression.

            v. Elevation.

            vi. Medications may also be utilized.

                • Analgesics.

                    – Very helpful in reducing pain.

                    – A good choice in first 24 to 48 hours as NSAIDs may increase bleeding/swelling early on.

                • NSAIDs.

        b. Maintenance of range of motion.

            i. Start the patient moving the ankle as early as pain will allow.

            ii. All planes of motion need to be included.

            iii. Writing the alphabet with the foot is an excellent exercise.

        c. Maintenance of strength.

            i. Isotonic and isometric strength programs are both helpful.

            ii. Use of resistance bands is especially helpful.

        d. Balance and position sense training.

            i. An important component of rehabilitation.

            ii. May be helpful in reducing the risk of recurrent sprain.

      iii. One-foot balancing drills.
- Stand with eyes open.
- Move through ankle and knee range of motion with eyes open.
- Stand with eyes closed.

    e. Sport-specific activities and return to sport.

Knee Injuries

A. More common in skiers than in snowboarders.

B. Cruciate and collateral ligament injuries have been associated with falling at high speeds, collisions with objects, and falling while loading and unloading from the lift with one leg unhooked from the binding.

C. For full discussion of ligamentous knee injuries, see Chapter 5, Alpine Skiing.

AXIAL INJURIES

Spine Injuries

A. General.
1. Account for 2–4 % of injuries and are among the most devastating of injuries to snowboarders.
2. Levy et al. (2002) showed that of 43 spinal injuries that required hospital admission, 12% had cervical injuries, 40% thoracic injuries, 53% lumbar, and 4% sacral.
   a. Many athletes had injuries to multiple sites.
   b. Cervical fractures have a higher risk of associated neurological injury than thoracolumbar fractures.
   c. There were also a significant number of associated abdominal and thoracic injuries in these cases.
3. Many of these injuries occur due to axial loading from falls or errors while jumping and landing.
4. Prevention efforts focus on emphasis on proper techniques of jumping with clear takeoff and landing.

B. General evaluation recommendations.
1. History.
   a. Pain.
      i. Typically acute onset of discomfort after a fall.
      ii. Often midline.
      iii. Neurological complaints may or may not be present.
2. Physical examination.

      a. A complete musculoskeletal examination of the affected areas is critical.

      b. Neurological examination.

      c. Mental status examination.

         i. If athlete is unconscious, assume spinal injury is present.

      d. Vascular examination.

      e. Abdomen and thorax.

3. Transport.

      a. If initial assessment raises suspicion of spine injury, transport to an appropriate medical facility is required.

         i. Initial transport may be to the base of the mountain.

         ii. May require air ambulance.

      b. Stabilize the spine appropriately prior to transport.

         i. C-spine stabilization.

            • Cervical collar.

            • Blocks on sides of head.

            • Spine board.

         ii. Thoracic and lumbar spine.

            • Spine board.

4. Diagnostic studies.

      a. Consider radiographs in any athlete with:

         i. Significant pain.

         ii. Midline tenderness.

         iii. Decreased range of motion.

         iv. Decreased mental status or other neurological symptoms.

      b. CT and MRI scans should be considered in particular circumstances.

         i. High suspicion of fracture despite negative X-rays.

         ii. To further evaluate fracture seen on X-ray.

         iii. To evaluate the spinal cord when significant neurological deficits are present.

5. Treatment is dependent upon diagnosis.

C. Treatment of sprains and strains.

      a. Relative rest.

         i. May require supportive device.

            • Cervical collar.

            • Lumbar corset.

      b. Ice often recommended early (first 24 to 48 hours).

      c. Heat can be added to treatment program to relieve muscle aches and spasm and to increase blood flow to the injured area.

      d. Medications.

      i. Analgesics.

      ii. NSAIDs.

      iii. Muscle relaxants sometimes needed.

   e. Rehabilitation.

      i. Home rehabilitation programs often adequate to improve motion, strength, and general function.

      ii. Formal PT sometimes required.

D. Thoracolumbar compression fractures.

   1. These injuries are most commonly seen in the region of the thoracolumbar junction.

   2. Mechanism of injury.

      a. Axial load from falls on the buttocks.

         i. Both feet fixed to the board and hips and spine flexed.

         ii. Force of impact is transmitted along the spine and is absorbed at the relatively stiff thoracolumbar junction.

      b. Other variations of axial loading and flexion to the spine can cause compression fractures.

         i. Falls on the thoracic spine and head (especially when inverted).

         ii. Collisions.

         iii. Hard landings on both feet.

   3. For a full discussion of thoracolumbar compression fractures, see Chapter 5, Alpine Skiing.

Chest Injuries

A. Chest injuries account for approximately 1–6% of all snowboarding injuries.

   1. Machida et al. (1999b) reviewed 96 cases of snowboarders with chest injuries who presented to a Japanese hospital for medical treatment.

      a. 6% of all injuries (N = 1579) over an eight-year period.

      b. Common injuries included:

         i. Rib fracture: 55.2%.

         ii. Contusion: 37.5%.

         iii. Sternum fracture: 3.1%.

         iv. Pneumothorax/hemothorax: 3.1%.

         v. Pneumomediastinum: 1.1%.

   2. Mechanism of injury.

      a. Riding mistake while jumping: 50%.

      b. Fall to the snow: 43%.

      c. Collision: 7%.
         i. With tree in 5%.
         ii. With another person in 2%.
      d. Beginners with less than one week of experience accounted for 45% of these injuries.
   3. The evaluation of chest trauma in a snowboarder begins with a primary survey and stabilization of the airway, breathing, and circulation status.
      a. Details of the injury can be determined after the primary survey.
   4. Chest radiographs are important in all but the most minor injuries.
      a. If abnormalities are present or suspicion is high, a chest CT may be indicated.
   5. Treatment depends on the specific injury.
      a. Immediate ability to decompress the chest in the event of a tension pneumothorax is important.
      b. Access to an appropriate facility for chest tube drainage for pneumothorax and hemothorax is important.

Abdominal Injuries

A. Account for 2–7% of snowboarding injuries.
   1. There appears to be a higher abdominal injury rate in snowboarders than in skiers.
B. Mechanism.
   1. Falls (53%).
      a. Rider falls forward on his or her outstretched hand and may strike the abdomen with his or her elbow and suffer significant blunt trauma to the abdomen.
         i. The common snowboarding stance of left foot forward places the athlete in a left arm and spleen forward position.
         ii. In a series of four spleen injuries, three athletes described falling on their own left arms with the left elbow striking the abdomen.
            • Two of these three required emergency splenectomy.
   2. Mistake during jumping (32%).
   3. Collisions (16%).
C. For discussion of abdominal injuries, see Chapter 5, Alpine Skiing.

Genitourinary Injuries

A. GU injuries are uncommon in snowboarding.
   1. Account for < 2% of all injuries.
   2. Higher incidence in females.

B. The most concerning injury pattern is lacerations and hematomas to the vulva in female snowboarders who fall on the bindings of their own boards.

    1. Kanai et al. (2001) reported a series of 65 vulvar injuries in snowboarders with more than 80% describing falling on the upright heel support of their binding.

        a. Most typically occur when unloading the lift chair and riding down the exit ramp with only one foot fixed to the board.

        b. Other common events:

            i. Fall while waiting in lift line.

            ii. While loading the chair lift.

    2. In the Kanai series, 69% required surgical treatment.

C. Prevention strategies.

    1. Turning down the back of the binding when the foot is out.

    2. Using flat, step-in bindings.

    3. Providing fixed railings in lift lines for support.

    4. Providing safe, gradual exit slopes from the chair lift.

CONCLUSION

A. The pattern of snowboarding injuries is distinctly different from that of skiing injuries.

B. The unique style and stance of the snowboarder is important to understand in order to properly care for these athletes.

C. It is helpful for the physician caring for snowboarders to be aware of the unique aspects of injuries to snowboarders to assure proper diagnosis and treatment.

D. The following recommendations are general guidelines for snowboarders.

    1. Wear a helmet.

    2. Wear wrist braces when learning to snowboard.

    3. Snowboard in control, and do not leave the area boundary.

    4. Dress appropriately and without loose-fitting clothing such as scarves that could get caught in the lift or tow rope.

    5. Snowboard in pairs so you are able to get help if you get hurt.

Suggested Readings

Blatt G, Tobias B, Lichtman DM. Scapholunate injuries. In: Lichtman DM, Alexander AH, eds. *The Wrist and Its Disorders*. 2nd ed. Philadelphia: WB Saunders Co.; 1997:268–306.

Crane L, Snowboard History Timeline, EXPN.com. Accessed November 2000.

Fukuda O, Takaba M, Saito T, Endo S. Head injuries in snowboarders compared with head injuries in skiers: A prospective analysis of 1076 patients from 1994 to 1999 in Niigata, Japan. *AJSM* 2001;29(4):437–40.

Funk JR, Srinivasan SCM, Crandall JR. Snowboarders talus fracture experimentally produced by eversion and dorsiflexion. *AJSM* 2003;31(6):921–28.

Idzikowski JR, Janes PC, Abbott PJ. Upper extremity snowboarding injuries: Ten-year results from the Colorado Snowboard Injury Survey. *AJSM* 2000;28(6):825–32.

Kanai M, Osada R, Maruyama K, Masuza wa H, Shih H, Konishi I. Warning from Nagano: Increase of vulvar hematoma and/or lacerated injury caused by snowboarding. *J Trauma* 2001;50(2):328–31.

Kirkpatrick DP, Hunter RE, Janes PC, Mastrangelo J, Nicholas RA. The snowboarder's foot and ankle. *AJSM* 1998;26(2):271–77.

Kocher MS, Dupre MM, Feagin JA Jr. Shoulder injuries from alpine skiing and snowboarding: Aetiology, treatment and prevention. *Sports Medicine* 1998;25(3):201–11.

Levy AS, Hawkes AP, Hemminger LM, Knight S. An analysis of head injuries among skiers and snowboarders. *J Trauma* 2002;53(4):695–704.

Machida T, Hanazaki K, Ishizaka K, et al. Snowboarding injuries of the abdomen: Comparison with skiing injuries. *Injury* 1999a;30(1):47–49.

Machida T, Hanazaki K, Ishizaka K, et al. Snowboarding injuries of the chest: Comparison with skiing injuries. *J Trauma* 1999b;46(6):1062–65.

McCrory P, Bladin C. Fractures of the lateral process of the talus: A clinical review—"Snowboarder's ankle." *CJSM* 1996;6(2):124–28.

Mehlhoff TL, Noble MS, Bennett JB, Tullos HS. Simple dislocation of the elbow in the adult. *JBJS(A)* 1988;70(2):244–49.

Nakaguchi H, Fujimaki T, Ueki K, Takahashi M, Yoshida H, Kirino T. Snowboard head injury: Prospective study in Chino, Nagano, for two seasons from 1995 to 1997. *J Trauma* 1999;46(6):1066–69.

Reckling FW. Unstable fracture-dislocations of the forearm (Monteggia and Galeazzi lesions). *JBJS(A)* 1982;64A(6):857–63.

Ronning R, Ronning I, Gerner T, Engebretsen L. The efficacy of wrist protectors in preventing snowboarding injuries *AJSM* 2001;29(5):581–85.

Stiell IG, Greenberg GH, McKnight RD, et al. Decision rules for the use of radiography in acute ankle injuries: Refinement and prospective validation. *JAMA* 1993;269(3):1127–32.

Takagi M, Sasaki K, Kiyoshige Y, Ida H, Ogino T. Fracture and dislocation of snowboarder's elbow. *J Trauma* 1999;47(1):77–81.

Tarazi F, Dvorak MF, Wing PC. Spinal injuries in skiers and snowboarders *AJSM* 1999;27(2):177–80.

U.S. Consumer Product Safety Commission. *Skiing Helmets: An Evaluation of the Potential to Reduce Head Injury.* Washington, DC: U.S. Government Printing Office; 1999. Available at www.cpsc.gov.

7

FREESTYLE SKIING

Jim Macintyre

INTRODUCTION

General

A. Freestyle skiing is an exciting sport practiced around the world in alpine (and some non-alpine) areas.
  1. It has evolved with time, and has become one of the most exciting spectator events in skiing.
  2. Its relatively small competition venue gives good spectator visibility; this combines with its spectacular nature to make it a popular spectator sport.
B. It shares many of the medical concerns of other skiing events, with its own unique issues due to its inherent demands.

History of Freestyle Skiing

A. Developed in the 1960s and 70s as an offshoot of the original "hot dog" skiers.
  1. Early attempts plagued by high injury rates.
  2. Safety issues prompted formation of standards for competition.
B. Initially three disciplines:
  1. Aerials.
  2. Moguls.
  3. Ballet.
C. 1980s—World Cup competitions introduced, sanctioned by FIS as governing body.

D. 1988—Moguls and aerials introduced as demonstration sports at Olympic Games (Calgary).
E. 1992—Mogul skiing becomes a full medal sport at Albertville Games.
F. 1994—Aerials became a full medal sport at Lillehammer Games.
G. Late 1990s—Ballet dropped as a World Cup sport.
   1. Never introduced as an Olympic event.

Epidemiology

A. Very few studies of injury patterns exist, none in the last ten years.
   1. In moguls, injuries resemble traditional alpine skiing.
   2. In aerials, injuries are unique and share features with skiing, gymnastics, and contact/collision sports.
B. Given the lack of published studies, this discussion is based on the author's experience of over ten years of National Team coverage for the U.S. and Canadian Freestyle Teams, including World Cup, World Championships, and Olympics. Valuable input was received from Kim Nelson, PT, AT-C, who has served as a therapist with the U.S. National Team for over ten years, including several Olympics.

Special Concerns and Aspects of the Sport

A. Moguls.
   1. Venue.
      a. Steep, fairly narrow course set in the fall line.
         i. Initially courses developed naturally as skiers descended the pitch.
      b. Maximum course length is 860 feet.
      c. Moguls are machine-made and are uniform regarding configuration and spacing.
      d. Three lanes down the fall line: right, center, and left.
         i. Skier comes out of the start gate and selects a lane to ski.
         ii. Once chosen, the skier skis the same lane for practice and competition.
      e. Two jump zones (upper and lower) in each of the three lanes.
         i. Specially constructed jumps are present in each jump zone, where the skiers will become airborne and perform various acrobatic maneuvers.
            • Skier may achieve a height of 3–4 m above the landing zone and carry 4–5 m, all done at full speed.

- Landing zone is flat and free of moguls.
  - Landing long results in a hard landing at full speed in the midst of a mogul field.
2. Typical maneuvers (no inverted aerials are permitted).
   a. Spread-eagles.
   b. Daffys.
   c. Twisters.
   d. Iron Crosses.
   e. 360° and 720° spins.
   f. Off-axis rotational flips recently introduced.
      i. Invented by Jonny Moseley, jump termed the "Dinner Roll."
      ii. Feet never go above the skier's head.
3. Competition format.
   a. Single moguls.
      i. Skiers perform semifinal runs that are, in effect, the qualifications for the finals.
      ii. Top 16 skiers advance to the finals.
   b. Dual moguls.
      i. World Cup only (not Olympics).
      ii. Competitors are seeded, then compete side by side and head to head on two parallel courses.
      iii. Single elimination format; loser goes home.
4. Scoring.
   a. Judged on three criteria; total score is calculated.
      i. Turns.
         - 50% of total score.
         - Rated on consistency and form.
      ii. Air.
         - 25% of total score.
         - Rated on form (height and distance), landing, and degree of difficulty.
      iii. Time.
         - 25% of total score.
         - Rated on elapsed time relative to a pacesetter with greater points for faster times.
   b. Highest score wins.
5. Equipment.
   a. Skis—regular alpine skis, slightly shorter lengths.
   b. Poles—Regular alpine poles.
   c. Bindings—Regular release bindings, usually set quite tightly to enhance ski retention.
   d. Helmets.
      i. Many, but not all, are now wearing helmets.

B. Aerials: on snow.
   1. Venue.
      a. Aerial competition takes place on specially designed and prepared jumping slopes.
      b. Five components/areas of the venue.
         i. In-run.
            • Allows the skier to attain the speed necessary to perform the planned aerial maneuver.
            • Up to 250 feet long.
            • The slope has an angle between 20 and 25°.
            • Skiers regulate their approach speed by varying the starting height and acceleration distance.
            • More complex and difficult jumps require greater height off the jump and therefore a greater in-run speed.
               – Achieved by starting higher up the hill.
            • Changing snow or wind conditions can lead to miscalculation of the required in-run velocity, and can lead to crashes.
         ii. Transition area/knoll.
            • Located at the bottom of the in-run.
            • Flat area with its length proportional to the slope of the in-run, measuring the same number of meters as the angle of the in-run.
            • The jumps sit on the knoll.
         iii. Launch area.
            • Constructed out of snow that is blown into a form to solidify and is then precisely contoured to specific angles to provide the appropriate amount of lift.
            • The jumps are carefully shaped and maintained by the athletes themselves.
            • There are commonly six jumps at World Cup events, with contours for single, double, and triple jumps.
            • The jumps themselves are up to 4 meters high.
            • The edges of the jumps are spray-painted to aid in visibility.
         iv. Landing area.
            • Steep slope for landing.
            • 115 feet in length and flattens out at the bottom where the competitors come to a halt.
            • The snow on the hill is chopped into small pieces frequently during the competition to soften it and reduce the impact of landing.

- Small pieces of pine branches often mixed with the snow in the landing area to provide contrast and assist in depth perception.
  v. Run-out.
2. Format.
   a. During practice and warm-up, the competitor performs progressively more difficult jumps.
      i. Speed on the in-run is carefully monitored for optimum performance.
         - If speed is too fast, the skier may get excessive height and over-rotate, leading to falls.
         - If speed is too slow, the skier may not complete the required moves and may land short.
         - If speed is wrong, the skier will raise or lower the start position slightly on the next jump to optimize takeoff speed.
         - Variable weather can have significant impact on in-run speed, and can lead to accidents.
         - Skiers generally leave a small flag on the side of the in-run to mark their optimum start position.
      ii. Competitions consist of morning qualifications with the top 12 male and female skiers carrying on to the finals.
3. Jumps.
   a. The skier will reach a maximum height of 4 meters from the top of the jump (8 meters above the level of the knoll), and will usually land 4–6 meters down the landing zone, a total drop of 12–14 meters from the maximum height.
   b. They have about 4 seconds in the air to perform their maneuvers.
   c. The jumper is exposed to several different forces during the jump.
      i. Vertical forces due to the effects of gravity, with the final landing velocity dependent on the height of the jump, and therefore the distance of the fall.
      ii. Rotational forces due to the somersaults and twisting involved.
         - The higher the number of twists or somersaults, the greater the angular velocity required to complete the jump before landing.
      iii. All inverted aerials are variations of the backward somersault.
         - At lower experience levels, they are performed in layout or in the tuck position.
         - At a higher level, they are combined with twists.

      iv. Aerial competition has evolved over the past decade with the competitors performing increasingly difficult jumps.
- In the late 1980s, the most complex jumps were double back somersaults with 2 or 3 twists.
- Male competitors now regularly perform triple back somersaults with 4 twists.
  - Some male aerialists are now doing quadruple back somersaults in exhibitions, but they are not permitted in competition at this time.
  - Some performing triple somersaults with 5 twists.
- Women generally do not attempt such big jumps.
  - Women have no trouble with the air and twisting portion of the jumps, but lack the considerable strength needed to safely land the jumps.
  - While some women perform triple somersaults, triple twisting double somersaults are more commonly performed.

  4. Judging.
    a. Judges sit in an elevated booth situated on the knoll, which allows accurate viewing of the takeoff, the execution of the maneuver, and the landing.
    b. Each trick has a degree of difficulty assigned to it.
      i. The higher the level of complexity of the trick, the greater the degree of difficulty.
      ii. It is better to do a less difficult trick well than to do a more difficult trick with poor form, or to crash on the landing.
    c. Judged on three criteria.
      i. Takeoff and execution—50% of score.
      ii. Air—20% of score.
      iii. Landing—30% of score.
    d. Points are multiplied by the degree of difficulty to give the final score.
    e. There are two jumps in the final with the highest cumulative score winning.

  5. Equipment.
    a. Skis—specially reinforced, short length.
    b. Bindings—set very tightly.
    c. No poles.
    d. All competitors must wear helmets and mouth guards.

C. Aerials: summer training.
  1. Venue.
    a. Preseason training performed at specialized training facilities.

       i. Trampoline training.
      ii. Water ramp training.
    b. Trampolines with harnesses allow the athlete to attempt new tricks.
      i. Once the new trick is mastered on the trampoline, athlete is allowed to attempt it on a water ramp.
    c. Water ramps.
      i. In-run covered with an artificial plastic, low-friction surface and ramps configured similarly to those on the World Cup circuit.
      ii. The athletes perform their tricks in the air, then land in the water.
        • The skis land flat on the water, which does not exactly simulate the on-snow landing on a steep hill with the ski tips pointed downward.
        • Surface tension of the water is reduced by jets of bubbles released from the bottom of the pool.
2. Format.
    a. The trick format is identical to that performed on snow, with the exception of the landing position as detailed above.
    b. Before athletes are cleared to attempt a maneuver on-snow, they must perform the trick 100 times on the water ramp and then be judged as they perform the jump flawlessly on five consecutive attempts.
3. Judging.
    a. Performed by the coaches on a day-to-day basis.
    b. Summer competitions have judging criteria similar to those of on-snow competitions.
4. Equipment.
    a. Dry suits.
    b. Life preservers.
    c. Reinforced jumping skis.
    d. Regular release bindings.
    e. Helmets and mouth guards.

EXERCISE PHYSIOLOGY

Moguls

A. Runs are 25–35 seconds long, which primarily utilizes the phosphocreatine and anaerobic energy systems.
B. Dry-land and preseason training emphasize anaerobic speed and endurance, as well as explosive power for performing jumps.

C. Eccentric strength of the quadriceps, hamstrings, and glutei is essential to absorb the impact of striking the moguls at full speed.

D. Core stability is critical to remain centered over the skis, to recover when off-balance, and to assist in control of the rotational forces in the twisting and jumping maneuvers.

Aerials

A. An anaerobic event.

B. Explosive power for takeoff is essential.

C. Core stability is critical to remain centered over the skis, to rotate, and to control the forces of the twisting and jumping maneuvers.

D. Eccentric strength of the quadriceps, hamstrings, and glutei is essential to absorb the impact of landing.

TRAUMATIC FREESTYLE INJURIES

Moguls

A. Two main mechanisms of injury.
  1. Mechanism similar to traditional skiing injuries.
     a. Usually occur with a fall.
     b. Usually affect the extremities.
  2. Injuries due to problems with the bumps.
     a. Skier loses control in the air or falls at landing.
     b. May lead to blunt trauma to the chest or abdomen.

B. Specific injuries.
  1. Knee is the most commonly affected body area.
     a. Anterior cruciate ligament tears. For full discussion of ACL tears, see Chapter 5, Alpine Skiing.
     b. Medial collateral ligament tears. For full discussion of MCL tears, see Chapter 5, Alpine Skiing.
     c. Meniscus tears. For full discussion of meniscus tears, see Chapter 5, Alpine Skiing.
  2. Upper extremity injuries are also common.
     a. Shoulder dislocations. For full discussion of shoulder dislocations, see Chapter 6, Snowboarding.
     b. Acromioclavicular sprains. For full discussion of AC sprains, see Chapter 11, Ice Hockey.
     c. Clavicle fractures. For full discussion of clavicle fracture, see Chapter 11, Ice Hockey.
  3. Blunt abdominal trauma.
     a. Can rarely lead to rupture of the spleen.

      b. Can rarely lead to renal contusion.

      c. For discussion of abdominal injuries, see Chapter 5, Alpine Skiing.

  4. Head and spinal injuries are uncommon.

Aerials

A. Main mechanisms of injury include:

  1. "Slap back crash."

      a. Athlete unable to overcome the angular velocity of the somersaults and continues to rotate posteriorly after the ski tails have contacted the snow. Skier lands hard on his or her back, neck, or head.

  2. The other mechanisms can lead to side impacts, whereby the skis contact the snow first and the skier then rotates sideways with the head and neck striking the snow last, or to the relatively rare frontal impact. These include:

      a. Skier lands too early (midway through a twist or somersault).

      b. Skier lands too late (over-rotates).

      c. Skier becomes disoriented in the air and lands awkwardly.

B. Closed head injuries.

  1. Can range from the minor "ding" in which there is momentary confusion and loss of cortical function, right up to the catastrophic head injury with prolonged unconsciousness and severe structural damage.

  2. Minor concussions are often unrecognized by the medical or coaching staff, and unreported by the athletes.

      a. Subtle disturbances of cortical function can persist with impaired information processing, which might not present a great problem in some circumstances, but may put the aerialist at significant risk if he or she is about to attempt a difficult jump.

  3. There is a serious risk for recurrent concussion and permanent sequelae in the athlete who returns to competition while remaining symptomatic from a previous minor or moderate concussion.

  4. For full discussion of concussions, see Chapter 11, Ice Hockey.

C. Spine injuries.

  1. Range in severity from minor ligamentous sprains to spinal cord concussions, transient quadriparesis, and cervical, thoracic, and lumbar spine fractures.

  2. Any unconscious athlete should be assumed to have a spinal cord injury.

    a. Appropriate immobilization and stabilization of the cervical spine are mandatory prior to evacuation from the hill.

3. Transient quadriparesis.

    a. Mechanism of injury.

       i. Symptoms typically develop after an axial load injury to the neck.

       ii. Can occur due to a fall or bad landing from a jump.

    b. History.

       i. Neck pain may or may not be present.

       ii. Numbness, tingling, and/or paralysis of all four extremities.

         • May last seconds to hours.

         • Most symptoms fully resolve within 15 minutes.

    c. Physical examination.

       i. By the time the skier is evaluated, physical examination may be completely normal.

       ii. Tenderness to palpation of the neck may be present.

       iii. Focal neurological deficits of the extremities may be noted.

    d. If the history and physical examination findings are indicative of transient quadriparesis, the athlete should be immobilized and transported to an appropriate medical facility for further evaluation and treatment.

       i. Full cervical, thoracic, and lumbar spine immobilization.

       ii. Full immobilization is necessary even if the symptoms have fully resolved prior to transport.

       iii. A positive history alone is enough to warrant full immobilization.

    e. Diagnostic studies.

       i. X-rays should be obtained in all cases.

         • 5-view series including AP, lateral (consider flexion and extension views), oblique, and odontoid views.

         • Cervical collar should not be removed until the cervical spine is felt to be free of fracture and instability.

       ii. MRI scan should be performed to assess for the presence of spinal stenosis in all cases.

    f. Treatment is supportive.

       i. Symptoms typically clear spontaneously without sequelae.

    g. Return to sport.

       i. If no spinal stenosis is present, the athlete may return to all activities without a known increased risk of spinal cord injury.

- There must be no residual symptoms.
- Neurological exam must be completely normal.
  ii. If spinal stenosis is present, the athlete may be disqualified from contact and collision sports as well as other high-risk activities.
  - Consultation with a spine specialist is recommended.
D. Maxillofacial injuries.
1. Facial and dental injuries are not uncommon.
2. Injuries include facial abrasions and contusions, mandible and maxillary fractures, dental or molar fractures, and tongue bite lacerations.
3. For discussion of dental injuries, see Chapter 11, Ice Hockey.
E. Extremity injuries.
1. Knee and shoulder injuries already mentioned in the moguls section are also common in aerials.
2. Femoral fractures.
   a. Mechanism of injury is typically a hard fall or very hard landing.
   b. History.
      i. Immediate thigh pain.
      ii. Unable to bear weight.
   c. Physical examination.
      i. Non-weight-bearing.
      ii. Gross deformity may be present.
      iii. Swelling may be present.
         - A significant amount of blood can leak into the thigh before swelling is obvious.
      iv. Pain on thigh palpation.
   d. When history and physical examination are suspicious for femur fracture, stabilize the athlete and transport for further evaluation and treatment.
   e. Diagnostic tests.
      i. X-rays must be obtained in all cases of suspected femur fracture.
   f. Treatment.
      i. Orthopedic surgery referral should be considered in all cases.
   g. Fat embolism syndrome.
      i. A rare complication (< 1% in retrospective reviews) of femur fracture that can be fatal.
      ii. Etiology is poorly understood.
         - Marrow fat embolizes into the blood stream, potentially causing end organ damage.

      iii. Fat embolism is more common with polytrauma.

      iv. Clinical evaluation may reveal:

- Respiratory distress.
- Altered mental status.
- Tachycardia.
- Fever.

      v. Treatment is supportive with respiratory assistance.

3. Hip dislocation.

  a. The majority of hip dislocations are in the posterior direction.

  b. Mechanism of injury.

    i. Hard fall causing axial loading of the hip joint.

    ii. Hip is usually slightly flexed.

    iii. Rotational forces may also play a role.

  c. History.

    i. Immediate pain in the hip or thigh.

    ii. Unable to bear weight.

  d. Physical examination.

    i. Non-weight-bearing.

    ii. Pain with any attempt at active or passive motion.

    iii. The affected extremity may appear:

- Shortened.
- Internally rotated.
- Adducted.

    iv. Neurovascular status should be documented.

  e. When history and physical examination are suspicious for hip dislocation, stabilize the athlete and transport for further evaluation and treatment.

    i. On-field attempts at reduction are rarely necessary.

  f. Diagnostic tests.

    i. X-rays should be obtained in all cases of suspected hip dislocation.

    ii. MRI scan rarely necessary at this stage.

  g. Treatment.

    i. Orthopedic surgery referral should be obtained.

    ii. Closed reduction can be performed under conscious sedation but often requires general anesthesia.

  h. Complications.

    i. Avascular necrosis.

- MRI scan can be helpful in the workup of this potential complication.

    ii. Post-traumatic arthritis.

    iii. Sciatic nerve damage from stretch injury or direct trauma as the femoral head is displaced posteriorly.

4. Elbow dislocation. For discussion of elbow dislocation, see Chapter 6, Snowboarding.
5. Patellar tendon rupture.
   a. Mechanism of injury.
      i. Sudden, severe contraction of the quadriceps musculature in an eccentric fashion.
      ii. Most commonly occurs when landing a jump.
   b. History.
      i. Sudden, acute pain.
         • Anterior knee.
         • Described as a tearing sensation.
      ii. Unable to stand.
      iii. Unable to actively extend knee.
   c. Physical examination.
      i. Unable to ambulate.
      ii. Unable to palpate patellar tendon.
      iii. Patella located superiorly.
      iv. Loss of ability to extend knee.
   d. Diagnostic testing.
      i. Radiographs should be obtained.
         • Look for associated fracture.
         • Compare patella height to uninjured side on the lateral view (Figure 7-1).
   e. Treatment.
      i. Surgical repair is necessary.
         • Should be performed within seven days if possible.
      ii. Postsurgical rehabilitation course may take up to nine months.
      iii. Some residual disability is common.
6. Achilles tendon rupture.
   a. Mechanism of injury.
      i. Sudden, severe contraction of the calf musculature in an eccentric fashion.
      ii. Most commonly occurs when landing a jump "short."
         • Full, final rotation does not take place.
         • Ankle in extreme dorsiflexion at time of impact.
   b. History.
      i. Sudden, severe pain in the Achilles region.
      ii. "It felt like someone kicked me in the back of the leg" is a common description.
      iii. Painful plantar flexion with reduced strength.
   c. Physical examination.
      i. Antalgic gait.
      ii. Palpable defect in the Achilles tendon.

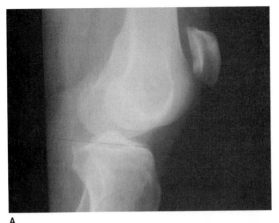

A

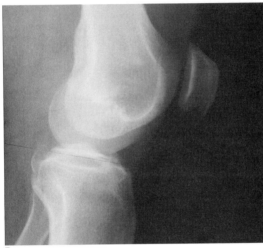

B

FIGURE 7-1 Lateral radiographs of a patient with left patellar tendon rupture. The patella on the injured side (a) is positioned superiorly in comparison to the uninjured right knee (b).

- The plantaris tendon may be palpable, leading the practitioner to believe that the Achilles injury is only a partial tear.
iii. Decreased plantar flexion strength.
- The athlete will be unable to perform a single-leg toe raise on the injured side.
iv. Positive Thompson test.
- Have patient lie prone.
- Flex knee to 90°.
- Squeeze the calf.

– If the ankle plantar flexes, the Achilles is, at least, partially intact.
– No plantar flexion means that the Achilles is completely ruptured.

   d. Diagnostic testing.

     i. Radiographs are commonly obtained but are rarely helpful.

     ii. MRI or ultrasound can be obtained if the diagnosis is in question.

   e. Treatment.

     i. Treatment of the more commonly encountered Achilles tendon rupture is controversial as both conservative and surgical treatment can result in acceptable outcomes.

     ii. In the younger, vigorously active population, and particularly in freestyle skiers who want to return to the sport, surgical management is recommended.

     iii. Postsurgical treatment includes:
- Immobilization for 4 to 8 weeks.
- Initiation of weight bearing in a cast.
- Cast removal and initiation of physical therapy.

F. Visceral injuries.

  1. Serious internal/visceral injuries are uncommon.

  2. Pulmonary contusions.

   a. Not an uncommon finding following a significant slap-back injury.

  3. Pneumothorax.

   a. Rare.

   b. May be spontaneous or traumatic.

   c. Spontaneous pneumothorax.

     i. Result of a congenital bleb on the surface of the visceral pleura that ruptures.

     ii. Typically seen in young, thin males between the ages of 20 and 40.

     iii. May occur at rest or with exertion.

     iv. Symptoms may include:
- Mild to moderate dyspnea.
  - More common with a small pneumothorax (< 15–20%).
  - Severe dyspnea often associated with a larger (> 20%) pneumothorax.
- Acute pleuritic chest pain.
- Cough.

    v. Physical examination.
- Athlete may appear anxious.
- Tachypnea.
- Tachycardia.
- Absent (or reduced) breath sounds on the affected side.
- Wheezing and poor air exchange on inspiration and expiration may be noted.

    vi. When pneumothorax is suspected based on history and physical examination findings, the athlete should be transported to an appropriate medical facility for workup and treatment.

    vii. Diagnostic tests.
- Radiographic evaluation.
  - PA chest X-ray at full, forced expiration.
  - Lateral decubitus view with the suspected side uppermost.

    viii. Treatment.
- Pneumothorax of 15–20% or less can often be treated conservatively:
  - Observation.
  - Supplemental oxygen.
  - Rest.
  - Repeat chest X-rays until clear.
- Pneumothorax of 20% or greater collapse typically requires hospitalization and chest tube placement.
  - Most leaks seal spontaneously within 24 hours.
  - Continued reexpansion must be demonstrated following clamping of the chest tube before removal can be attempted.

  d. Traumatic pneumothorax.

    i. Typically results from a direct blow to the chest or a fractured rib that pierces the lung.

    ii. The injury may present as a simple pneumothorax with dyspnea and chest pain, or a tension pneumothorax (see below).

    iii. History, physical examination findings, diagnostic testing, and treatment follow the same guidelines as noted for spontaneous pneumothorax.

  e. Tension pnuemothorax.

    i. Increased intrapleural pressure develops due to a parenchymal tear and a subsequent one-way air flow valve permitting free air to enter the pleural space during respiration.

- Increasing pressure reduces lung expansion and shifts the mediastinum toward the opposite side.
  - ii. Signs and symptoms.
    - Acute respiratory distress.
    - Tachypnea.
    - Tachycardia.
    - Hypotension.
    - Absent breath sounds on the affected side.
    - Tracheal deviation away from the affected side.
  - iii. Treatment should be initiated as soon as possible.
    - Insertion of a 14- to 18-gauge needle in the second intercostal space at the mid-clavicular line of the affected side.
    - Transport to an emergency room facility for chest tube placement is indicated to stabilize and prevent further expansion of the pneumothorax.
- **4.** Visceral contusions or ruptures.
  - **a.** Rare.
  - **b.** It is important to note that these athletes are highly trained, and an athlete may have internal bleeding and a relative compensatory tachycardia, yet still have a pulse of less than 100 bpm.
    - **i.** If there is any question, check for a postural change in heart rate or blood pressure and always err on the side of caution.

Aerials: Summer Training Injuries

- **A.** Trampoline injuries are uncommon.
  - **1.** Failure to use a harness when attempting new tricks can lead to serious injury.
  - **2.** Falls from the trampoline can cause the sort of visceral, head, and spinal injuries that would be expected with blunt trauma.
  - **3.** Fractures, dislocations, contusions, and ligament injuries can occur.
- **B.** Water ramp training can lead to usual musculoskeletal, head, and internal injuries.
  - **1.** Tympanic membrane rupture is not uncommon and can preclude training for a time.
  - **2.** Near drowning has occurred, especially if there is an associated loss of consciousness.

OVERUSE INJURIES

Overuse injuries arise mainly from the dry land and off-season training, but several injuries can occur with on-snow training and competition.

A. Patellar tendinopathy and patellofemoral pain are fairly common in mogul skiers.

    1. Discussion of these injuries can be found in Chapter 13, Speed Skating.

B. Back pain.

    1. Very common in freestyle skiers.

    2. Cause of back pain is multifactorial.

        a. Repeated hard landings.

        b. Back slaps with direct trauma.

        c. Hyperextension and twisting injuries during jumps and falls.

    3. Many sites and structures are involved.

        a. True herniated nucleus pulposus is relatively rare.

        b. Discogenic pain from annular tears or internal disc disruption is fairly common and can be disabling.

        c. Mechanical low-back pain from sacroiliac joint dysfunction or facet dysfunction and arthrosis is very common.

    4. Mechanical thoracic and rib pain are common in aerialists due to the twisting involved.

    5. Treatment requires the identification of the specific pain generator, as nonspecific diagnosis leads to a nonspecific treatment result.

        a. Local modalities, while of limited use in the ongoing treatment of many back pain patients, are valuable in treating freestyle skiers, due to the ongoing demands of continued participation in their sport.

        b. Restoration of normal mechanical SI joint and facet mobility is critical.

        c. Occasional epidural steroid injections are employed for discogenic pain.

        d. Core stability is critical to the success of the rehabilitation program.

C. Stress fractures.

    1. Repeated landing impacts have led to tibial and calcaneal stress fractures.

    2. Risk factors:

        a. Female athlete triad.

        b. Inadequate calcium intake.

        c. Inadequate lower leg strength.

3. History.
    a. Athlete presents with pain in either the shin or heel.
        i. Worse with impact-loading activities.
          • Landing jumps.
          • Skiing moguls.
          • Running (cross-training).
        ii. Relieved by rest.
4. Physical examination.
    a. Tibia.
        i. Tender on direct palpation.
        ii. May be tender with percussion hammer tapping.
        iii. May be tender with tuning fork testing.
          • Felt to be a specific though not very sensitive test.
        iv. No gross deformities.
        v. Nontender resisted strength testing.
        vi. Neurovascular status intact.
    b. Calcaneus.
        i. Tender to squeeze.
        ii. Examination is generally unremarkable otherwise.
5. Diagnostic tests.
    a. X-rays are usually negative.
    b. Tibia X-rays may show:
        i. Periosteal elevation.
        ii. Cortical thickening.
        iii. Lucent fracture line.
6. Treatment includes:
    a. Protection from further injury.
        i. May require cast or ROM walker immobilization.
        ii. Eliminate impact-loading activities.
    b. Correction of the underlying factors.
    c. Nutritional guidance.
    d. Lower leg strengthening.
    e. Total treatment time may be 6 to 8 weeks.

ON-SITE EVENT COVERAGE

Preparation

Health care professionals providing coverage for freestyle events should have an awareness of the types of injuries that they may encounter, and be prepared to handle catastrophic life- and limb-threatening injuries.

Competition Venue Medical Team

A. Ski patrollers.
B. Physicians.
C. Emergency medical technicians.

Position of Team Members

A. A medical team member should be stationed at the bottom of the jumping hill at the exit from that landing area corral in order to perform a quick mental status assessment of any athlete who has slapped back or fallen.
B. Disoriented athletes are withdrawn until fully assessed.

Equipment

Aside from general medical equipment, the following special equipment should be available on-site for training and competition.
A. Spine immobilization equipment.
    1. Cervical collar.
    2. Backboards.
    3. Splints.
B. Airways, oxygen, and ambu bags.

Transport

Transporting injured athletes from the slope is an important consideration. Modes of transportation may include:
A. Sleds.
B. Snowmobiles.
C. Helicopter airlift.
    1. The FIS mandates that a helicopter be on site for medical evacuations at all major competitions.

Preparing for an Event

A. Make a facility plan that outlines various procedures.
    1. Stabilization.
    2. Evacuation.
    3. Transport.

SUMMARY

A. Freestyle skiing is a spectacular and exciting event.

B. An understanding of the demands of the events will assist the physician in adequately diagnosing and treating freestyle injuries.

C. Traumatic injuries are the most common.

    1. Similar to those found in recreational and competitive skiers.

D. Serious injuries are rare.

    1. Must be recognized and appropriately treated in order to avoid serious sequelae.

E. Moguls incorporate traditional skiing with various upright maneuvers.

F. Aerial competition involves the performance of various acrobatic stunts after jumping from a specially prepared and configured jump.

G. Medical issues are also present for off-season aerials training, which is conducted on trampolines and in specially constructed pool facilities with ramps.

Suggested Readings

Cantu RC. Functional cervical spinal stenosis: A contraindication to participation in contact sports. *Med Sci Sports Exerc* 1995;25(9):1082–84.

Jordan BD, Warren RF, Tsairis P, Ghelman B. How to evaluate transient quadriparesis. *PSM* 1992;20(2):83–90.

Maffulli N. The clinical diagnosis of subcutaneous tear of the Achilles tendon. *AJSM* 1998;26:266–70.

Matthews BD. Fatal cerebral fat embolism after open reduction and internal fixation of femur fracture. *J Trauma* 2001;50(3):585.

Mello A. Fat embolism. *Anaesthesia* 2001;56(2):145–54.

Rudman N, McIlmail D. Emergency department evaluation and treatment of hip and thigh injuries. *Emer Med Clin North Am* 2000;18(1):200.

Soldatis JJ, Goodfellow DB, Wilber JH. End-to-end operative repair of Achilles tendon rupture. *AJSM* 1997;25:90–95.

8

TELEMARK SKIING

Carol S. Federiuk

INTRODUCTION

General

A. Description.
- **1.** Telemark skiing is a graceful form of skiing with origins in nineteenth-century Norway.
- **2.** This style of skiing uses specialized equipment to allow a skier to walk uphill on skis as well as ski down steep slopes.
  - **a.** Walking is possible because the heel of the boot is not attached to the ski.
  - **b.** Descent of difficult terrain is accomplished using parallel and telemark turns.

B. Telemark turn.
- **1.** The unique telemark turn is the hallmark of telemark skiing.
  - **a.** Body weight is evenly distributed between the skis as they are steered into the turn.
  - **b.** The skier slides the outside leg forward while the inside ski slides back with the knee flexed in a position known as the telemark stance.
- **2.** The telemark position provides front-to-back stability and works well in ungroomed snow.

C. Other terms for telemark skiing.
- **1.** Free-heel skiing.
- **2.** Nordic downhill skiing.

      a. This term emphasizes the ability to both walk on skis like Nordic (cross-country) skiers and to ski down slopes like alpine (downhill) skiers.

History of Telemark Skiing

A. Early history.
    1. Telemark skiing originated in the Telemark region of Norway in the mid-nineteenth century.
      a. Sondre Norheim, a skier from the Telemark district, introduced the technique to the country during the first Norwegian national ski competition in 1868.
      b. Norheim used innovative equipment for his time, including short skis with sidecut and bindings that went around the heel of the boot.
    2. Became popular in Europe in the early 1900s.
    3. Brought to the United States when Norwegian skiers immigrated.
B. Mid-twentieth century.
    1. Telemark technique fell out of favor with advances in alpine skiing methods and equipment.
      a. The introduction of alpine bindings that attached the boot heel to the ski in the 1950s meant that the telemark turn was no longer used as an alpine technique.
    2. Alpine and Nordic skiing divided into two schools.
      a. Alpine skiers with fixed heel bindings used parallel turns to rapidly descend slopes.
      b. Nordic skiers with free-heel bindings used the diagonal stride technique to travel cross-country.
        i. Nordic skiing was best suited for traveling on relatively flat terrain due to limited ability to turn the narrow, lightweight skis quickly.
      c. Telemark technique was used only by the relatively few skiers practicing ski mountaineering.
C. Late twentieth century to present.
    1. Interest in telemark skiing was revived in the 1970s.
      a. Stein Eriksen, a Norwegian Olympic champion, wrote about the telemark turn in a book and brought his skills to the United States as an instructor.
      b. Telemark technique was revitalized as a method to use free-heel skiing to travel in more mountainous terrain.
        i. The opportunity to ski in the wilderness and avoid the crowds at established ski resorts was enticing to many skiers.

2. Telemark ski racing was introduced in the 1980s.
    a. Telemark racing has two disciplines, the classic and giant slalom races.
        i. Classic races include cross-country and downhill segments.
            • Made up of three sections: giant slalom, super telemark (high-speed section), and cross-country.
        ii. Giant slalom requires a telemark turn at each gate, and includes a jump of 5–25 m that must be landed in the telemark position.
3. Telemark skiing has continued to gain followers in recent years.
    a. Telemark skiers have become common at lift-served ski areas as well as in the back country.
    b. There has recently been a huge leap in the development of specialized equipment for telemark skiing.

Epidemiology

A. Demographics.
    1. Location.
        a. Telemark skiing is most widely practiced in the mountainous regions of the western United States and Canada, as well as in Europe.
        b. Because of the ability to climb uphill and ski downhill, telemarkers are able to ski both on ski-lift served slopes and on back country terrain.
            i. Telemarkers are twice as likely to be injured when skiing at lift-served areas compared to skiing in the back country.
                • One retrospective study reported that 75% of telemark injuries are sustained at lift-served areas.
                • This is likely attributable to the greater vertical distances skied in a day at the lifts.
    2. Age.
        a. Telemark skiers tend to be older than snowboarders or alpine skiers.
            i. Mean age reported to be 24 to 33 years in studies from ski area clinics in the United States (Oregon), Sweden, and Norway.
            ii. Telemark skiers who take lessons or belong to ski organizations tend to be even older, with mean ages of 40 to 43 years.

      b. Many participants take up telemark skiing after learning alpine skiing when young.

  3. Male:female ratio is approximately 2:1.

  4. Experience level of injured skiers.

      a. Beginners have been reported to have higher injury rates than more experienced skiers.

      b. Expert skiers, skiers with more years of skiing experience, and those who ski more frequently are more likely to have been injured at some time.

  5. Most injuries occur in the afternoon around 3:00 p.m. Reasons for this may include:

      a. Skier fatigue.

      b. Snow conditions.

B. Injury rates.

  1. Injury rates traditionally reported as injuries per 1000 skier days, but this is difficult to extrapolate to telemark skiing.

      a. Skier days data based on lift ticket sales.

      b. Ski areas do not distinguish between tickets sold to alpine and telemark skiers. Therefore, the number of telemark skiers can only be estimated.

  2. Several small studies have estimated telemark injury rates based on the proportional usage of the lifts by telemarkers compared to alpine skiers and snowboarders.

      a. Accomplished by counting the number of each type of user on the lifts.

      b. These studies suggest that telemark injury rates are comparable to or perhaps slightly higher than alpine rates, but lower than snowboarder rates.

         i. Estimated injury rates of 0.9 to 4.1 per 1000 skier days have been reported.

         ii. Attempts to quantify telemark injuries in studies that do not use the ski lift data have been fraught with sample selection bias.

C. Injury mechanisms.

  1. The telemark turn is a factor in most injuries with the majority of injuries occurring due to a fall while turning.

      a. In two Oregon studies, > 90% of skiers were performing a telemark turn at the time of injury.

  2. The mechanism of a fall while performing a telemark turn is different from that of a fall while downhill skiing in several respects.

      a. The genuflection position of the telemark turn places the skier's center of gravity closer to the ground.

   b. The ability of the heel to lift off the ski allows movement at the foot, ankle, and knee with the potential to distribute the force of the fall.
 3. Overall, falls occurring in telemark skiing may be less dangerous than falls while alpine skiing.
   a. Made et al. (2001) found that telemark skiers fell over twice as often per ski run than alpine skiers, although their injury rates were not proportionally elevated.
 4. Less than 15% of injury events involve collisions with other people or fixed objects.
 5. Overuse injuries from climbing and repetitive turning also occur.

Equipment

A. Boots.
 1. Telemark boots have evolved from soft leather models to stiff plastic boots that bear a resemblance to alpine boots and allow faster skiing on telemark gear.
 2. All telemark boots flex at the forefoot for performance of the telemark turn.
 3. Boots come in several styles designed for different types of skiing.
   a. Shorter, lighter plastic boots are used with lighter skis for trekking in the back country.
   b. Higher, stiffer plastic boots are rigid torsionally and provide good lateral control.
     i. Designed for aggressive skiing on heavy skis.
     ii. Often used for lift-served skiing.
   c. Leather and combination leather/plastic boots are still used by some skiers.
     i. These boots are softer and generally lighter than plastic boots.
     ii. Best suited for back-country touring on light skis.
B. Bindings.
 1. Telemark bindings allow the foot to plantar flex and the heel to come up off the ski.
   a. The concept is similar to Nordic (cross-county) ski binding design, but telemark equipment is constructed to withstand the higher forces associated with quick turns and rapid descent.
 2. Telemark bindings use various mechanisms to attach the skis to the boots.

    a. Classic three-pin bindings attach the front of the boot to the ski with pins that fit into pinholes in the boot toe.

      i. Still used with leather boots by some skiers.

      ii. Not strong enough for use with most modern boots and skis.

    b. Cable bindings loop around the back of the boot to attach the entire boot to the binding.

      i. These bindings are stronger and more rigid to control heavier boots and skis and are used by many telemarkers.

      ii. Tension spring bindings expand when flexing the boot.

      iii. Compression spring bindings compress when flexing the boot, and are designed to drive heavy boots and skis.

3. Several models of releasable bindings have been marketed, including releasable bindings that meet German DIN standards.

    a. Releasable bindings are used by < 30% of telemarkers.

    b. The issues that prevent telemarkers from using releasable bindings include concerns with reliability, safety, ease of use, weight, and price.

      i. Releasable bindings released during < 20% of injury events in the Oregon studies.

      ii. It is therefore likely that the skis will remain attached to the skier during a fall.

      iii. No direct correlation between attached skis and types of injury has been made for telemark skiing, although it is likely that there is an increased risk of lower extremity injuries because the ski can act as a lever to twist or bend the leg.

      iv. The free heel may reduce the risk of some lower extremity injuries when the skis remain attached.

      v. The bindings available at the time of the studies were not DIN-certified and the settings were chosen by the user.

        • Newer releasable bindings are certified, but there is no data available yet regarding the use of these bindings and injury rates.

C. Skis.

  1. Modern telemark skis have become wider and resemble alpine skis, but are generally lighter.

  2. Different skis are now made for different types of snow and terrain.

    a. Lightweight touring models.

    b. Wide downhill boards.

      i. Require high plastic boots and substantial bindings to turn them.

    c. All telemark skis are alpine-cambered with metal edges and a large sidecut for turning.

      i. Camber refers to the flex of the ski.

- Alpine-cambered skis distribute weight over the entire ski when flexed.

      ii. Sidecut is the concave arch in the middle of a ski that causes the ski to turn when weighted.

- More sidecut makes the waist of the ski narrower than the tip and tail.

    d. Variations in flex, shape, and width make skis better suited for particular snow conditions and types of use.

D. Skins.

    1. Lengths of plastic or synthetic plush fabric with an adhesive backing that adhere to the bottom of the skis.

    2. The fabric gives traction on steep snow surfaces, allowing skiers to hike up hills on their skis.

BIOMECHANICS AND EXERCISE PHYSIOLOGY

The Telemark Turn

A. The telemark turn is an action unique to the sport. The motion of telemark skiing is a fluid, up-down repetitive activity.

B. As one telemark turn is completed, the back leg slides forward, the opposite knee flexes, and the next turn is initiated.

Lack of Studies

A. No specific studies related to the exercise physiology of telemark skiing have been published.

B. Telemark utilizes a combination of alpine and cross-country skiing techniques, and a great deal of exercise physiology data exists for both of these sports.

    1. For a discussion of alpine skiing exercise physiology principles, see Chapter 5, Alpine Skiing.

    2. For a discussion of cross-country skiing exercise physiology principles, see Chapter 9, Cross-Country Skiing.

MEDICAL ISSUES

General

There are no published reports regarding medical problems commonly encountered in telemark skiing.

Head Injuries

Head injuries may occur from the head striking the snow or a fixed object, or from a collision with another skier.

A. Helmets are infrequently worn by telemarkers.
B. For full discussion of concussion, see Chapter 11, Ice Hockey.

MUSCULOSKELETAL ISSUES

Knee Injuries

A. Reported to occur slightly less frequently and tend to be less severe than those seen in alpine skiing.
    1. The ability of the heel to lift off the ski allows greater freedom of movement of the leg and might afford some protection to the knee.
    2. Leather boots have been proposed to be protective against knee injuries compared to plastic boots, but no correlation between boot type and knee injuries has been noted in the few studies that exist.
B. Injuries to the ACL, MCL, and LCL as well as meniscus tears do occur in telemarkers. For a full discussion of these injuries, see Chapter 5, Alpine Skiing.
C. Patellar fracture.
    1. General.
        a. Not an uncommon injury in telemark skiing.
        b. The telemark position allows the knee to come forward and impact the ski or snow with a forward fall.
    2. Fractures can be treated conservatively if:
        a. Nondisplaced.
        b. Extensor mechanism remains intact.
    3. Conservative treatment includes:
        a. Immobilization.
            i. Extension immobilizer splint.
            ii. Cylinder cast.
        b. Range of motion exercises.
            i. May begin in 3 to 4 weeks, after the fracture has had time to initiate healing.
            ii. Degree of motion is added gradually.
        c. Quadriceps strengthening.
    4. Surgical treatment required when:
        a. Fracture is displaced.
        b. Quadriceps mechanism is not intact.

D. Patellar dislocation.
   1. General.
      a. Most patellar dislocations are lateral in direction.
      b. Often confused with ACL injury based on history.
   2. Mechanism of injury.
      a. May occur in a fall where the tibia is externally rotated relative to the femur.
   3. History.
      a. Knee pain.
         i. Typically anteromedial but may be described as global.
      b. May describe a "pop" at time of injury.
      c. Swelling.
      d. May describe instability.
         i. In many cases, the patella dislocates and spontaneously reduces in the field.
   4. Physical examination.
      a. If still dislocated:
         i. Knee partially flexed.
         ii. Patella visibly located along lateral knee.
      b. If reduction has taken place:
         i. Antalgic gait.
         ii. Effusion.
            • May be significant.
         iii. Apprehension test positive.
            • Supine position with knee in extension or slightly flexed over a pillow.
            • Examiner moves patella in lateral direction.
            • Examination positive if:
               – Patient shows apprehension (indicates a fear or feeling that the kneecap is about to dislocate).
               – Patella dislocates.
         iv. Ligament examination negative.
            • Excursion equal to contralateral knee.
            • Solid end points.
   5. Diagnostic tests.
      a. X-rays should be obtained to rule out fracture.
      b. MRI typically not necessary unless other pathologies are considered.
         i. Ligamentous injury.
         ii. Meniscus injury.
         iii. Occult fracture.
         iv. Chondral fracture.
   6. Treatment.

    a. Patella dislocated:
      i. Check neurovascular status.
      ii. Reduction on the field usually appropriate.
- Explain the procedure to the patient, try to get the patient to relax his/her musculature as much as possible.
- Extend the knee while simultaneously manipulating the patella medially.

    a. Patella reduced:
      i. Knee immobilizer (extension splint).
- Can be discontinued in favor of a patella stabilizer knee sleeve once swelling has subsided.

      ii. Assisted ambulation early on; the athlete may wean the use of crutches as tolerated.
      iii. Ice.
      iv. Elevation.
      v. Medications.
- Analgesics preferred in first 24 to 48 hours.
- NSAIDs.

      vi. Begin active rehabilitation after swelling and pain under good control. This may take several days.
- Active and passive ROME.
- Patella stabilization exercises.
- Balance and proprioception exercises.

Femur Fractures

Femur fractures have been reported. This injury is a result of the high speeds attainable on telemark gear. For description of femur fracture, see Chapter 7, Freestyle Skiing.

Lower Leg and Ankle Injuries

A. Among the most common telemark injuries, ankle injuries appear to be decreasing in recent years, probably because of the increased stiffness of modern boots and bindings.
    1. Made et al. (2001) found that high boots were protective against ankle injuries.
    2. Federiuk et al. (1997) reported that severe ankle injuries were more likely in leather boots compared to plastic.
B. Ankle sprains. For full discussion of ankle sprains, see Chapter 6, Snowboarding.
C. Distal fibula and combined tibia/fibula fractures have been noted but are not common.

Shoulder Injuries

A. Anterior shoulder dislocations can occur when a ski pole gets caught, forcing the arm into external rotation and abduction.
  1. For full discussion of anterior shoulder dislocation, see Chapter 6, Snowboarding.
B. Falls on the shoulder can result in acromioclavicular separations or clavicle fractures in young people or humerus fractures in the older skier.
  1. For full discussion of AC separations, see Chapter 11, Ice Hockey.
  2. For full discussion of clavicle fracture, see Chapter 11, Ice Hockey.
C. Rotator cuff injuries may also occur due to blunt trauma in the older athlete. For discussion of rotator cuff injuries, see Chapter 5, Alpine Skiing.

Wrist and Hand Injuries

A. Fractures of the distal radius occur with falls on the wrist.
  1. For discussion of distal radius fractures, see Chapter 6, Snowboarding.
B. Thumb ulnar collateral ligament (UCL) injuries.
  1. Injuries of the ulnar collateral ligament of the metacarpophalangeal joint of the thumb are common in telemarkers.
     a. The mechanism of injury is forced abduction of the thumb against the ski pole.
     b. For full discussion of UCL injuries, see Chapter 5, Alpine Skiing.

Overuse Injuries

A. There are no studies evaluating overuse injuries in telemark skiers.
B. The telemark turns place great demands on the quadriceps, hamstring, and gluteal muscles, and it is possible that partial muscle tears or tendinopathy may occur from overuse.
  1. Patellofemoral knee pain. For full discussion of patellofemoral knee pain, see Chapter 13, Speed Skating.
  2. Patellar tendonitis/tendinosis
  3. Quadriceps tendonitis/tendinosis.

Axial Injuries

These injuries are not common in telemark skiing.

A. Spine injuries.
  1. Cervical, thoracic, and lumbar muscle strains have all been reported.
B. Trunk injuries.
  1. These injuries are due to blunt trauma.
  2. Chest wall contusions and rib fractures have been reported.

SUMMARY

A. Telemark skiing is a form of skiing practiced primarily in mountainous areas.
B. The sport is enjoying increased popularity in recent years.
C. Injury patterns may be evolving as equipment changes.
  1. Further studies are needed to elucidate the effects of equipment and technique on injury patterns.

Suggested Readings

Federiuk CS, Mann NC. Telemark skiing injuries: Characteristics and risk factors. *Wilderness Environ Med* 1999;10:233–41.

Federiuk CS, Zechnich AD, Vargyas GA. Telemark skiing injuries: A three-year study. *Wilderness Environ Med* 1997;8:204–10.

Jorgsholm P, Bauer M, Ljung BO, Lerner A. Downhill skiing is developing: Snowboard and telemark skiing give new injury patterns. *Lakartidningen* 1991;88:1589–92.

Made C, Borg H, Thelander D, Elmqvist L. Telemark skiing injuries: An 11-year study. *Knee Surg, Sports Traumatol Arthrosc* 2001;9:386–91.

Parker P. *Free Heel Skiing: Telemark and Parallel Techniques for All Conditions.* 3rd ed. Seattle, WA: The Mountaineers; 2001.

Ronning R, Gerner T, Engebretsen L. Risk of injury during alpine and telemark skiing and snowboarding. *Am J Sports Med* 2000;28:506–8.

Tuggy ML. Telemark skiing injuries. *J Sports Med Phys Fitness* 1996;36:217–22.

Tuggy ML, Ong R. Injury risk factors among telemark skiers. *Am J Sports Med.* 2000;28:83–89.

CROSS-COUNTRY SKIING

Janus D. Butcher

INTRODUCTION

History

A. Cross-country skiing is one of the three Nordic skiing disciplines along with ski jumping and Nordic combined (jumping and skiing).

B. Cross-country skiing evolved in Scandinavia as a convenient form of transportation and has evolved into an integral part of Scandinavian and Finnish life.

C. Cross-country skiing had remained relatively unchanged from its remote beginnings until dramatic changes in equipment and technique were introduced over the past 20 years.

D. Currently, two very distinct techniques are used.

    1. The diagonal stride or classic technique.

    2. The ski-skating or freestyle technique.

    3. Most competitors train and race in both the classical and skating techniques.

Competition

A. Historical.

    1. The history of competitive skiing can be traced back to the Norwegian military in the late eighteenth century. Subsequently, civilian ski clubs formed to promote the sport and competition.

    2. The most famous ski race, the Holmenkollen, takes place each March in Oslo, Norway, and traces its roots back to these club competitions in 1879.

B. Elite level competition.

    1. Governing body: The International Ski Federation (FIS) governs international competition. The FIS establishes race rules, schedules, doping control systems, athlete injury surveillance, and most other aspects of World Cup and World Championship racing.

    2. The specific events held at elite competitions are varied in both distance and technique. Formats include: sprint (1 km), sprint relay, middle distance (5 km, 10 km, 15 km), team relay (4 × 5 km, 4 × 10 km), long-distance (30 km, 50 km), classic/skate pursuit, and others.

    3. One unique aspect of elite cross-country skiing is that the athletes frequently compete as both sprinters (1 km) as well as marathon skiers (30 or 50 km) within the same race schedule.

C. Nonelite competition.

    1. In recent years marathon distance races have been organized in all countries of northern, central, and eastern Europe as well as Japan, North America, and Australia.

    2. In the United States a full calendar of local, regional, and national marathon races are scheduled throughout the winter months. The largest of these, the American Birkebeiner, is 52 km long with over 7000 participants.

    3. High school and college cross-country ski teams are common in the Northeast, the upper Midwest, and the western states. These competitions include races of 5 to 15 km in length with both classic stride and skating formats.

Injury Epidemiology and Pathophysiology

A. Overall incidence.

    1. Historically, injury rates of between 0.1 and 5.63 injuries per 1000 skiers were reported. The true incidence is difficult to determine due to lack of confined population.

    2. In the limited data available from more confined circumstances, such as endurance races, the incidence was found to be substantially higher, at 10 to 35 per 1000 skiers.

B. Changing injury patterns.

    1. As the technique and equipment have changed, several equipment–injury relationships have been suggested.

        a. Increased pole length, which accentuates demands on the shoulder and elbow.

    b. Stiffer bindings and rigid boot construction with heel-ski fixation devices, which may increase the risk of ankle and knee injuries.

    c. The equipment–injury relationships are largely anecdotal at this point as few studies have compared injury patterns in the two techniques.

  2. The biomechanics of the new technique are also suggested in the changing injury patterns.

    a. The skating stride places significantly greater demands on the hip adductors and external rotators.

    b. A greater emphasis on upper body strength in the double-poling action has been implicated in increasing upper extremity overuse injuries.

  3. Comparison of techniques.

    a. Initial reports suggested greater incidence of injury in the skating technique. However, this remains unsubstantiated.

    b. Several relationships have been shown.

      i. Low back pain is more common in the classical technique.

      ii. Lower extremity complaints are more common in the skating technique.

      iii. In a recent report of injuries occurring during a long-distance event in which the skating technique was the dominant style used, the injury rate was found to be higher than reported for similar races in the pre-skating period. This report, however, did not specifically compare injuries between the two techniques.

C. Injury distribution.

  1. Studies describing the distribution of musculoskeletal injuries in mass participation events demonstrated that lower extremity injuries are somewhat more common than upper extremity injuries (55% vs. 35%).

  2. The distribution of injuries.

    a. Sprains/twists 40.4%, fractures 27.4%, contusions 16.4%, lacerations 9.3%, dislocations 5.8%, other 0.7%.

    b. The most frequently encountered acute orthopedic complaints include thumb ulnar collateral ligament sprain, knee medial collateral ligament sprain, and plantar fascia strain.

    c. The most common overuse injuries include sacroilliitis, first MTP DJD/synovitis, lateral ankle pain, and wrist tendinitis.

D. Medical problems.

  1. Common medical illnesses reported include exhaustion/dehydration, cold injury, GI symptoms, photokeratitis, and bronchospasm.

BIOMECHANICS

Technique

A. Diagonal (classic) technique.
1. The diagonal stride technique has been used for centuries and remains a popular style for ski touring and back-country skiing.
2. In the diagonal stride, forward propulsion is accomplished through alternating kick and glide actions of the skis (Figure 9-1).
   a. This requires a full stop of the "kick" ski to propel the skier forward.
   b. Backward slip of the planted ski is limited by the application of high-friction kick wax on the cambered portion of the ski surface.
3. The requirement to plant the ski to generate thrust limits the maximum speeds obtainable.
4. In the diagonal stride the poles are used primarily for balance but can contribute up to 30% of forward thrust in higher-level skiers.
5. Double-poling (planting both poles simultaneously) is utilized as increasing tempo limits the effectiveness of the kick and glide action.

B. Skating technique.
1. Developed in the late 1970s, this new technique has rapidly evolved and become the method of choice for most recreational skiers. Skating is the only technique used in both biathlon and Nordic-combined competitions.
2. The skating technique generates forward momentum by driving the skis at an angle to the direction of travel in a motion analogous to speed skating (Figure 9-2).
   a. There is no kick phase and thus no stopping of the ski during the cycle.
   b. Several different strides (V1 skate, V2 skate, marathon skate) are utilized depending on terrain and skier tempo.

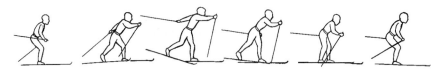

FIGURE 9-1   Diagram of the kick and glide actions of the classic skiing technique. Artwork produced by the Eisenhower Medical Center medical illustration section, Ft. Gordon, Georgia.

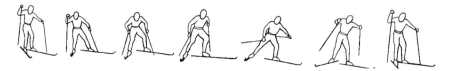

FIGURE 9-2 Diagram shows the skating technique in which propulsive forces are due to the ski pushing out at an angle to the forward motion. Artwork produced by the Eisenhower Medical Center medical illustration section, Ft. Gordon, Georgia.

    3. Double-poling is used in most skating strides to transfer upper body energy to the skiing surface and can provide up to 60% of the forward propulsive force.

C. Biomechanical comparison of the techniques.
    1. Skating is much more energy-efficient than the diagonal stride technique.
    2. In addition, with skating there is no need for a high-friction kick wax, so low-friction glide waxes can be used along the entire surface of the ski.
    3. These factors combined with the use of extremely lightweight construction materials such as carbon fiber and Kevlar as well as improvements in skiing surface preparation have resulted in a 10–30% increase in average speed since the 1950s.

MEDICAL ISSUES

Exercise-Induced Bronchospasm (EIB)

A. Highest incidence found in cross-country skiers.
B. For full discussion of EIB, see Chapter 2, Pulmonary Pathophysiology.
C. Doping control.
    1. Care must be taken to ensure compliance with doping control measures in elite-level skiers.
    2. Most asthma medications are restricted and appropriate procedures for documenting their use are required. Recently, the IOC and FIS have begun requiring documented testing of these athletes prior to the use of asthma medications.
    3. The United States Anti-Doping Agency (USADA) hotline is a useful resource for any questions regarding the use of these medications (1-800-223-0393).

LOWER EXTREMITY MUSCULOSKELETAL ISSUES

Sacroiliitis

A. The sacroiliac joint is a biconcave articulation of the hemipelvis to the sacrum.
  1. It has relatively small rotational motion and functions primarily to transmit force from the lower extremity to the spine.
  2. Sacroiliac dysfunction is the most common cause of low back pain in the cross-country skier.
B. Injury can result from direct trauma associated with a fall, but more commonly arises from repetitive loading. Contributing factors in this injury include:
  1. SI joint hypermobility.
  2. Excessive shear forces.
  3. Relative core strength deficits.
C. History.
  1. Symptoms stem from inflammation in the SI joint, including local pain at the SI joint.
  2. Often have associated lateral hip pain, and pain at the gluteal prominance.
  3. Radicular symptoms are unusual and are associated with piriformis spasm, facet irritation, or concomitant disk disease.
D. Examination.
  1. Tenderness at the SI joint, and relative hypomobility on the affected side with a standing knee-to-chest test.
  2. FABER test (**f**lexion, **ab**duction, and **e**xternal **r**otation) usually elicits symptoms.
    a. With the athlete supine, the hip is abducted with the knee in flexion and the leg externally rotated.
    b. This produces pain in the ipsilateral SI joint.
  3. Neurologic examination is normal.
E. Diagnostic testing.
  1. Radiographs may demonstrate arthrosis or degenerative disease of the lower spine.
  2. MRI is useful if disk disease is suspected.
F. Treatment.
  1. Pain relief strategies include oral analgesics/antiinflammatory medications, manipulation treatment, ice, massage, and stretching.
  2. Long-term management aims at improving SI function through core stabilization and muscle balance training (Theraball program, Pilate's method, or similar).
  3. Technique and equipment issues should also be reviewed.

Piriformis Syndrome

A. Anatomy.
　1. The piriformis muscle originates at the sacrum and inserts into the greater trochanter.
　2. It functions primarily in external rotation of the lower extremity.
　3. The sciatic nerve lies deep in the muscle and may pass through the muscle belly in up to 15% of athletes.
B. Mechanism of injury.
　1. Injury may be acute such as a fall or eccentric muscle overload but is more commonly an overuse injury.
　2. It occurs most frequently in sitting sports (biking, rowing) but may be encountered in any athlete.
　3. Symptoms arise from piriformis muscle spasm, insertional inflammation, or irritation of sciatic nerve.
C. History.
　1. Typically the athlete will complain of an aching pain in the buttocks often associated with sciatica.
　2. Symptoms may subside with skiing but will be worse at rest or with prolonged sitting.
D. Examination.
　1. Marked tenderness over the gluteal prominence.
　2. Pain can be reproduced with:
　　a. Resisted abduction and external rotation of the hip.
　　b. Passive internal rotation of the hip (examined with the patient lying supine and the knee in full extension).
　3. The athlete will have a normal neurologic examination but may have a positive straight leg raise.
E. Diagnostic testing.
　1. Usually none is indicated.
　2. MRI is useful to rule out associated disk disease.
F. Treatment.
　1. The principles of PRICEMM may be useful to alleviate the muscle spasm and inflammation.
　　a. Protection.
　　b. Rest.
　　c. Ice.
　　d. Compression.
　　e. Elevation.
　　f. Medications
　　g. Modalities.
　2. Deep-tissue massage such as Rolfing may be helpful.
　3. Manipulation treatments are also frequently beneficial.

4. Definitive treatment involves physical therapy directed at improving flexibility and correcting any associated underlying SI dysfunction.

Greater Trochanter Bursitis

A. Anatomy.
   1. Trochanteric bursitis results from irritation of any of three bursae overlying the superior margin of the greater trochanter.
   2. These bursae lie between the tensor fascia lata/IT band and the greater trochanter of the femur.
B. Mechanism of injury.
   1. Injury occurs from either direct trauma or chronic overuse in the setting of sacroiliac joint dysfunction.
   2. Associated etiologic factors include:
      a. Tightness in the tensor fascia lata/IT band.
      b. Leg length discrepancy.
      c. Gait anomalies.
      d. Shortened hip abductors or external rotators.
      e. Increased varus angulation of the hip.
      f. Broad pelvic structure.
C. History.
   1. Skiers typically complain of a deep, aching, lateral hip pain that may extend into the buttocks or down into the lateral knee.
   2. The pain is aggravated by activity, local pressure, or stretching, and is often worse at night.
D. Examination.
   1. Palpation over the bony prominence of the greater trochanter and slightly inferiorly or posteriorly elicits tenderness.
   2. Pain is often reproduced with resisted hip abduction and external rotation.
   3. A functional or anatomic leg length discrepancy is common.
   4. Findings of SI dysfunction including tenderness and restricted motion are almost universal.
   5. Ober's test is often helpful.
      a. The patient lies on the unaffected side; both hips and knees are initially flexed.
      b. The affected hip and knee are extended, stressing the soft tissues over the greater trochanter.
      c. This test will demonstrate poor flexibility in the IT band and allow focal palpation of the affected bursa.
E. Diagnostic testing.
   1. Usually none indicated.
   2. Plain radiograph may be useful to evaluate for associated degenerative joint disease.

      a. MRI or three-phase bone scan should be done if there is concern about stress fracture or avascular necrosis.

F. Treatment.

  1. Begins with pain management, usually with antiinflammatory medications, and activity modification to limit symptoms.

  2. The local injection of corticosteroid is often effective in relieving symptoms (see Appendix).

  3. Definitive treatment usually involves rehabilitative exercises aimed at improving flexibility of the illiotibial band, SI function, and hip rotator strength.

  4. A comprehensive core stabilization program designed to improve strength and function of the low back, pelvis, and bilateral lower extremities should accompany this.

  5. Weight loss, conditioning, and proper lifting technique can aid in preventing recurrent or chronic injury.

Patellofemoral Knee Pain

This is also known as patellofemoral dysfunction (PFD) or retropatellar knee pain.

A. This term refers to a painful condition resulting from a wide spectrum of injuries to structures deep in the patella.

  1. Synovium.

  2. Synovial plica.

  3. Articular cartilage.

  4. Bursae.

  5. Other soft tissues of the anterior knee.

B. Pathoetiology.

  1. This is the most common cause of chronic knee pain in the skier.

  2. PFD usually develops as an overuse injury in the setting of knee malalignment.

  3. Etiologic factors in PFD are described as both intrinsic (those related to anatomy, strength, and function) and extrinsic (external factors).

    a. Intrinsic factors include:

      i. Patellar malalignment.

        • Increased Q angle.

        • Patella alta or baja.

        • Lateral patellar tilt.

      ii. Quadriceps muscle imbalance.

      iii. Poor hamstring and quadriceps tendon flexibility.

      iv. Iliotibial band tightness.

      v. VMO hypoplasia.

      vi. Foot biomechanics.

    b. Extrinsic factors include:
      i. Inappropriate ski equipment.
      ii. Precipitous changes in training volume.
      iii. Poor training technique.
C. For full discussion of PFD, see Chapter 13, Speed Skating.

Patellar or Quadriceps Tendinitis

A. Symptoms are due to inflammation of either of the knee extensor tendons, most commonly at the insertion of the inferior pole of the patella.
B. Pathophysiology.
    1. Extensor tendinitis is associated with similar underlying intrinsic and extrinsic factors as found in PFD (as noted above).
    2. More common in classic technique.
C. History.
    1. The athlete complains of anterior knee pain.
    2. Symptoms are typically precipitated by eccentric overload and usually resolve at rest.
    3. Stiffness is common after rest.
D. Physical examination.
    1. Tenderness is localized to the patellar or quadriceps tendon and may be associated with:
      a. Mild swelling.
      b. Erythema.
      c. Warmth.
    2. Malalignment is typically seen.
      a. Increased Q angle.
      b. Lateral patellar tracking.
    3. The posterior muscle/tendon chain and the extensor group are generally tight.
E. Diagnostic testing.
    1. Usually not necessary to make diagnosis.
    2. MRI indicated if disruption of the extensor mechanism is suspected.
F. Treatment.
    1. Directed toward symptom relief initially.
      a. Activity modification.
      b. NSAIDs.
      c. Ice.
      d. Elevation.
    2. Definitive therapy aims at correcting the functional malalignment and tightness through structured physical therapy.

    a. The patient should be advised to continue in alternative, nonpainful activities while in rehabilitation.
  3. Eccentric loading exercise is the cornerstone of treatment for this condition.
  4. Infrapatellar straps have been advocated for symptom relief and may be useful in some individuals.

Iliotibial Band Friction Syndrome (ITBFS)

A. Anatomy.
  1. The illiotibial band (ITB) arises from the tensor fascia lata muscle in the lateral buttocks and runs along the lateral leg.
  2. Inserts at Gerdes tubercle on the anteriolateral tibia.
B. Pathophysiology.
  1. Tightness in the ITB leads to friction irritation at the lateral femoral condyle resulting in inflammation and pain.
    a. When knee extended, ITB is anterior to the lateral femoral condyle.
    b. When knee flexes, the ITB moves to a position posterior to the lateral femoral condyle.
  2. Predisposing factors include:
    a. Genu varum.
    b. Leg length discrepancy.
    c. Excessive foot pronation.
  3. More common with the skating technique.
C. History.
  1. Lateral knee pain that is usually worse with skating or running.
  2. Pain frequently described as aching over the lateral femoral condyle.
D. Physical examination.
  1. Marked tenderness and mild swelling along the distal course of the ITB as it crosses the lateral femoral condyle.
  2. Ober's test (see description above) will usually demonstrate tightness in the ITB.
E. Diagnostic testing.
  1. Generally not indicated.
F. Treatment.
  1. Pain relief and antiinflammatory measures follow the general guidelines of PRICEMM.
  2. Corticosteroid injection is useful for symptom relief (see Appendix).
  3. Physical therapy is directed at improving ITB flexibility through stretching exercise.

4. Treatment should also address any foot biomechanical issues and underlying sacroiliac dysfunction.

Chronic Exertional Anterior Compartment Syndrome

A. Pathophysiology.
   1. Precipitated by exercise-induced swelling of the soft tissue in the confined compartment, which leads to ischemic pain in the affected muscle.
   2. Most common with skating technique whereby the foot is dorsiflexed and everted during ski recovery.
      a. Was prevalent when the technique was first introduced due to the excessive length of the ski and the relatively soft binding used with the classic stride.
      b. As equipment has been developed specifically for the skating technique, this has become less common.
      c. Now most commonly seen with the use of combination equipment (designed for both skating and classic technique) and with poorly fitting equipment.
B. For full discussion of chronic exertional anterior compartment syndrome, see Chapter 13, Speed Skating.
C. Other treatment ideas that may be helpful for the cross-country skier include equipment modifications.
   1. Use a skating-specific boot-binding-ski system.
   2. Use a stiffer binding.
   3. Use shorter skis.

Peroneus Tendon Injury

A. Anatomy.
   1. The peroneus tendons (longus and brevis) travel in a common sheath through the osseous groove at the posterior and inferior aspect of the lateral malleolus. The groove is covered by a retinaculum.
   2. Distal to the osseous groove, the tendons split.
      a. Brevis attaches to the proximal fifth metatarsal.
      b. Longus inserts on the first metatarsal/cuneiform.
B. Pathophysiology.
   1. Injury to the peroneus tendons can occur with an acute inversion/dorsiflexion injury or can develop through repetitive overload that leads to tendinitis.
   2. With an acute injury, the peroneus tendons can be torn or may be subluxed from the fibular groove with disruption of the overlying retinaculum.

3. Acute injuries occur with both classic and skating techniques, whereas chronic tendinitis is usually seen with the skating technique.

C. History.
   1. Acute injuries.
      a. Present with pain, swelling, and bruising along the posterior and inferior fibula.
      b. The athlete often reports a "pop" in association with an appropriate mechanism.
      c. Following the acute phase, a chronic clicking sensation may be present representing subluxation of the peroneal tendon.
   2. Chronic or overuse injury.
      a. Peroneal tendinitis usually presents with pain and swelling along the posterior and inferior fibula.
         i. Pain is worse after skiing and interferes with other activities such as running and walking.

D. Physical examination.
   1. May demonstrate subluxation of the affected peroneus tendon when compared to the contralateral ankle.
   2. The athlete complains of pain with active or resisted eversion of the ankle.
   3. Resisted eversion of the foot produces pain.

E. Diagnostic testing.
   1. In most acute injuries, an ankle X-ray is useful to rule out associated fracture.
   2. In an acute peroneal tear or subluxation, MRI evaluation may be helpful to evaluate the extent of injury.

F. Treatment.
   1. Acute strain injuries without a complete tear.
      a. Immobilization (either casting or CAM walker boot depending on extent of injury).
         i. This is typically continued for 4 to 6 weeks.
      b. After immobilization phase, active rehabilitation is initiated.
         i. Passive stretching.
         ii. Eccentric overload exercises.
   2. Complete tear of the tendon or avulsion of the retinaculum is best managed surgically.
   3. Tendinitis.
      a. Temporary immobilization in a CAM walker may be necessary.
      b. Active rehabilitation incorporating passive stretching and eccentric overload exercise.
      c. Antiinflammatory medications may be helpful for pain management.

    d. Corticosteroid injection may also address the athlete's discomfort.

    e. An ankle brace or taping may allow the athlete to continue active training during the rehabilitation process.

Skier's Toe

A. Anatomy.
    1. Skier's toe is a term frequently used to describe pain in the first MTP joint.
    2. This may represent either an acute injury (turf toe or acute sesamoid injury) or chronic problem (hallux rigidus, MTP synovitis, or sesamoiditis).

B. Pathophysiology.
    1. In skiers, the chronic form stemming from degenerate joint disease and synovitis is most common and is associated almost exclusively with the classic technique.
    2. The mechanism of injury is repetitive extreme extension of the MTP joint.

C. History.
    1. Pain at first MTP joint associated with:
        a. Swelling.
        b. Limited motion.
    2. Symptoms are exacerbated with classic skiing, running, and other activities involving repetitive forced extension of the toe.

D. Physical examination.
    1. Inspection may reveal obvious degenerative changes.
    2. Tenderness and erythema are common.
    3. Pain is exacerbated with passive extension/flexion.

E. Diagnostic testing.
    1. Radiographs will typically demonstrate first MTP degenerative disease.
    2. If a stress fracture or sesamoiditis is suspected, bone scan or limited MRI study may be useful.
    3. Analysis of joint aspirate may demonstrate uric acid crystals if degeneration is due to gouty arthritis.

F. Treatment.
    1. Temporary exclusion of the classic technique will help to alleviate symptoms.
    2. Modifying nonskiing footwear to eliminate flexion with a spring steel insert or rigid orthotic is also beneficial.
        a. Severe cases may require temporary use of a rocker-bottom boot.

3. NSAIDS are often helpful.
4. In cases with substantial degeneration the athlete may benefit from surgical intervention.

UPPER EXTREMITY MUSCULOSKELETAL ISSUES

Rotator Cuff Tendinitis (Tendinosis) and Impingement

A. Relatively uncommon in cross-country skiing.
  1. Most often seen in skiers using excessively long poles, usually with the skating technique.
B. These problems typically arise secondary to functional instability with the forces applied on the glenohumeral joint exceeding the intrinsic strength of the rotator cuff.
C. History.
  1. Athletes complain of an insidious onset of pain as they transition into the ski season.
  2. Pain localized to the anterior or lateral shoulder.
     a. Exacerbated with abduction or forward flexion of the arm.
     b. Pain at night is common.
D. Examination.
  1. Typical findings of impingement:
     a. Hawkins' and/or Neer's test reproduces pain.
     b. Active motion may be restricted due to pain.
  2. Typical findings of rotator cuff tendonitis.
     a. Manual motor testing of the specific rotator cuff component exacerbates the athlete's pain and usually defines the specific muscle/tendon involved.
        i. Abduction in scapular plane ("empty can") tests supraspinatus.
        ii. External rotation tests infraspinatus and teres minor.
        iii. Internal rotation tests subscapularis.
E. Diagnostic tests.
  1. Plain radiographs may demonstrate subacromial spurring or AC joint arthrosis.
  2. MRI arthrogram should be considered if symptoms persist after treatment. This test is ideal for evaluating for cuff tears or labral injuries.
F. Treatment.
  1. Pain management.
     a. Relative rest.
     b. Ice.

    c. Oral NSAIDs.

    d. Corticosteroid injection may also be effective.

  2. Functional rehabilitation to increase stability of the shoulder complex.

    a. Gradual rotator cuff strengthening program encourages healing of the injured tendon and improves intrinsic strength of the rotator cuff.

      i. Therapy should address associated scapulothoracic dysfunction through aggressive upper thoracic strengthening.

      ii. Off-season conditioning should be encouraged to maintain rotator cuff strength and allow a problem-free transition to skiing.

Lateral Epicondylitis

A. This refers to tendonitis (tendinosis) of the origin of the extensor carpi radialis brevis at the lateral epicondyle.

  1. Relatively uncommon but affects skating technique more frequently than classic technique.

  2. This problem was common for a brief time when horizontal pole grips were more widely used.

B. Mechanism of injury usually involves repetitive strain with eccentric overload due to resisted wrist extension.

  1. May also arise with a direct blow to the lateral epicondyle.

  2. May arise from a single macrotraumatic wrist flexion injury (against active wrist extension).

C. History.

  1. The skier complains of lateral elbow pain exacerbated by active extension of the wrist.

    a. This is seen with pole recovery as the athlete lifts the pole forward.

D. Examination.

  1. Tenderness at the lateral elbow.

  2. ROM is usually preserved.

    a. The athlete frequently complains of discomfort with passive flexion of the wrist with the elbow fully extended.

  3. Pain with resisted wrist extension is nearly universal.

E. Diagnostic tests.

  1. Radiographs and other diagnostic tests are generally not indicated.

F. Treatment.

  1. Pain management.

     a. Oral NSAIDs or acetaminophen.
     b. Ice massage.
     c. Physical modalities.
        i. Ultrasound.
        ii. Electrical stimulation.
 2. Rehabilitation.
     a. Home stretching is usually effective.
        i. Elbow extended.
        ii. Passive wrist flexion/forearm supination.
     b. Eccentric strengthening program.
        i. The athlete should be educated on the gradual improvement to be expected with this problem.
     c. Wrist bracing or a counterforce forearm brace may be useful adjuncts to allow the skier to continue skiing.
     d. Corticosteroid injection may be helpful (see Appendix).
     e. Instruction on proper technique to avoid pole overgripping and excessive wrist extension is also important.

DeQuervain's Tenosynovitis

A. The repetitive gripping and ulnar/radial deviation motion associated with double-poling can lead to tendinitis of the extensor pollicis brevis or abductor pollicis longus.
 1. Both tendons occupy the first dorsal wrist compartment and are generally both involved.
B. Symptoms can be insidious in onset or may arise acutely with a traumatic event.
C. Chronic pain is common if untreated.
D. For full discussion of DeQuervain's tenosynovitis, see Chapter 15, Curling.

Intersection Syndrome

A. Intersection syndrome describes a tendinitis/tenosynovitis involving the intersection of extensor pollicis brevis, abductor pollicis longus, and the wrist extensors.
 1. A relatively common complaint early in the ski season as the athlete transitions into skiing.
B. The injury typically arises from repetitive overuse associated with gripping and wrist extension.
C. For full discussion of intersection syndrome, see Chapter 15, Curling.

Extensor Carpi Ulnaris (ECU) Tendinitis

A. Anatomy.
  1. The ECU is contained in the sixth dorsal wrist compartment.
  2. Travels just volar to the ulnar styloid.
  3. Inserts on the dorsal proximal fifth metacarpal.
B. Pathophysiology.
  1. Acute strain.
    a. Resulting from eccentric radial deviation.
  2. Subluxation.
    a. Resulting from hypersupination of the wrist.
  3. Most commonly occurs with a fall forward with the pole planted.
    a. May develop as a result of overuse.
      i. Poor poling technique (tight gripping of the pole).
      ii. Using poles with an inferior pole extension that applies pressure to the ulnar aspect of the wrist.
C. History.
  1. The athlete complains of pain at the ulnar wrist.
    a. Exacerbated by wrist extension or resisted ulnar deviation.
    b. The pain often extends into the ulnar forearm.
  2. Athlete may note swelling along the ulnar wrist and hand.
D. Examination.
  1. Tenderness at the ulnar wrist that extends into the distal forearm.
  2. Pain is reproduced with:
    a. Resisted ulnar deviation.
    b. Passive radial deviation.
    c. Resisted wrist extension.
E. Diagnostic testing.
  1. Plain radiographs are useful in acute injuries to rule out fracture.
  2. MRI arthrogram is often necessary if symptoms persist after treatment, to rule out TFCC tear.
F. Treatment.
  1. PRICEMM.
  2. NSAIDs may be useful for analgesia and swelling.
  3. In acute injuries, a brief period of casting (2–3 weeks) may be helpful.
    a. Protective bracing with the wrist in neutral or slight dorsiflexion is usually indicated.
  4. Physical therapy addresses inflammation and early mobilization.
  5. Surgical treatment is rarely indicated for ECU tendinitis but is frequently required with a TFCC tear.
  6. Corticosteroid injections are useful in the subacute phase to speed the athlete's return to activity (see Appendix).

Skier's Thumb (Ulnar Collateral Ligament Injury)

A. Mechanism of injury.
  1. Injury results from valgus stress to the thumb MCP.
     a. Usually associated with a fall on an outstretched hand resulting in a hyperabduction injury at the MCP and a partial or complete tear of the ulnar collateral ligaments.
B. For full discussion of skier's thumb, see Chapter 5, Alpine Skiing.

Suggested Readings

Anderson SD, Daviskas E. The mechanism of exercise-induced asthma is.... *J Allergy Clin Immunol* 2000 Sep;106(3):453–59.

Beate-Claudia F. Verletzungsrisiko, uberlastungsbeschwerden und prophylaktische Moglichkeiten beim skilanglauf. *Sportverl Sportschad* 1995; 9:103–8.

Bovard R. The new ski-skating poles: A role in fracture risk? *Phys Sport Med* 1994;22:41–47.

Boyle JJ, Johnson RJ, Pope MH. Cross-country ski injuries: A prospective study. *Iowa Orthop J* 1981;1:41–48.

Butcher J, Brannen S. Comparison of injuries in classic and skating Nordic ski techniques. *Clin J Sport Med* 1998 Apr;8(2):88–91.

Carlsen KH, Engh G, Mork M. Exercise-induced bronchoconstriction depends on exercise load. *Respir Med* 2000 Aug;94(8):750–55.

de Bisschop C, Guenard H, Desnot P, Vergeret J. Reduction of exercise-induced asthma in children by short, repeated warm-ups. *Br J Sports Med* 1999 Apr;33(2):100–4.

Dorsen P. Overuse injuries from Nordic ski skating. *Phys Sport Med* 1986; 14:34.

Eggleston PA. Methods of exercise challenge. *J Allergy Clin Immunol* 1984 May;73(5 Pt 2):666–69.

Eriksson K, Nemeth G, Eriksson E. Low back pain in elite cross-country skiers: A retrospective epidemiological study. *Scan J Med Sci Sports* 1996; 6:31–35.

Garcia de la Rubia S, Pajaron-Fernandez MJ, Sanchez-Solis M, et al. Exercise-induced asthma in children: A comparative study of free and treadmill running. *Ann Allergy Asthma Immunol* 1998;80(3):232–36.

Hoffman MD, Clifford PS. Physiological responses to different cross-country skiing techniques on level terrain. *Med Sci Sports Excerc* 1990; 22(6):841–48.

Larsson K, Ohlsen P, Larsson L, Malmberg P, Rydstrom PO, Ulriksen H. High prevalence of asthma in cross-country skiers. *BMJ* 1993 Nov 20;307(6915):1326–29.

Lawson SK, Reid DC, Wiley JP. Anterior compartment pressures in cross-country skiers. *Am J Sports Med* 1992;20:750–53.

Lindsay DM, Meeuwisse WH, Vyse A, Mooney ME, Summersides J. Lumbosacral dysfunction in elite cross-country skiers. *JOSPT* 1993; 18(5):580–85.

Mannix ET, Manfredi F, Farber MO. A comparison of two challenge tests for identifying exercise-induced bronchospasm in figure skaters. *Chest* 1999 Mar;115(3):649–53.

Ogston J, Butcher J. A sports-specific protocol for the diagnosis of exercise-induced asthma. *Clin J Sports Med* 2002;12(5):291–95.

Randolph S, Fraser B, Matasavage C. The free-running athletic screening test as a screening test for exercise-induced asthma in high school. *Allergy Asthma Proc* 1997;18(5):311–12.

Renstrom P, Johnson RJ. Cross-country skiing injuries and biomechanics. *Sports Med* 1989;8(6):346–70.

Rundell KW, Wilber RL, Szmedra L, Jenkinson DM, et al. Exercise-induced asthma screening of elite athletes: Field versus laboratory exercise challenge. *Med Sci Sports Excerc* 2000;32(2):309–16.

Schelkun PH. Cross-country skiing: Ski skating brings speed and new injuries. *Phys Sports Med* 1992;20(2):168–74.

Sherry E, Asquith J. Nordic skiing injuries in Australia. *Med J Australia* 1987; 146:245–46.

Smith GA. Biomechanical analysis of cross-country skiing techniques. *Med Sci Sports Excerc* 1992;24(9):1015–22.

Street GM. Technological advances in cross-country ski equiptment. *Med Sci Sports Excerc* 1992;24(9):1048–54.

Sue-Chu M, Larsson L, Bjermer L. Prevalence of asthma in young cross-country skiers in central Scandinavia: Differences between Norway and Sweden. *Respir Med* 1996 Feb;90(2):99–105.

Vaage and Kristensen, eds. *Holmenkollen: History and Results.* Oslo: De norske Bokklubbene; 1992.

10

BIATHLON

Jim Carrabre
Sami F. Rifat

GENERAL INFORMATION

History

A. The word "biathlon" comes from the Greek prefix "bi" meaning dual and "athlon" meaning contest.

B. Norwegian rock carvings from 4000 years ago of hunters on skis depict the earliest origins of the biathlon.

C. The first modern biathlon took place in 1767 along the Swedish–Norwegian border, between border patrol troops.

D. Initial competitions involved the use of high-powered rifles on shooting ranges of 150 m.

    1. The rifles were generally heavy and ammunition was expensive.

    2. Due to the range of bullet travel, safety was an early concern and therefore events had to be held in rural locations.

    3. Many of the first participants were military personnel who had access to the equipment and ranges.

E. In 1978, international rules changed the rifles from large-caliber to a smaller .22-caliber rifle. This not only improved safety but facilitated access to competition venues and enhanced participation in the sport.

Competitive Biathlon

A. The International Biathlon Union (IBU) is the sport's governing body.

1. An association of the national federations around the world and other organizations representing and interested in the sport of biathlon.
2. The IBU sponsors several competitive events:
   a Biathlon World Championship.
   b. Biathlon World Cup.
   c. Biathlon Continental Championships.
   d. Biathlon Continental Cups.
A. Olympic competition.
   1. Biathlon became an official Winter Olympic sport in 1954, and the first men's Olympic competition took place in 1960 at the Squaw Valley games.
   2. Women's Olympic competition began in 1992 in Albertville, France.
   3. There are currently eight (four men's, four women's) Olympic biathlon events.
      a. Sprint: In the sprint, women race 7.5 km and men race 10 km. The competitors stop twice and shoot five targets with five bullets. The competitor must ski a 150-m penalty loop for each target missed. The top 60 competitors qualify for the pursuit.
      b. Pursuit: In the pursuit, women race 10 km and men race 12.5 km. The competitors start at intervals based on their finishing time in the sprint competition. The contestants stop four times and must hit five targets with five bullets. A 150-m penalty lap is assessed for each target missed.
      c. Individual: In the individual competition, women race 15 km and men race 20 km. The competitors stop four times and must hit five targets with five bullets. A 1-minute penalty is added to their total time for each target missed.
      d. Relay: The relay is a team event covering 30 km. Each team is composed of four members who each race a 7.5-km leg. Each team member stops twice to attempt to hit five targets. Each competitor is allowed three extra bullets for a total of eight. Extra bullets must be loaded one by one. Competitors ski a 150-m penalty lap for each missed target.

EPIDEMIOLOGY

Most injuries and medical conditions in the biathlon have three main causes.

A. Injures associated with the training process.
B. Injuries associated with the environment.
C. Injuries associated with muscle-strength and flexibility deficits.

Injuries Associated with the Training Process

A. These injuries are best understood if the process is broken down into four key areas:
  1. Physiological training.
  2. Psychological training.
  3. Technical training.
  4. Tactical training.
B. Physiological training.
  1. Generally biathletes demonstrate high levels of fitness, often exceeding distance runners and cyclists with Vo_2 max reaching 90 mL/kg/minute in elite males and up to 80 mL/kg/minute in elite females.
  2. To achieve this level of fitness, biathletes devote several hundred hours to training each year.
  3. To maximize training, biathletes, like many other athletes, break down the year into segments in a process called periodization (Figure 10-1).
    a. The training year can be divided into several sequential but interdependent periods known as macrocycles. Each macrocycle can be further divided into mesocycles (monthly training) and microcycles (weekly training).
    b. Training is scheduled this way so as to enhance and focus the conditioning of the athlete toward the next sequential period, eventually achieving a peak in performance during the competitive season.
    c. A periodized year contains at least six mesocycles.
      i. Strength phase.

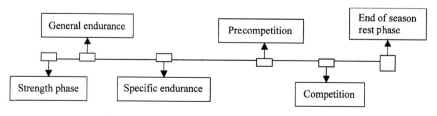

FIGURE 10-1   A periodized (macrocycle) year.

- This phase lasts 6 to 8 weeks.
- The athlete primarily works to correct or improve strength deficits.
- Most injuries sustained during this phase are secondary to improper strength training techniques.

ii. General endurance phase.
- This phase lasts approximately 12 weeks.
- The athlete works to improve fitness with high-volume training. The goal is to improve the athlete's base fitness.
- Cross-training is often employed to meet volume demands. For the biathlete, this training often takes place during the summer, utilizing roller skiing and biking.
- Injuries are usually secondary to overuse during this phase.

iii. Specific endurance training.
- This phase lasts 6 to 12 weeks.
- Training volume increases and becomes sport-specific. The biathlete increases roller skiing and early snow skiing (if available).
- Overuse injury, particularly when the biathlete returns to the snow, can occur.

iv. Precompetition phase.
- This phase lasts about 4 weeks.
- Total training hours are gradually decreased, but the percentage of high-intensity training increases.
- The goal of this phase is to build up in order to peak in the competition phase.
- The high-intensity training of this phase often predisposes the athlete to viral illness. Proper rest and nutrition are essential during this phase.

v. Competition phase.
- This phase usually lasts 8 to 12 weeks.
- The training loads are at their lowest of the year (except the rest phase).
- The athlete remains fit by competing.
- Physical and emotional stress are high and may lead to mood disorder.

vi. Rest phase.
- This phase is often very short, lasting only a few weeks.
- The focus is on recovery.

- The athletes typically go on a holiday, perform any equipment modifications, and train for fun (e.g., fun runs, hiking, etc).
- New injuries are unlikely in this phase but rehabilitation from the season can be ongoing.

SPECIAL CONCERNS IN BIATHLON

The Rifle

A. Rifle safety.
  1. Rifle safety has always been a high priority for biathlon.
  2. The risk of accidental shooting is exceedingly low. The rules of the sport have been designed to maximize safety.
     a. Athletes can remove the rifle only when at their range position.
     b. Rifles can be loaded only when pointed down range.
     c. The rifle is never loaded when skiing.
     d. Most athletes travel with their rifle bolts separate from the rifle, so the rifle cannot be used if stolen.
B. Rifle carrying position.
  1. Biathlon is a closed kinetic chain activity in which the rifle is carried on the back.
  2. The added weight of the rifle places greater stress on the kinetic chain.
  3. This carrying position also raises the athlete's center of gravity and subsequently leads to a greater risk of injury primarily because of an increased risk of falling.

The Skate Ski Technique

A. The differences between the traditional and skate ski techniques are discussed in Chapter 9, Cross-Country Skiing.
B. Although most biathletes are proficient in both of these techniques, biathlon races exclusively use the skate technique.
C. The skate technique places greater demand on the athlete's core strength conditioning.
  1. Core strength refers to the strength of the central musculature of the abdomen, back, hips, pelvis, and buttocks.
  2. In biathletes, although not technically correct, the ankle also may be thought of as one of the "core" muscle groups (particularly the peronei and ankle dorsiflexors).

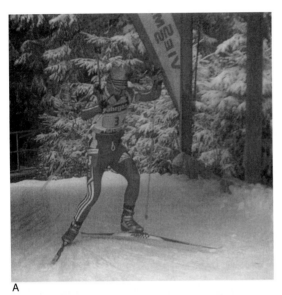

A

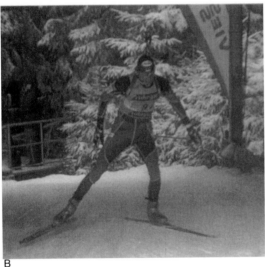

B

FIGURE 10-2
Inadequate core conditioning can lead to mechanically inefficient skating technique (a). When the skier maintains correct alignment of ski, leg, and torso (b), efficiency is maximized. Photo courtesy of Jim Carrabre, MD.

D. Without adequate core conditioning, mechanically efficient skating motion is impossible.
1. Core weaknesses manifest as a rotation of the body from the pelvis upward around the fixed gliding ski leg.
2. This appears as if the knee actually rotates inward (Figure 10-2a).
3. The resulting loss of biomechanical alignment over the gliding ski leads to decreased glide, loss of ski speed, and suboptimal performance.

4. When the athlete can maintain correct alignment of ski, leg, and torso (Figure 10-2b), efficiency is maximized.
5. It is important for the practitioner to recognize this common biomechanical problem, as it often predisposes to injury.
B. Addressing the problem.
1. Coaches need to address and correct technique.
2. Core muscle weakness may be corrected with an intense course of training or physical therapy.

Doping

A. General doping issues are discussed in Chapter 4, Doping.
B. In biathlon, the IBU is active in the fight against doping.
1. A multinational committee of five physicians monitor and test athletes both in and out of competition.
2. Biathlon follows the World Anti-Doping Agency (WADA) anti-doping list and code.
C. Beta-blockers.
1. Biathlon does not ban beta-blockers, contrary to all other shooting sports.
2. In biathlon, the negative performance effect of beta-blockers would more than offset any potential gain in shooting accuracy.

Ski Wax Safety

A. The Nordic sports have witnessed many technical advances since the 1980s, but the most important has been the introduction of fluorocarbon-based ski waxes.
1. These waxes have a much lower coefficient of surface friction, thereby greatly increasing ski speed.
2. This technology is similar to that used in nonstick cookware.
3. Fluorocarbon waxes are not unique to Nordic ski events like biathlon; they are also used in the alpine disciplines, sailing sports, and other sports where friction-reducing waxes are of benefit.
B. Fluorocarbon-based products are potentially toxic.
1. Many skiers are unaware of the potential danger.
2. The problem arises when waxes are heated above 300°C and start to smoke.
   a. When this happens, the fluoropolymers are released into the air as free fluorine.
   b. Since they are less than 2 microns in diameter, they reach the alveoli in the lung periphery.

    c. Here they combine with water to form hydrofluoric acid (HF).

    d. The resultant reaction can range from coughing to full-blown adult respiratory distress syndrome (ARDS).

C. Prevention of injury.

    1. Waxing should always been done in well-ventilated areas.

    2. Properly fitting, well-maintained respirators with adequate filter media should be worn.

    3. The Medical Committee of the IBU has developed a wax-room ventilation system that will be offered to all sites hosting IBU-sanctioned events.

    4. Although we are uncertain of the long-term effect of hydrocarbon and fluorocarbon wax exposure, preliminary sporadic reports in the emergency medicine literature agree with the fluorocarbon industry reports that it is not benign.

MEDICAL ISSUES

Cold-Weather Inhalation Injury

A. Inhalation of extremely cold air can cause injury to the lungs. A complete discussion of pulmonary pathophysiology in the cold-weather athlete is found in Chapter 2, Pulmonary Pathophysiology.

B. IBU rules specify that no competition can take place under –20°C; consequently, thermal lung injuries in competition are rare.

Cold-Weather Corneal Injury

A. General considerations.

    1. Prolonged cold exposure can freeze the superficial layers of the cornea, leading to edema and focal pain.

    2. This is more likely to occur during long technical descents when the athlete always keeps his or her eyes open.

    3. The risk of this injury is increased when the ambient temperature is below –20°C.

B. Diagnosis.

    1. The signs and symptoms are similar to corneal abrasion (see Chapter 11, Ice Hockey).

    2. The athlete may complain of pain, blurred vision, and foreign body sensation.

C. Management.

    1. Corneal cold injury is treated much like a corneal abrasion, with corneal protection and topical antibiotics.

2. The injured cornea(s) tend to be light-sensitive and increased tearing is present. Symptoms tend to clear in 1 to 2 days with no sequelae.
3. In a biathlete, however, the ensuing blurring of vision could mean a competition missed or training opportunities canceled.
4. Prevention.
   a. Athletes should be counseled to blink often in subzero temperatures, especially on long technical downhill descents.
   b. Eye protection should be encouraged. Several manufacturers now produce sport goggles that ventilate well (therefore, do not fog) and protect the athletes' eyes from injury.

Snow Blindness (Ultraviolet Keratitis)

A. General considerations.
   1. Prolonged exposure to reflective light can lead to corneal damage similar to sunburn.
   2. The damage is caused by ultraviolet (UV) light.
   3. It is especially a problem at high altitudes and in the polar regions.
   4. Although not a typical finding in biathlon, athletes training on glaciers for long periods are at risk for developing this problem.
B. Diagnosis.
   1. The athlete has a history of exposure to ultraviolet light without adequate protection.
   2. The athlete often complains of pain.
   3. A foreign body sensation (grittiness) is often reported.
   4. Blurred vision.
   5. Photophobia.
   6. Corneal injection.
   7. Rarely corneal opacification.
C. Treatment.
   1. First aid.
      a. Prevent further UV exposure.
      b. Patch eye.
   2. Refer for emergent clinical evaluation.
   3. Like most injuries caused by exposure, prevention is key. The athlete should use eyewear with UV protection whenever training conditions necessitate.

Depression

A. General considerations.
1. Depression is a principal disorder of affect and mood.
2. Though generally thought to be rare in elite endurance athletes, depression may occur in active individuals of all ages and levels.
3. More common at the end of the season, particularly if the season's goals have not been met.
4. Also may occur when athletes leave their sport or retire.
5. Team physicians need to be aware of the warning signs of depression and be ready to initiate treatment and/or make appropriate referral.

B. Diagnosis.
1. Insidious onset of dysphoric (depressed) mood.
2. Symptoms of: loss of pleasure, suicidal thoughts, appetite loss, sleep disturbance, lack of energy, and feelings of guilt.
3. In children, somatic symptoms and psychomotor agitation are more common.
4. In adolescents, one sees more frequent anorexia, weight loss, excessive sleepiness, and hopelessness.

C. Management.
1. Referral to a mental health practitioner is often warranted.
2. Psychotherapy.
3. Antidepressant medication.
4. Combination treatment of pharmacotherapy and psychotherapy often produces the quickest improvement in symptoms.

Overtraining Syndrome

A. General considerations.
1. Overtraining, sometimes referred to as "staleness," is a poorly understood condition in which the athlete's training program exceeds the body's ability to adapt.
2. Overtraining in athletes is common.
3. It is seen more often in those earlier in their careers who have yet to learn their training limits.
4. It is also seen in athletes rebounding from an injury, eager to "make up lost time."

B. Diagnosis.
1. Clinical indicators include both physiological and psychological parameters.
2. Psychological indicators.
   a. Fatigue.
   b. Increased irritability.

    c. Decreased training and competition motivation.

    d. Lack of concentration.

    e. Loss of confidence.

    f. Poor sleep.

    g. Poor appetite.

    h. Overt depression.

3. Physiological indicators.

    a. Increased resting heart rate (more than 10 beats over baseline).

    b. Weight loss.

    c. Postural hypotension.

    d. Delay in heart rate recovery after exercise.

    e. Frequent illnesses (usually respiratory).

    f. Nagging musculoskeletal injuries.

        i. Muscle soreness.

        ii. "Heavy" legs.

    g. Excessive thirst.

    h. Breakdown in technique (skiing or shooting in the biathlete).

4. Laboratory evaluation.

    a. Diagnosis is usually clinical but some laboratory abnormalities may exist.

    b. Elevated CPK levels indicating excessive muscle breakdown.

    c. Decreased testosterone levels.

    d. Increased cortisol.

    e. Decreased testosterone to cortisol ratio may indicate anabolic/catabolic imbalance and warn of overtraining.

5. Management.

    a. Prevention.

        i. Proper coaching and training techniques can prevent overtraining syndrome from occurring.

        ii. Training should be individualized and balanced.

    b. Treatment.

        i. Short periods of active relative rest, from a few weeks to several months.

          • Performance may actually improve in overtrained athletes after a period of rest.

          • Length of rest period depends on the severity of the condition.

        ii. Absolute rest may be required in severe cases.

    c. Early indicators of recovery usually are represented by normalization of personality (not irritable), restful sleep, and improved motivation.

Acute Upper Respiratory Infection

A. General considerations.
   1. Common in all athletes.
   2. Often manifests during physically and emotionally stressful periods.
   3. Viral etiology.
B. Diagnosis.
   1. Fever.
   2. Chills.
   3. Myalgias.
   4. Cough.
   5. Nasal congestion.
   6. Sore throat.
   7. Fatigue.
C. Management.
   1. Supportive treatment.
      a. Rest.
      b. Fluids.
      c. Analgesics.
      d. Decongestants, but use caution not to prescribe or advise a banned substance.
   2. Prevention.
      a. Frequent hand washing.
      b. Rest.
      c. Adequate nutrition.
   3. Return to play.
      a. Afebrile.
         i. It is not recommended that athletes participate if fever > 38°C (100.4°F).
         ii. Myocarditis secondary to viral illness may lead to heart failure and has been reported to cause sudden death.
      b. Improvement/resolution of myalgias.
      c. Some mild viral illnesses may cause a delay in return to normal performance.
D. Mononucleosis: For full discussion, see Chapter 11, Ice Hockey.

TRAUMATIC INJURY

Abrasions (Road Rash)

A. General considerations.
   1. Traumatic injury to the skin in which the top layer(s) is (are) removed.

    2. In the winter sport athlete, usually occurs secondary to a fall on the ice.
B. Diagnosis.
    1. History of trauma.
    2. Painful wound with serous exudates.
    3. Signs of infection (erythema, redness) may be present.
C. Management.
    1. The wound needs to be cleaned and any foreign body removed.
    2. Nonviable tissue should be debrided.
    3. Topical or oral antibiotics (for gram-positive coverage) would be appropriate for deep or especially dirty wounds.

Metatarsal Stress Fracture

A. General considerations.
    1. A stress fracture is a focal structural weakness that results from bone remodeling as a consequence of repeated stress.
    2. Mechanism.
        a. Stress from activity invokes bony remodeling.
        b. If the osteoclastic activity (bone breakdown) exceeds osteoblastic activity (new bone formation), microfracture(s) develop.
        c. If stress continues, the microfracture propagates and a symptomatic stress fracture develops.
    3. Originally described in military recruits.
    4. The tibia is the most common site of stress fracture in runners; however in biathletes and cross-country skiers, the metatarsal bones are most commonly injured.
        a. The second metatarsal is most commonly affected, followed by the third and the fourth.
        b. Fifth-metatarsal stress fractures can also occur and are generally more complicated lesions.
        c. First-metatarsal stress fractures rarely occur.
    5. Changes in training frequency, intensity, duration, or combinations of the above predispose to injury.
    6. In the winter athlete, changes in weather predispose to injury.
        a. In temperatures above freezing (particularly in new snow conditions) and in temperatures below $-20°C$ (particularly in old snow conditions), the ability of the ski to glide greatly diminishes.
        b. This forces athletes to get up higher on their toes during the push-off phase.
        c. This action places greater stress on the metatarsals and predisposes them to stress injury.

B. Diagnosis.
   1. History of activity or change in activity.
   2. Pain relieved by rest.
   3. Localized pain, worse with weight bearing.
   4. Swelling sometimes present.
   5. Point tenderness.
   6. Pain with percussion or tuning fork testing.
   7. X-rays.
      a. Often initial films are negative.
      b. Only half ever show radiographic changes.
      c. When present, periosteal elevation and cortical thickening are signs of stress injury.
      d. Specific, but not sensitive for stress fracture.
   8. Bone scan.
      a. "Gold standard."
      b. Very sensitive.
      c. Not always clinically useful.
   9. Magnetic resonance imaging (MRI).
      a. Able to detect many stress injuries.
      b. No radiation exposure.
      c. Usually more expensive.
C. Management.
   1. Second through fourth metatarsals are generally treated conservatively.
      a. Relative rest.
         i. Initially may need supportive measures such as crutches and/or post-op shoe.
         ii. Cessation of weight-bearing activity.
      b. Ice.
      c. Analgesics.
      d. Analyze technique/training program, and correct as needed.
      e. Gradual return to activity as symptoms allow.
   2. Fifth-metatarsal stress fracture (Jones fracture).
      a. Stress fracture of the proximal metatarsal shaft.
      b. High rate of delayed union or nonunion with conservative treatment.
      c. Nonoperative treatment.
         i. Non-weight-bearing cast immobilization until symptoms resolve (2–3 weeks).
         ii. Then may begin weight bearing in cast (i.e., walking cast) if symptoms allow.
         iii. A total of 6 to 12 weeks of immobilization is often necessary.

    d. Operative treatment.
        i. Initial surgical fixation with an intermedullary screw may allow earlier return to sport.
        ii. Necessary for those with delayed or nonunion fractures.

Low Back Injury

A. Lumbar strain.
    1. General considerations.
        a. Acute nonradiating back pain of muscular origin.
        b. Cause.
            i. Trauma.
            ii. Overuse.
            iii. Often no known precipitating event.
    2. Diagnosis.
        a. Local low back pain.
        b. Usually limited range of motion.
        c. Neurological examination is normal.
    3. Management.
        a. Activity as tolerated.
        b. Ice/ice massage.
        c. Analgesics or antiinflammatories.
            i. Avoid long-term use of narcotic medications if possible.
        d. Short-term (1 week) use of muscle relaxants if muscle spasm is evident.
        e. Rehabilitation.
            i. Cornerstone of treatment.
            ii. Improve flexibility.
            iii. Address core strength deficiency.
        f. Return to activity as symptoms allow.
B. Sacroiliac sprain.
    1. General considerations.
        a. The sacroiliac (SI) joints are sturdy joints with limited movement.
        b. The SI joints are lined with a synovial membrane and are held together with strong ligaments.
        c. The rotational movement of the pelvis on the leg during the skating motion creates shear forces on the SI joint that can lead to injury.
        d. The added weight of the rifle contributes to this problem.
    2. Diagnosis.
        a. A history of trauma is sometimes present.
        b. Pain usually unilateral, localized to the SI joint.

      c. Tenderness over the SI joint.

      d. FABER test may produce pain.

      e. Gaenslen's test usually produces pain.

      f. Neurological examination is usually normal.

      g. X-rays usually normal.

  3. Management.

      a. Relative rest.

      b. Ice.

      c. Analgesics/antiinflammatory medication.

      d. Radiographic guided injection.

      e. Return to activity as symptoms allow.

Suggested Readings

Guide to the Safe Handling of Fluoropolymer Resins. 3rd ed. Washington, DC: The Society of the Plastics Industries, Inc.; 1998.

Koutedakis Y, Budgett R, Faulmann L. Rest in underperforming elite competitors. *Br J Sports Med* 1990;24(4):248–52.

Niinimaa, VM. *Double Contest Biathlon: History and Development*. Manitoba: DW Friesen; 1998.

www.biathloncanada.com

www.biathlonworld.com

www.fasttechnologies.com

www.IOC.org

www.skinnyski.com

www.Usbiathlon.com

www.WADA.org

11

ICE HOCKEY

James L. Moeller
Michael R. Bracko

GENERAL INFORMATION

History

A. Ice hockey appears to have evolved from hurling, an Irish field game played with sticks and a ball.

   1. Early 1800s: Hockey-like game played by the Micmac Indians in Nova Scotia, Canada. This game was played with a "hurley" (stick) and a square wooden block. "Hoquet" means "shepherd's stick" in French.

   2. British soldiers and Irish immigrants spread the game throughout Canada in the early 1800s.

B. Game moved from frozen fields to frozen ponds at King's College in Windsor, Nova Scotia. There were no skates and no goalies, and teams consisted of 30 to 50 players per side on the pond at the same time.

C. 1870: James Creighton introduces game to Montreal, Quebec, Canada.

   1. First organized game played on an enclosed rink, on skates, nine players per side.

   2. "Halifax Rules" written.

D. 1885: First organized league started in Kingston, Ontario. It consisted of four teams.

E. 1892:

   1. Lord Stanley of Preston, the governor general of Canada, donates a silver bowl to be awarded to the best amateur hockey team in Canada.

   2. The first organized women's game was played in 1892.
F. Hockey and the Olympic Games.
   1. 1920: First men's Olympic ice hockey tournament.
   2. 1998: Women's ice hockey debuts as a medal sport.

Injury Statistics

A. There are many studies reporting on injury rates in ice hockey, though comparing studies is difficult due to lack of consistency regarding many factors such as the definition of injury, calculation of incidence (injuries per season vs. injuries per player exposures vs. injuries per hours played, etc.). There are, however, noticeable trends among the various reports.
   1. Age group and level of play differences exist, and these will be explored in Competitive Categories in Ice Hockey.
   2. The general trends noted in studies of male ice hockey players are also noted in studies of female players.
B. Level of play: Injury incidence increases as level of play increases, right up to the professional level.
C. Game versus practice: Injury rates are significantly higher in game situations compared to practice.
   1. In most reports ~ 90% of injuries take place during games.
   2. Injuries are 20–25 times more likely to occur during a game.
D. Timing.
   1. Games: Injuries are most likely to occur during the third period (over 40%) compared to the second (30–35%) and first (20–25%) periods.
   2. Practice: Injuries are more likely to occur during early-season practices compared to mid- and late-season sessions.
E. Type of injury: Sprains and strains (listed as a single injury type in most studies) are the most common injury type encountered.
F. Cause of injury: Contact (with the boards, ice, pucks, or sticks) and collision with another player are consistently the most common causes of injury in ice hockey at all levels of play.

Competitive Categories in Ice Hockey

A. Youth hockey is divided by age.
   1. Injury is fairly uncommon at the younger age levels including Mite (age 7–8 years), Squirt (age 9–10), and Pee Wee (age 11–12).
      a. Helmet with full facial protection is required for all practices and game situations.

      b. Body checking not allowed in most countries until the Pee Wee level.

  2. Injury incidence begins to increase at the Bantam (age 13–14) and Midget (age 15–16) levels.

      a. Helmet with full facial protection is required for all practices and game situations.

      b. Body checking allowed unless otherwise specified by individual league rules.

  3. Junior (16- to 20-year-olds).

      a. Play under the same rules as professional leagues.

      b. Different leagues have different rules regarding the use of head/facial protection. All leagues require helmet use with either a half-shield or full facial protection.

         i. Injury rates of up to 96.1 injuries/1000 player game hours (nearly 25 times higher than the 3.9/1000 player practice hours).

         ii. Facial injuries are very common, particularly in leagues that do not require full facial protection.

         iii. Acromioclavicular sprains are the most common musculoskeletal injury encountered.

  4. Fair-play rules have been advocated in an attempt to reduce injury rates in youth hockey.

      a. Points are added to final standings of teams that are penalized below a preestablished limit of team penalties per game.

      b. Points are subtracted from final standings for teams that are penalized above the same preestablished limit.

      c. Fair-play rules have been shown to decrease total penalty minutes and number of injuries in youth ice hockey tournaments where both sets of rules were used (fair-play rules in preliminary rounds, standard rules in play-offs).

         i. 136 injuries/1000 player game hours in standard rules play.

         ii. 51.4 injuries/1000 player game hours under fair-play rules.

B. Interscholastic programs have not been as widely studied as youth programs, but injury statistics are similar.

  1. High school injury statistics are similar to Midget level statistics.

  2. Collegiate ice hockey injury statistics are similar to those seen in Junior leagues that require full facial protection.

C. Adult leagues.

  1. In most adult leagues, some type of facial protection is mandatory.

  2. Leagues for older players (> 30 years) are usually "no check" leagues.

3. Injury rates are similar to those seen in Bantam and Midget ages (12/1000 player game hours).

    a. Head and facial injury rates higher than in youth hockey due to the option of half-shield facial protection.

    b. Sprains and strains are still the most common type of injury.

    c. Contact/collision is the main mechanism of injury even in the "no check" leagues.

D. Professional.

  1. The highest level of North American professional hockey is the National Hockey League (NHL). In Europe there are several professional or "elite" leagues.

    a. North American players believed to be more violent than European players.

    b. In the 1995–96 season, North American–born NHL players (80.5% of the players) accounted for a significantly higher proportion of penalty minutes than the European-born players (86.4% vs. 13.6%).

      i. This study did not account for the violent nature of the penalties (e.g., slashing is more violent than tripping, spearing is more violent than hooking, etc.).

  2. NHL.

    a. Injury rates of up to 129/1000 player game hours have been reported.

      i. 89% of injuries occur during game situations.

    b. Strains and sprains are the major injury types (25% and 20%, respectively).

      i. Knee ligament sprains are the main cause of missed games.

      ii. AC separations are the most common shoulder injury.

      iii. Strains of the groin, hip flexors, and thigh musculature are very common, but often do not lead to missed time.

  3. European elite leagues.

    a. Injury rates of 46.8–83/1000 player game hours have been reported.

      i. 75–80% of injuries occur in second and third periods.

    b. Lower extremity, particularly knee, injuries are more common than upper extremity and head injuries.

Special Considerations and Demographics

A. Ice rink conditions may not be optimal for the health and performance of the skater due to cold temperatures, poor ventilation, and potentially poor air quality.

1. For a complete discussion of cold injury and cold-weather cardiac and pulmonary physiology, see Chapters 1 to 3.
2. Carbon monoxide (CO) and nitrogen dioxide (NO_2) exposure produced by the ice resurfacing machine.
   a. Symptoms of CO poisoning include: headache, nausea, vomiting, weakness, tachypnea, and incoordination.
   b. Symptoms of NO_2 poisoning include: cough, hemoptysis, dyspnea, chest pain, sweating, nausea, dehydration, weakness, and anxiety.

BIOMECHANICS AND PHYSIOLOGY

Introduction

A. "Hockey is uniquely stressful in ways scientists don't really understand. The heat and humidity of the protective gear, the high level of coordination required, the repeated demands made on the muscles with little rest and the 'astounding' requirement that it's played while balancing on skate blades are all factors in fatigue." (personal communication, January 17, 2003, Oral, Howie Green, PhD, University of Waterloo, Canada).
B. There are many factors to consider when trying to understand the physiology of ice hockey:
   1. The "shift": Time when a player is on the ice competing.
      a. An individual shift lasts 30–90 seconds.
         i. The length of a shift depends on age level, skill level, conditioning, game/team strategy, and whether a player is a high or low point scorer.
         ii. Shifts are repeated 3–8 times during a 20-minute playing period.
            • Each game consists of three periods.
            • Periods last from 10 to 20 minutes depending on the level of play.
         iii. Some shifts are more strenuous than others. Some shifts have micro-breaks for rest either when a whistle is blown to stop play, or when the game strategy does not cause the player to have a high-intensity work load.
      b. Rest between shifts is passive, and lasts between 30 seconds and 5 minutes.
      c. Rest between periods ranges from 3 to 20 minutes depending on the level of play.
   2. The equipment, especially the helmet, retains heat.

3. Environment.
   a. Hockey arenas can be hot and humid.
   b. Pollutants in the air such as CO, NO_2, sulphur dioxide, and mold.
4. Individual player factors.
   a. Fitness level of the hockey player.
   b. Position of the hockey player.
      i. Defensemen do not have as high a workload during a shift as forwards.
         • Defensemen shifts are considered aerobic.
         • The shift of a forward is considered anaerobic.
      ii. Goalies are on the ice for the entire game (unless they are replaced by the backup goalie). Their physiologic demands are different from those of defensemen and forwards, yet have not been studied in depth.
   c. High point scorers versus low point scorers:
      i. High point scorers spend up to 20 seconds longer per shift on the ice than low point scorers.
         • Translates to 42.2 more minutes on the ice over a sample of 12 games (and 17 more shifts over 12 games).
         • It is hypothesized that high point scorers could be considered aerobic players since they stay on the ice longer than their low point anaerobic teammates.
C. Hockey is characterized by repeated low-, medium-, and high-intensity skating, gliding on two feet, and body contact.
   1. Ice hockey is considered a high-static, high-dynamic demand activity.
   2. Upper body movements such as shooting, passing, puck handling, and contact with other players are combined with static and dynamic contractions of the legs.

Anaerobic Demands

A. Anaerobic demands are a result of short-duration, high-intensity shifts on the ice, especially for forwards.
B. The main source of energy during play is anaerobic metabolism. Because of the near-maximal effort on the ice, hockey players must limit the length of a shift to avoid fatigue.
C. It has been speculated that anaerobic glycolysis and the ATP-PC energy systems account for 69% of the energy demand of ice hockey.
   1. The ATP-PC energy system is important in hockey because during a shift, a player has short (1–3 seconds) bouts of maximal effort through high-intensity skating and body contact.

    a. Glycolysis is important because a hockey player can be on the ice, using high-intensity muscle contractions, for upward of 60 seconds.

    b. After a shift, muscle fatigue is due, in large part, to muscle phosphagen depletion and lactate/H^+ ion accumulation.

D. When comparing elite to nonelite female hockey players, two of the distinguishing factors of elite players are the ability to perform a repeat sprint skate test faster than nonelite players, and predicted anaerobic capacity.

    1. When investigating the off-ice fitness variables that predict skating performance, 40-yard dash time, a measure of anaerobic power, was found to be the strongest predictor of skating speed in female hockey players 8 to 16 years old.

Aerobic Demands

A. It can be argued which is more important in hockey: the training that is done to prepare a hockey player for his or her performance on the ice, or the training for recovery during rest to prepare for the next shift.

B. It has been speculated that 31% of the energy demand in ice hockey is provided by oxidative phosphorylation.

C. The main source of energy between shifts and between periods is the aerobic system.

    1. The ability to replenish energy stores during rest after a shift is important for repeated high-performance efforts during the game. The recovery process involves the resynthesis of ATP-PC.

    2. The efficient resynthesis of ATP-PC relies on the oxidative energy system.

Recovery between Shifts

A. Traditionally, hockey players spend the entire recovery phase between shifts sitting on the bench in passive recovery.

B. Early research with hockey players and other athletes found active recovery superior to passive recovery to facilitate lactate removal, while other studies found the opposite. More recent research found no difference between active and passive recovery on lactate concentration and subsequent performance in repeated on-ice work bouts.

    1. The only drawback to this study is that the work-to-rest ratio did not simulate actual gamelike time motion analysis.

2. It is hypothesized that active recovery leads to a reduced blood lactate level; therefore, subsequent performance in the next work bout would be expected to be enhanced when compared to a passive recovery. However, no performance enhancement was noted even when there were statistically significant decreases in blood lactate concentrations.

C. Another study has shown that athletes who sit on a bench after warming up (passive rest) demonstrate increased spine stiffness (back extension and lateral flexion) compared to active rest situations.

1. It is suggested that spine stiffness may be linked not only to poor low back health but possibly to decreased performance as well.

2. Sitting in a flexed spine position (the posture hockey players assume on the bench) is not only linked to disk herniation and other injury mechanisms, but is contraindicated for athletes with back problems.

Lactate Removal after Games and Practices

A. It has become the practice in professional and elite hockey for players to participate in what is referred to as a "flush ride" on a stationary bike after games, in the attempt to clear lactic acid quicker.

1. The theory behind such rides, as described by some team coaches and strength and conditioning coaches, is that clearance of lactic acid will enhance recovery, prevent muscle soreness, and prepare players for the next game or practice.

   a. Post-game active recovery is based on anecdotal evidence and needs further research to be justified.

2. It is important that the "flush ride" be below 55% of the player's maximal capacity for aerobic metabolism because blood lactate accumulates and increases at exercise intensities above this percentage.

3. Players must also be careful that the "flush ride" does not promote further dehydration, weight loss, glycogen depletion, and general fatigue.

B. Elimination of lactate from the blood has a half-life of 15 minutes during passive recovery; therefore, lactate is eliminated from the blood even if a player is at rest after a game.

1. Players are never totally at rest after games because they are active as they remove their equipment, move through the dressing room to a shower, and put their clothes on.

C. It has been shown that the production of lactic acid does not cause delayed onset muscle soreness (DOMS). Prevention of DOMS is more of an issue of muscle fitness and muscle activity.

D. It may behoove players to prepare for their next game by hydrating and replenishing glycogen stores instead of exercising after a game.

Muscle Fitness Requirements

Hockey players need a combination of muscle strength, hypertrophy, power, and endurance.

A. Muscle strength is important at all levels of play.
  1. Youth hockey.
    a. Players need strength to generate force for skating, maintaining balance, body contact, and handling the puck.
    b. Although body checking is not allowed at very young and young ages (generally speaking, body checking is allowed starting at ages 12 to 13, depending on regional area of North America), there is body contact.
      i. After ages 12 to 13, when body checking is allowed, muscle strength takes on added importance.
      ii. The ability to give and receive a body check is in large part due to motor coordination, skill acquisition, emotional self-esteem, skating ability, and muscle strength.
    c. All organized hockey, regardless of age, gender, or skill level, uses the same size puck (vulcanized rubber, 6 ounces [170g], 3 inches across, 1 inch thick). Young players need sufficient strength in the upper body to handle, pass, and shoot the puck.
      i. Observation of male and female youth hockey games and practices suggests that young hockey players do not have the strength to handle, pass, and shoot the regulation puck with great accuracy and high velocity.
      ii. It seems that for young players, the weight of the puck in relation to the size and strength of the players creates a disadvantage in puck control.
        • Some speculate that a change in the size of the puck in relation to age will enhance performance and skill.
    d. Good muscle strength can be advantageous as a fitness base for the production of the other components of muscle fitness.
  2. Elite hockey.
    a. Body checking, body contact, and struggling for the puck or position account for approximately 10% of the total time

on the ice. As such, muscle strength plays a major role in the success or failure of a player at a higher level of hockey.

3. Women's ice hockey.
   a. The effects of lightweight pucks in women's ice hockey have been studied.
      i. Pucks weighing 4.5, 5.0, and 5.5 ounces were tested with 171 subjects ranging in age from 9 to 33 years old. The ability levels of the players ranged from youth players to members of the Canadian Women's National Team.
         • Skill tests; 3-D film analysis of the wrist shots; surveys completed by players, referees, and parents; and game statistics were used to collect data.
      ii. Based on the results of the study, use of a 5-ounce puck for women's ice hockey was recommended.
         • Players, parents, coaches, and referees felt the 5-ounce puck could be shot and passed with greater velocity.
         • Skill tests showed that the 5-ounce puck was most conducive to puck-handling control and a higher scoring percentage.
      iii. All study subjects except the Canadian National Team felt that a lighter puck would be a social disadvantage to the game because others would view it as being too easy to play with a lighter puck.

B. Muscle hypertrophy.
   1. A hockey player's off-ice training should be periodized, concentrating on all components of fitness in the appropriate proportions for the demands of hockey.
   2. In a contact sport like ice hockey, lean body mass is important for success in all aspects of the game; therefore, it would behoove a hockey player to spend some time specifically developing muscle size.

C. Muscle power.
   1. Muscle power is a requisite requirement for hockey players because the game is characterized by short (1–3 seconds) bursts of high-intensity muscle exertion.
      a. These bouts of effort can be in the form of high-intensity skating, body contact, struggling for the puck or position, or shooting.
      b. Workouts focused on high strength output over a short period of time are beneficial in building muscle power.

D. Muscle endurance is perhaps the most underrated and underdeveloped component of muscle fitness in hockey players.

1. Due to a lack of understanding of the physiology of hockey, many hockey players and strength and conditioning coaches neglect muscle endurance.
2. Muscle endurance is important in hockey because the work bouts are repeated every 4–5 minutes during a period and 12–15 times during a game.
   a. Some teams play over 100 games spanning the preseason, regular season, play-offs, and tournaments.

Women's Ice Hockey

A. Physical characteristics/anthropometrics.
   1. Novice players (~ 9.1 years) are at or just above the reference medians for height (HGT), weight (WGT), and body mass index (BMI) and were slightly higher for the sum of 5 skin fold areas compared to controls.
   2. Pee Wee (~ 12.3 yrs) and Midget (~15.9 yrs) players were heavier, heavier for their height, and had higher skin fold measurements than reference data.
   3. Female hockey players across a wide range of ages tend to be heavy for their height.
      a. The composition of excess weight appears to vary with level of maturity and playing ability.
      b. Excess weight for height may not pose a hindrance to performance as long as players can move their weight effectively while skating.
B. Off-ice fitness.
   1. Bracko and George (2001) fitness tested female hockey players between the ages of 8 and 16 years old to determine what off-ice fitness variables predict skating performance.
      a. Forty-yard dash was the strongest predictor of skating speed.
      b. Players had the following fitness measures:
         i. Vertical jump—31.29 cm.
         ii. 40-yard dash—7.19 seconds.
         iii. Push-ups/minute—29.00.
         iv. Sit-ups/minute—33.00.
         v. Sit-and-reach flexibility—38.83 cm.
   2. Effect of a season of play on the fitness level of female hockey players has been studied.
      a. There are no significant differences between preseason and postseason fitness scores, indicating one of two things:
         i. Practices and games are of sufficient intensity, duration, and frequency to maintain fitness.

      ii. Practices and games are not of sufficient intensity, duration, and frequency to improve fitness.

  3. Physiological testing on female hockey players with a mean age of 19.4 years reveals:

    a. Mean Vo_2 max of 45.51 mL · kg · min^{-1}.

    b. Peak anaerobic power of 8.60 W · kg^{-1}.

    c. Mean bench press weight of 53.80 kg.

    d. Trunk flexibility of 43.93 cm.

Biomechanics and Kinematics of Hockey Skating

A. Forward skating.

  1. Forward striding is triphasic.

    a. Single-support propulsion phase.

      i. Propulsion starts approximately halfway through the single-support phase and continues through the entire double-support phase.

      ii. Propulsion ends in the double-support phase, after which the propulsion skate becomes the recovery skate.

      iii. Propulsion is produced by knee extension and hip abduction/extension. The hip also externally rotates at the start of the propulsion phase.

        • Therefore, the primary muscles of the legs involved in hockey skating include the quadriceps, hip abductors, and gluteus maximus.

        • The quadriceps develop the largest contractile forces when extending the knee during the propulsion phase of hockey skating.

    b. Double-support propulsion phase.

      i. The double-support phase starts when the recovery skate returns to the ice.

    c. Single-support glide phase.

  2. Skating characteristics of fast skaters when compared to slow skaters:

    a. Greater left stride width.

    b. Greater right stride width.

    c. Greater width between strides.

    d. Greater hip abduction angle.

    e. Quicker recovery time after push-off (the recovery foot should be brought forward close to the ice).

    f. Greater knee flexion angle prior to propulsion/push-off.

    g. Quicker knee extension during propulsion.

    h. Greater hip–skate forward inclination.

    i. Greater forward lean of the trunk.

3. An essential technical aspect of skating is the fact that the direction of the push-off is perpendicular to the gliding direction of the skate; in other words, the propulsion skate pushes to the side (hip abduction with extension, at the end of the propulsion phase).

   a. This unique characteristic of the propulsion phase of skating results in the sinusoidal (wave-like) trajectory of the body when skating straight.

4. When Newton's law of action-reaction is applied to hockey skating, it becomes apparent that when the hips abduct and adduct during the propulsion and recovery phases, the glenohumeral joints must also abduct and adduct for the player to maintain balance, create momentum, and increase velocity. This is particularly true when a hockey player has two hands on the stick.

   a. As velocity increases, the player's trunk must increase its forward lean, causing the glenohumeral joints to change from abduction adduction with the trunk upright (at slow speeds and gliding) to horizontal or transverse abduction/adduction.

5. Full knee extension during propulsion is not as important as a powerful stride.

   a. Power range of the knee is between 130 and 170°.

   b. A "full" stride is impossible at high speeds, when the length of the stride is determined by the quickness of returning the "recovery" skate to the ice.

6. Hockey skating is the opposite of speed skating in regard to stride rate and stride length.

   a. Hockey skating velocity is dependent on high stride rate and negatively related to stride length.

7. Acceleration.

   a. Acceleration is characterized by a high stride rate and significant forward lean of the trunk.

   b. Significant hip external rotation of the push-off skate during the first and second strides causes more hip extension, after which less external rotation takes place and more hip abduction.

      i. Horizontal movements (T-start or thrust start) instead of vertical movements (crossover or hopping start) are conducive to fast acceleration.

8. Two-foot gliding.

   a. NHL forwards spend 40% of the time on the ice gliding in a two-foot balance position, interspersed with left and right turns.

      i. The gliding is not sustained.

      ii. The average length of time spent in a skating character-
istic was 1.5 seconds.

   b. Skates should be approximately shoulder-width apart, slight
trunk, hip, and knee flexion and ankle dorsiflexion.

      i. A good two-foot gliding or balance position prepares a
player for acceleration, body contact, and/or puck contact.

  9. Turning.

   a. Gliding turns.

      i. Weight must be on the outside skate to maintain bal-
ance.

        • Inside knee is flexed and outside knee is extended.

      ii. Centrifugal force will "pull" the body away from the
turn; therefore, the outside skate maintains the cen-
tripetal force, pulling the player into the turn.

   b. Crossover turns.

      i. Outside leg moves in front, inside leg moves behind.

      ii. Horizontal movements should be emphasized.

        • Vertical movements (hopping around a corner)
increase recovery time, therefore slowing the player.

      iii. A study of NHL forwards showed that they execute more
left turns than right turns.

 10. Maturity.

   a. Below ages 8 or 9, hockey players generally skate more
upright without fluid hip and trunk rotation and have vertical, rather than horizontal, movements of the skates.

      i. The basic ice skating pattern/technique has been devel-
oped by age 10.

      ii. Young hockey players have difficulty coordinating the
movements of their arms with their legs.

        • Skill training should concentrate on the coordination
of arm and leg movement, which will enhance performance.

   b. Young or inexperienced players characteristically have vertical movements with their skates and a narrow stride.

      i. High-performance skaters have horizontal movements
with their skates and wide strides.

B. Backward skating.

  1. Backward striding.

   a. Similar to forward striding in that the hip movement for
propulsion is abduction and adduction.

   b. The body position for backward striding is: slight trunk,
hip, and knee flexion and ankle dorsiflexion.

      c. "C-cuts."
         i. Both skates stay on the ice.
         ii. Propulsion phase during which the hip abducts and the skate pushes off to the side.
         iii. Short glide phase while the propulsion skate recovers and is positioned under the hip.
      d. During acceleration from a stationary position, the hips internally rotate for the first 1–3 strides. After the third stride, the movement is hip abduction adduction.
      e. Shoulder movement corresponds with hip movement.
         i. As the hips abduct and adduct, so do the glenohumeral joints.
  2. Backward crossover.
      a. Body position: trunk, hips, knees, and ankles are flexed/dorsiflexed.
      b. The player will abduct the hip to push off to the side with the outside skate, after which there is a short glide phase. The leg/hip of the inside skate will adduct with the skate pushing behind the outside skate.
      c. In game-performance skating, 1 to 3 crossover strides are typical for a defensive maneuver.
      d. Game-performance backward skating is characterized by "c-cuts" or crossovers for acceleration, followed by a defensive player skating backward using a combination of "c-cuts," crossovers, and two-foot backward gliding.
C. Game-performance skating.
  1. Bracko et al. (1998) identified the skating characteristics of NHL forwards, and the time and frequency of the characteristics during a game (Table 11-1).
  2. Game-performance skating is characterized by gliding on two skates, interspersed with short bouts of low-, medium-, and high-intensity skating and "cruising" strides that last 1–3 seconds with left and right gliding and crossover turns.
      a. The most common sequential pattern of skating characteristics for 30 seconds after the start of play from a face-off is given in Table 11-2.
  3. All skating characteristics evolve from a two-foot glide position, and eventually a player will go back into a two-foot glide position.
      a. The ability to move into other skating characteristics from a two-foot glide position is important for hockey players, as the nature of the game is "stride—glide—stride—glide."

TABLE 11-1

Characteristics of game skating in **NHL** players.

Timed Skating Characteristics	% of Total Time on Ice	Frequency Skating Characteristics	% of Total Occurrences
Two-Foot Glide	40%	L-Crossover Turn	20%
Cruise Strides	16%	Gliding L-Turn	17%
Medium-Intensity Skating	10%	R-Crossover Turn	17%
Struggle for Puck/Position	10%	Gliding R-Turn	16%
Low-Intensity Skating	8%	Stop & Start	10%
High-Intensity Skating	5%	Fwd Bkwd	7.6%
Backward Skating	5%	Bkwd Fwd	6%
2-Foot Stationary	3%		

TABLE 11-2

Common sequence of skating characteristics in first **30** seconds after a face-off.

1. Struggle for Puck/Position	2 seconds
2. 2-Foot Glide (Gliding Left Turn, Gliding Right Turn)	2 seconds
3. Cruise Stride (Left Crossover Turn)	1 second
4. 2-Foot Glide (Gliding Left Turn)	2.5 seconds
5. Cruise Stride (Left Crossover Turn)	1 second
6. 2-Foot Glide (Gliding Left Turn)	2.5 seconds
7. Cruise Strides (Right Crossover Turn)	1 second
8. 2-Foot Glide (Gliding Left Turn, Gliding Right Turn)	2 seconds
9. Struggle for Puck/Position	2 seconds
10. Medium-Intensity Skating (Left Crossover Turn)	2.5 seconds
11. 2-Foot Glide (Gliding Right Turn)	1.5 seconds
12. Medium-Intensity Skating (Right Crossover Turn)	1 second
13. 2-Foot Glide (Gliding Left Turn, Gliding Right Turn)	1.5 seconds
14. Cruise Strides	1.5 seconds
15. Low-Intensity Skating (Left Crossover Turn)	3.5 seconds
16. 2-Foot Glide (Gliding Left Turn)	2.5 seconds

4. A great deal of skating and maneuvering is performed while under the influence of stick and/or body contact (struggle for puck or position).
  a. Increases energy expenditure.
  b. May cause fatigue in combination with intermittent high-intensity skating.

Efficacy of on-Ice Testing of Hockey Players

A. Skating performance: Many sports scientists question the accuracy of "field tests" because skill (player and tester) is required to perform well.
  1. Sports scientists want to eliminate the skill factor in exercise testing to produce objective results.
  2. Coaches are interested in a player's sport-specific fitness and game-performance skating ability.
  3. With the use of prediction equations, on-ice testing provides the opportunity to analyze both.
B. Anaerobic fitness testing.
  1. On-ice testing for anaerobic fitness may be more appropriate than using a Wingate cycle ergometer test for many reasons.
    a. In skating, external power is used to overcome air and ice resistance and to support body weight. During cycling, weight is supported and the requirements of external power are reduced.
    b. During skating the arms are used to maintain balance and aid in forward momentum; in cycling the arms are stationary.
  2. The most commonly used skating performance tests include:
    a. 6.10 m (20 feet) acceleration from a static position.
    b. 44.80 m (147 feet) speed.
    c. Agility cornering "S" turn.
      i. May be most representative of the way players skate during a game, and therefore it may be the best evaluation of game-performance skating.
      ii. Players must accelerate from a stationary position, maintain their balance during high-speed gliding and crossover turns, and accelerate from two-foot gliding and striding positions while turning and in a straight line.
        • During a game, professional hockey forwards execute a skating pattern similar to the one used during the agility skating test.
          – Stationary and dynamic acceleration.
          – Striding.
          – Gliding and crossover turns.

3. The test-retest reliability of on-ice skating tests has been evaluated:
   a. Acceleration: r = .80
   b. Speed: r = .76
   c. Agility: r = .64
4. Repeat sprint skate test (RSS), based on time-motion analysis of game-performance skating, was developed and has been used to evaluate the on-ice fitness of male and female, elite and nonelite players from 6 to 60 years old.
   a. Test protocol:
      i. Skate at full speed 54.86 m (180 feet), stop, change direction, and skate in the opposite direction 36.57 m (120 feet) to the finish line.
         • 30-second clock started as test begins.
      ii. Whatever time is left of 30 seconds after crossing the finish line is used for recovery before the next sprint starts on the 30-second mark.
      iii. Player performs three sprinting repeats in the same fashion.
      iv. Upon completion of the third sprint, the following data is collected:
         • Σ3 repeats.
         • Drop-off time: (3rd repeat −1st repeat).
         • Post-test heart rate.
         • Post-test lactate.
         • Recovery heart rate (4–5 minutes post-test, sitting).
         • Post-test recovery lactate (4–5 minutes post-test, sitting).
         • Post-test rating of perceived exertion.
         • Predicted anaerobic power.
            $$W = \frac{Mass\ (kg) \times Length\ (m)}{Time}$$
         • Predicted anaerobic capacity.
            $$Watts = \frac{Mass\ (kg) \times Length\ (m)}{Time}$$

Off-Ice Testing

A. Hockey skating is such a complex motor skill it is difficult to evaluate "hockey fitness" off the ice using standard testing protocols.
B. A combination of off-ice and on-ice testing can give sports scientists and coaches an excellent understanding of a player's fitness and skating ability.

Shooting

A. The hockey stick.
  1. Three component parts to a hockey stick:
    a. The blade.
    b. The shaft.
    c. The butt end.
  2. Hockey sticks are designed to withstand over 100 pounds of force and are made to be flexible yet strong.
    a. Wooden sticks.
      i. Made of rock elm, which is strong and flexible.
      ii. Most wooden sticks are reinforced with laminated fiberglass or graphite.
      iii. Made with the blade shaped into, and glued onto, the shaft.
      iv. Weight: 350–400 g.
    b. Aluminum, fiberglass, graphite, and Kevlar sticks are also available.
      i. Two-part sticks.
        • Shaft is made of material noted above.
        • Blade is wooden and plugs into the shaft.
      ii. The advantage of these sticks is that if the blade breaks, a player only has to replace the blade and not the entire stick.
      iii. Weight: 250–350 g.
    c. The newest style of stick is a one-piece carbon-composite stick.
      i. Weight < 250 g.
      ii. Felt to be more accurate than other sticks.
      iii. Shots estimated to be 10% faster.
B. The slap shot.
  1. Five phases to a slap shot:
    a. Windup (Figure 11-1a).
      i. Stick moves backward as the player abducts and adducts the shoulders.
        • Left-handed shooter abducts the left shoulder and adducts the right shoulder.
        • Right-handed shooter abducts the right shoulder and adducts the left shoulder.
      ii. Height of the windup depends on how quickly the player wants the shot to be released.
      iii. The top hand on the stick holds the very end of the stick and the bottom hand slides down so that it is positioned halfway or further down the shaft.

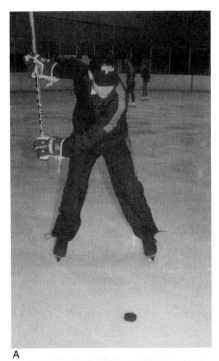

A

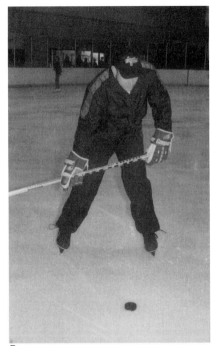

B

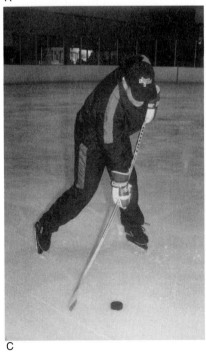

C

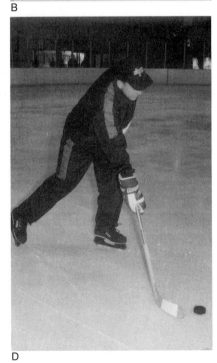

D

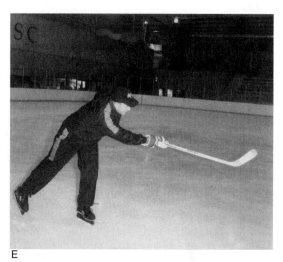

FIGURE 11-1 Slap shot: a) windup, b) acceleration, c) contact with the ice (note the flex in the stick shaft), d) the moment after contact with the puck, and e) follow-through. Photos courtesy of Frederick Moeller Jr.

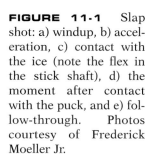

E

    iv. As the player brings the stick back in the windup there are also trunk flexion, lateral flexion and rotation, hip rotation, flexion of the hips and knees, and dorsiflexion of the ankles. The elbow of the arm that holds the top of the stick is flexed, and elbow of the arm holding the shaft of the stick is slightly flexed.

    v. Body mass is approximately evenly distributed on both skates.

  b. Acceleration (Figure 11-1b).

    i. Movement initiated with adduction of the top-hand shoulder, abduction of the bottom-hand shoulder, and rotation of the hips.

    ii. After initiation of movement, all the movements that occur in the windup are reversed, but with much greater velocity.

    iii. The arms and stick move at the same angular velocity about the pivot point located somewhere near the player's center of gravity.

    iv. During the acceleration phase body mass is transferred from even distribution on both skates to total mass on the front skate.

  c. Contact with ice (Figure 11-1c).

    i. Blade of the stick makes contact with the ice approximately 3–12 inches behind the puck.

    ii. When the blade hits the ice, the shaft of the stick bends, becoming loaded with potential energy.

- The greater the angular velocity of the acceleration phase, the greater the flex in the shaft, and the more potential energy that can be transferred to the puck.
  - Shaft can flex as much as 30°.
  iii. The bottom hand must be at least halfway down the shaft or further away from the player's center of gravity.
    - This puts more mass on the stick, making the shaft flex more and causing more potential energy to be stored in the shaft during ice contact.
  d. Contact with puck (Figure 11-1d).
  i. Contact time between the blade and the puck is estimated to be 0.013 second when the blade is traveling at 100 mph.
    - 0.022 second when blade traveling at 60 mph.
    - Stick returns to its original shape, transferring its potential energy to the puck.
  e. Follow-through (Figure 11-1e).
  i. Movements of the acceleration phase continue until reciprocal inhibition causes a slowing of the movement.
  ii. Body mass is transferred so that all the weight is on the front leg, with the back leg coming up off the ice.
  iii. At the very end of the follow-through a player may pronate the bottom hand and supinate the top hand to rotate the blade to get added velocity on the puck.
  2. The fastest slap shots have been recorded to be 100–105 mph. Average speed of the slap shots of professional male hockey players is approximately 90 mph.
C. Wrist shot and backhand shot.
  1. The biomechanics of a wrist and backhand shot are almost identical to those of the slap shot. Major differences include:
    a. No windup phase.
    i. Leads to a quicker release.
    b. Use more forearm pronation and supination for velocity.
    i. During a wrist and snap shot, the top hand supinates and the bottom hand pronates to rotate the blade for velocity on the puck.
    ii. When executing a backhand shot, the opposite movements of the wrists occur.
    c. Lower velocity than the slap shot.
    d. Higher accuracy than the slap shot.
  2. The puck starts at the heel of the blade and is transferred to the toe of the blade for release.

      a. Rotation of the puck creates velocity on the puck.

      b. Tape on the blade creates friction which can add velocity to the puck.

D. Snap shot.

    1. The snap shot is a hybrid of a wrist shot and a slap shot.

    2. Before shooting, a player pushes the puck slightly forward to start forward momentum, and then executes a snapping motion with the blade as the top hand rapidly supinates and the bottom hand pronates.

MEDICAL ISSUES

Concussion

A. Definition (Aubry et al. 2002): A complex pathophysiological process affecting the brain, induced by traumatic biomechanical forces. Several common features that incorporate clinical, pathological, and biomechanical injury constructs that may be used in defining the nature of a concussive head injury include:

    1. Concussion may be caused by a direct blow to the head, face, neck, or elsewhere on the body with an "impulsive" force transmitted to the head.

    2. Concussion typically results in the rapid onset of short-lived impairment of neurological function that resolves spontaneously.

    3. Concussion may result in neuropathological changes, but the acute clinical symptoms largely reflect a functional disturbance rather than structural injury.

    4. Concussion results in a graded set of clinical syndromes that may or may not involve loss of consciousness. Resolution of the clinical and cognitive symptoms typically follows a sequential course.

    5. Concussion is typically associated with grossly normal structural neuroimaging studies.

B. Incidence: As many as 10–12% of amateur hockey players sustain a documented concussion annually. It is likely that many more go unreported.

    1. Rate estimated at 4.63–5.95/1000 player game hours.

    2. In a study of Canadian amateur players, 60% of players had sustained a concussion at some time during their careers.

    3. 90% occur in game situations.

C. Mechanism of injury.
  1. The main cause of injury is contact with the boards and end glass.
  2. The second most common cause is contact with another player. Most of these contacts are thought to be illegal (e.g., elbow to head, elbow to jaw).
D. More common in forwards than defensemen and goalies, even more than predicted.
  1. Forwards make up 50% of on-ice players at any one time and account for ~ 60% of concussions.
  2. Defensemen (33% of players) account for 32–34% of injuries.
  3. Goalies (17% of players) account for 6–8% of injuries.
E. Severity. There are many grading scales used to assess the severity of concussion. No one system is perfect or universally endorsed. Severity of injury is based on many factors including:
  1. History.
      a. Of the injury itself. Important factors to note at time of injury are listed in Table 11-3.
      b. Of post-injury course. Important symptoms to note during the post-injury course are listed in Table 11-4.

TABLE 11-3

Important historical information to obtain at the time of sport-related head injury.

Was there loss of consciousness?
   Reported vs. witnessed
Is there neck pain?
Is there any numbness or tingling in the extremities?
Is there any post-traumatic amnesia?
   What does the athlete remember immediately following the injury?
Is there anterograde amnesia?
   What does the athlete remember leading up to the injury?
Headache?
Nausea?
Visual disturbance?
   Blurred vision
   Double vision
   Sensitivity to light
Hearing disturbance?
   Decreased hearing
   Sensitivity to noise
Drowsiness?

TABLE 11-4

Important historical information for the assessment of post-concussion course.

Headache
Nausea
Vomiting
Visual disturbance
   Blurred vision
   Double vision
   Sensitivity to light
Sensitivity to noise
Fatigue
Irritability
Extremity numbness or tingling
Sleep disturbance
   Drowsiness
   Sleeping more or less than usual
   Insomnia
Mentation disturbance
   Trouble concentrating
   Slowed thinking
   Troubles with schoolwork
   Trouble remembering
Dysequilibrium

2. Physical examination.
   a. Full neurological evaluation.
   b. Mini mental status evaluation.
3. Neuropsychological testing. An important component to any concussion evaluation and return-to-play decision making.
   a. Baseline testing is recommended.
   b. Neuropsychological tests are performed at intervals during the post-injury period to assess changes in cognitive function.
      i. A battery of various tests provides a more sensitive indication of function compared to a single test.
      ii. Neuropsychological tests are a more sensitive indicator of cognitive function than mini mental status exams or subjective reporting of symptoms.
   c. In most cases of mild traumatic brain injury from sport, these tests return to baseline levels in 5–10 days.

    4. Imaging studies.

      a. Generally contribute little to concussion evaluation.

      b. CT or MRI scan should be considered in cases in which suspicion of structural lesion exists.

        i. Downward progression of signs and symptoms.

        ii. Prolonged loss of consciousness.

        iii. Focal neurological findings.

        iv. Seizure.

        v. Persistent cognitive or clinical symptoms.

F. Management of concussion.

    1. If concussion is suspected, remove athlete from game/practice for evaluation.

      a. Serial evaluations necessary to assess progression/resolution of injury.

      b. Do not leave athlete alone.

      c. No athlete returns to play if post-concussion symptoms are present.

    2. Perform full evaluation in appropriate setting.

      a. If injury is considered severe on the sidelines, transport to an appropriate medical facility should be instituted.

        i. Assume C-spine injury if athlete is unconscious.

      b. Sideline evaluation is appropriate in mild and even moderate injury situations if the proper medical personnel are present.

      c. Appropriate post-game follow-up should be arranged with a practitioner with experience in the treatment of sport-related head injury.

G. Return to play.

    1. There are many return-to-play guidelines, none of which is perfect or universally accepted. Return-to-play decisions should be made on a case-by-case basis.

    2. It is agreed that athletes with continued symptoms or neurocognitive deficits (as determined by neuropsychiatric testing) should not be allowed to return to athletic participation.

    3. Once determined that an athlete is ready to begin his/her return to play, activities should follow a step-wise process. The speed of progression through this process is an area of debate.

      a. At the time of injury, the athlete is removed from sport activity including strenuous, noncontact activity.

      b. Once asymptomatic, light aerobic exercise can be initiated.

      c. Sport-specific training (i.e., skating).

      d. Noncontact training drills.

      e. Full-contact training after medical clearance.

      f. Game play.

  4. The recurrence of post-concussive symptoms at any stage of return should cause the athlete to return to the previous asymptomatic level.

H. Equipment effects on concussion.

  1. Helmet: It is well accepted that use of a properly fitted helmet will reduce the risk of severe head injury.

  2. Facial protection: Many believe that use of full facial protection will increase the severity of head injuries in ice hockey because players will feel "invincible" and will use a more aggressive style, but this has not been shown to be the case.

      a. Use of full-face shield (compared to half-shield) decreases the risk of facial and dental injuries without increasing the risk of concussion.

      b. Players sustaining a concussive injury while wearing a helmet with full-face shield lose less playing time than those who are injured while wearing a helmet with half-shield. This suggests that use of full-face shield may reduce the severity of concussive injury.

I. Prevention.

  1. Rules.

      a. Rule changes may reduce concussion risk.

      b. Enforcement of current rules is essential to reduce risk as evidenced by the common causes of injury.

  2. Equipment modifications such as improvement in helmets may continue to decrease the risk of head injury.

  3. Environmental factors: Some believe that certain types of boards and glass may increase risk of injury. This has not been proven.

Commotio Cordis (CC)

A. CC is a cause of sudden cardiac death due to blunt, nonpenetrating, typically low-velocity chest wall trauma.

  1. 128 cases of CC were registered in the United States through 2001.

      a. Age: 3 months–45 years (mean 13.6 ± 8.2 years)

         i. 44% < 12 years old.

         ii. 95% male.

B. It is believed that three major impact factors lead to sudden cardiac death from CC.

1. Location: The impact needs to be in the mid-chest area, usually directly over the precordium.
   a. Experiments in an animal model showed ventricular fibrillation (VF) would only be produced by chest impact directly over the heart (compared to noncardiac sites; $p < 0.0001$).
   b. Blows over the center of the heart were more likely to initiate VF than impacts at other precordial sites ($p = 0.02$).
2. Timing: In the cardiac cycle there is a vulnerable phase just before the peak of the T-wave during repolarization.
   a. 15–30 msec prior to T-wave peak.
   b. Impact to the heart during this vulnerable time can reproducibly cause instantaneous VF.
3. Force:
   a. This factor may not be as important as location and timing of impact.
   b. High-force (e.g., high-velocity impact with a hockey puck) and low-force (e.g., velocity force with a medium soft baseball) impacts may both cause CC if the location and timing of the impact are appropriate.

C. The trauma causing CC is sport-related in 83.6% of cases reported in the United States (107/128).
   1. Competitive sport-related in 79 cases, and recreational sport-related in 28.
      a. Baseball/softball accounted for 63.5% (68/107) of sport-related CC cases.
      b. Ice hockey accounted for 12% (13/107) of cases.
         i. CC in hockey was more likely to be from a high-velocity trauma, e.g., slap shot at close range.
      c. In over 80% of cases of sport-related CC, the chest wall trauma was imparted by a projectile (i.e., ball or puck) that is a standard implement of the game.
         i. Most projectiles had a solid core.
      d. In 22 of 79 (28%) cases reported in competitive sport, the athlete was wearing appropriate chest protection.
         i. 12 hockey players (2 goalies) are included in this group.
         ii. 3 lacrosse goalies and 2 baseball catchers also included in this group.
         iii. The majority of commercially available chest protectors do not appear to provide significant CC risk reduction. (Studies were performed on baseball chest protectors.)

D. Morbidity and mortality: 83.6% of registered CC cases in the United States (107/128) have been fatal. Of the 21 survivors:
   1. In 19 cases, resuscitative measures were instituted for cardiac arrest including 2 cases in which an AED was utilized.

      a. If resuscitative measures were initiated within 3 minutes of the event, chance of survival was ~ 25%.

      b. If resuscitative measures were initiated after 3 minutes, chance of survival was < 3%.

   2. There were two reported cases of spontaneous recovery including a professional hockey player struck by a slap shot during the Stanley Cup playoffs.

Eye Injury

A. Eye injuries in hockey used to be very common. The institution of face mask use in amateur hockey has effectively eliminated these injuries in certain age groups.

   1. All youth hockey requires full facial protection to be worn for all games and practices. Eye injuries are very rare in this group.

   2. Some Junior leagues require full facial protection while others allow the option of half-shield. Senior leagues also require some type of facial protection.

   3. Professional players have the option on facial protection. Most NHLers still opt for no facial protection.

B. In the pre–facial protection era, an average of nearly 300 eye injuries (32 blind eyes) annually were reported in Canadian hockey players.

   1. In the first year that masks were introduced, the total number of injuries dropped to 90 (12 blind eyes).

   2. In the post–facial protection era, the average annual number of injuries is 94 (16 blind). All injuries occurred in the absence of Canadian Standards Association certified eye protection.

C. Multiple studies have shown that use of facial protection significantly reduces the risk of eye injury as well as other facial injuries.

D. Cause of injury.

   1. In the 1970s, 75% of eye injuries were stick-induced, leading to new high sticking rules.

      a. Design standards include that no regulation stick blade can pass through any portion of the face mask.

   2. It was also noted in the 1970s that 38% of the injuries that caused blindness were puck-induced.

E. Specific injuries.

   1. Corneal abrasion.

      a. The most common sport-related eye injury.

         i. Makes up approximately 83% of all nonperforating anterior globe injuries.

      b. The cornea is a very thin structure with a normal central thickness of 0.5–0.65 mm. It is composed of five layers.

      i. Corneal abrasion is an injury to the epithelium, the outermost layer.

      ii. These injuries tend to heal well without scar formation.

         • Permanent scarring can result from injury to deeper layers.

  c. Chief complaint is a painful eye with or without foreign body sensation.

      i. Trauma may or may not be recalled.

      ii. Symptoms may include:

         • Increased lacrimation.

         • Photophobia.

         • Blurred vision.

         • Headache.

         • Blepharospasm.

  d. Physical examination.

      i. Assess visual acuity.

         • Acuity can be tested on the field by using a handheld eye chart.

      ii. Assess extraocular muscle activity and pupillary light reflex.

      iii. Evert lid to look for foreign body if history is suggestive.

      iv. Slit lamp or cobalt blue light examination.

         • Introduce fluoroscein strip in the pool of tears in the inferior cul-de-sac; the patient should then blink 2–3 times to spread the stain, and should remove excess tears prior to evaluation.

           – Anesthetic eyedrops may be used prior to staining if desired.

         • View eye using a cobalt blue light or Wood's lamp.

           – Magnification can help but is not absolutely necessary.

           – Corneal abrasion appears as a greenish-yellow fluorescent defect in the epithelium.

         • If there is a question as to the depth of the injury, or if there is suspicion of a penetrating or perforating injury, ophthalmologic consultation should be obtained without delay.

  e. Treatment: The three main objectives include controlling pain, decreasing the likelihood of secondary infections, and promoting reepithelialization of the cornea.

      i. Treatment of uncomplicated corneal abrasion generally includes:

         • Antibiotic eyedrops.

         • Follow-up within 24–36 hours.

    ii. The decision to use other medications such as oph-
thalmic nonsteroidal antiinflammatory drugs (NSAIDs)
or mydriatics is generally based on the individual athlete's pain level.
- Ophthalmic NSAIDs have been shown to decrease
pain, photophobia, and foreign body sensation and
allow for earlier return to work without causing significant adverse effects or delaying the healing
process.
- Anesthetic eyedrops should not be used for long-term
treatment of eye pain.
- Anesthetic eyedrops should not be given simply to
allow return to play.

    iii. Patches are not absolutely necessary to treat uncompli-
cated corneal abrasions.
- Some studies have shown that patients treated without eye patches may experience less pain and faster
healing over patients treated with eye patches.

  f. Return to play is allowed once there is no residual evidence
of abrasion and the eye examination is otherwise normal.

    i. This may only take 24–36 hours in some cases.

  g. Ophthalmology referral is recommended when:

    i. Deep corneal injury suspected (immediate referral).

    ii. Penetrating or perforating injury suspected (immediate
referral).

    iii. There is no improvement or there is worsening of the
appearance of the lesion at the 24- to 36-hour follow-up
visit.

2. Hyphema: The accumulation of blood in the anterior chamber;
may be caused by blunt or penetrating trauma.

  a. Injury is classified by the amount of blood in the chamber. Grade I injuries are most common; however, even a
small amount of blood may signify a severe intraocular
injury.

    i. Grade 1—< 33% of the chamber filled.

    ii. Grade 2—33–50% of chamber filled.

    iii. Grade 3—50% to nearly all the chamber filled.

    iv. Grade 4—entire chamber filled.

  b. History.

    i. Blunt trauma is usually caused by the puck but may be
caused by an elbow or fist.

    ii. Penetrating trauma is usually caused by the stick.

    iii. Time of the injury is very important as it will identify the
period of greatest risk for rebleeding.

     iv. Previous eye problems should be documented.

     v. All medications being used should be documented including dietary supplements.

  c. Examination.

     i. Assess visual acuity.

     ii. Assess extraocular muscle activity and papillary light reflex.

        • Afferent pupillary response (no response to direct light but consensual response maintained) suggests optic nerve or retinal damage but may be due to hyphema alone.

     iii. Evaluate for other injury such as lacerations, fractures, etc.

     iv. Evaluation for foreign bodies should be performed if suspicion exists.

     v. Size and shape of hyphema should be documented.

     vi. Gonioscopy should be delayed to avoid inducing rebleed and should be performed by an ophthalmologist.

  d. Treatment: The primary goal is to prevent rebleeding, corneal staining, and glaucoma.

     i. In mild cases, no treatment is required, and the blood is absorbed within a few days.

     ii. Bed rest.

        • Important to remain at inclined position so blood stays at inferior-most location.

     iii. Eye patching.

     iv. Sedation to minimize activity and reduce the likelihood of recurrent bleeding.

     v. Mydriatic eyedrops.

     vi. Removal of the blood by an ophthalmologist may be indicated, especially if the intraocular pressure is severely increased or the blood is slow to resorb.

     vii. Hospitalization may be required.

3. Traumatic iritis: Inflammation of the iris that develops shortly after blunt trauma.

  a. History.

     i. Pain in the eye or brow region.

     ii. Headache.

     iii. Blurred vision.

     iv. Photophobia.

  b. Physical examination.

     i. Erythema at the periphery of the iris.

     ii. Increased tearing.

  iii. Decreased visual acuity.
  iv. Constricted pupil.
  v. Shining light in the normal, unaffected eye causes pain in the affected eye due to consensual pupillary constriction.
  vi. Slit lamp examination reveals cells (white blood cells) and flares (particles of protein) in the aqueous humor.
  c. Treatment.
  i. Topical anesthetics do not relieve the pain associated with iritis.
  ii. Dilators.
  iii. Steroid drops.
  iv. If symptoms do not resolve in one week or if symptoms worsen during treatment, ophthalmology consultation should be obtained.

Facial Lacerations

A. Common in players who wear half-shields or no facial protection and uncommon in players who wear full facial protection.
  1. Risk is 2.31 times greater with half-shield versus full shield.
B. Common locations of laceration are different based on type of facial protection worn.
  1. Full shield.
    a. Chin: Most common location because the helmet rides back on the head, exposing the chin.
    b. Forehead.
  2. Half-shield.
    a. Lip.
    b. Eyebrow.
C. Mechanism of injury.
  1. Lacerations in full-shield wearers are primarily due to contact with another player or contact with a stick (40% each).
  2. In half-shield wearers, contact with the stick is the overwhelming cause of laceration (> 50%).
D. Laceration repair.
  1. Repair decisions are not significantly different for lacerations encountered from ice hockey compared to other situations, with some exceptions.
    a. In a game situation, suture repair is often performed in the training or medical room and the athlete returns to the ice.
    b. Initial repair is often focused primarily on hemostasis, with a more cosmetic, final repair performed after the game.

2. Preparation.
   a. Universal precautions and sterile technique should be employed and consent obtained.
   b. Skin prepped to decrease risk of infection.
      i. Isopropyl alcohol.
      ii. Betadine.
      iii. Chlorhexidine (Hibiclens).
   c. Irrigation of the wound may be necessary and should be performed with either sterile water or sterile saline.
   d. Anesthesia can be administered in a variety of ways.
      i. Topical: Generally not used for repair during game situations as it takes up to 20 minutes to achieve adequate anesthesia.
      ii. Local anesthetic infiltration.
         • Lidocaine is generally the anesthetic of choice.
            – Rapid onset.
            – Generally well tolerated.
            – May be used with epinephrine to decrease small vessel bleeding. (Do not use epinephrine at tip of nose.)
         • Longer-acting local anesthetics are available but are not generally needed for simple laceration repair.
      iii. Field block.
         • Creates a wall of anesthesia around the wound.
         • Especially useful when there are concerns of tissue distortion by the anesthetic.
         • Epinephrine not helpful in reducing bleeding.
      iv. Regional block.
         • Anesthetic administered to main sensory nerve branch affecting a large area of skin.
         • Effective for large or complex lacerations.
         • Does not distort injured tissues.
         • Reduces total volume of anesthetic needed for repair.
         • Epinephrine not helpful.
3. Choice of closure agent.
   a. Sterile wound closure tapes.
      i. Good choice for smaller, linear lacerations in nonbeard and low-hair areas.
      ii. May not remain adherent due to sweat.
      iii. Poor edge approximation and wound eversion may lead to larger scar.
   b. Skin adhesives.
      i. Used in nonhairy areas.
      ii. Should not be used around the eyes.

    c. Suture.
        i. Best choice for most facial lacerations, especially the longer and more complex lesions.
       ii. Suturing techniques are variable and each type has its pros and cons. The technique utilized is a product of physician preference and wound type.
- Simple interrupted.
  - Allows precise adjustment between stitches.
  - Quick, easy to perform.
  - Allows for selective stitch removal.
  - More likely to cause uneven tension of the wound.
  - Prone to "train track" scars.
- Running continuous.
  - Even tension.
  - Quick, easy.
  - Must be removed in entirety.
- Vertical mattress.
  - Increased wound eversion.
  - Increased wound strength.
  - Good dead space closure.
  - Time-consuming.
  - Edge approximation can be difficult.
  - Prone to prominent suture marks.
- Horizontal mattress.
  - Good wound eversion.
  - Good dead space closure.
  - Time-consuming.
  - Prone to suture scars.
  - Risk of epidermal necrosis.
- Subcuticular.
  - Best for edge approximation with limited tension.
  - Low incidence of suture scars.
  - Time-consuming.
  - Poor strength under tension.
  - Poor wound eversion.

  d. Staples.
    i. Excellent choice for wounds in which cosmetic outcome not as important, such as scalp wounds.
   ii. Quick, easy to apply and remove.

4. Post-repair instructions regarding antibiotic ointment use, bathing, dressings, and suture removal should be reviewed with the athlete.
  a. Different wounds require different post-repair instructions.

    b. Sutures can be removed in as little as 3 days in some cases but are typically left in for 5–7 days.

Dental Injury

A. Still very common despite the availability of full facial protection and dental protection (mouthguards).
    1. Consistent use of a well-fitted mouthguard has been shown to reduce the risk of dental injury.
        a. Boil-and-bite mouthguards.
            i. Pros: Inexpensive, readily available, can be made at home, generally well tolerated.
            ii. Cons: Occlusal thickness decreases dramatically during moulding, and fit is dependent on the individual and may not be adequate for optimal protection. Athlete may need to clench teeth to hold guard in place.
        b. Custom-made mouthguards.
            i. Pros: Custom fit, more comfortable, minimal interference with speech and breathing. Stay in place without clenching of teeth.
            ii. Cons: More expensive, difficult to replace, require dental appointment for construction/fitting.
        c. Despite knowledge that mouthguards are effective in reducing dental injury, many athletes still do not use them on a regular basis.
    2. Risk of sustaining dental injury is 9.9 times greater for players wearing a half-shield versus those wearing full facial protection.
B. Most injuries occur in game situations (69%) compared to practice (31%).
    1. Contact with a stick is the most common mechanism of injury (48.9%).
    2. Other common mechanisms include contact/collision with another player and contact with the puck.
C. Majority of injuries affect the maxilla (up to 80%).
    1. Upper central incisors account for nearly 50% of the damaged teeth.
    2. Injury to the incisors (upper, lower, central, lateral) make up nearly 90% of the dental injuries.
    3. Contact with another player typically results in injury to a single tooth. Contact with a stick or puck usually results in injury to multiple teeth.
D. Types of injury: The types and severity of maxillofacial and dental trauma encountered in ice hockey are highly variable.

Although these injuries make up a relatively small percentage of the total injuries seen, related costs are very high and disproportionate to the number of injuries.

    1. The most common injury is noncomplicated crown fracture (43.5%).

    2. Complicated crown fracture is much less common (14%).

    3. Other injuries include luxation, root fracture, and avulsion.

  E. Treatment of crown fracture.

    1. Chipped teeth and other noncomplicated crown fractures do not involve the tooth pulp.

      a. Dental referral should be made, but does not need to be immediate.

      b. Fragments should be collected, if found, and sent with the athlete to the dental office. Fragments should be handled on the enamel side only.

    2. Complicated crown fractures include pulp exposure.

      a. Pulp involvement is a more important indicator of severity of injury than amount of tooth affected.

      b. Pulp exposure can be very painful due to the presence of nerves and blood vessels in the pulp.

        i. Decreasing the exposure to air, saliva, and temperature changes can reduce pain.

        ii. Root canal can be sealed by a drop of "super glue" or cyanoacrylate.

      c. Dental referral is needed.

        i. Does not need to be immediate if pain is controlled but should not be delayed beyond 24 hours.

        ii. Save and send fragments.

  F. Treatment of luxation: Luxation (displacement of tooth at root level without removal from socket) can take three forms: extrusion, lateral displacement, and intrusion.

    1. An extruded tooth appears longer than surrounding teeth. A laterally displaced tooth will take a position either ahead of or behind the normal tooth row.

      a. Tooth may be repositioned on-site.

        i. Universal precautions.

        ii. Abort reduction attempt if too difficult or painful.

    2. An intruded tooth has been pushed into the gum and has a shortened appearance. It may be present along with lateral displacement.

      a. Repositioning on-site should not be attempted.

      b. Refer to dentist for repositioning.

  G. Treatment of avulsion: Tooth has been completely removed from socket.

1. For best outcome, reimplantation should take place in < 30 minutes. Delay of > 2 hours greatly decreases the chance of saving the tooth.
2. Handle the tooth by enamel only.
3. Gently cleanse the tooth with water or saline.
4. If the athlete is alert, reposition the tooth in the socket.
    a. The tooth may "click" into place.
    b. Immediate tooth replacement greatly increases the chance of successful healing.
    c. Be careful to replace tooth with the proper side facing forward.
    d. Splint tooth in place. Gum, Silly Putty, or aluminum foil can be used for splinting.
5. If the athlete is not alert or if repositioning is not possible, protect the tooth in a moist environment.
    a. Hank's Balanced Salt Solution.
    b. Save-A-Tooth kit (3M, St. Paul, MN).
    c. Cold milk.
    d. Saline-soaked gauze on ice.
    e. In the athlete's cheek or under tongue (only if alert).
6. Refer immediately to a dentist.

Tinea Pedis

A. Hockey players believed to be at high risk for tinea pedis.
    1. Occlusive footwear.
    2. Feet exposed to sweat-soaked socks for hours at a time.
    3. Community-style shower facilities.
B. Hockey players found to have no higher (and perhaps a lower) incidence of fungal foot infection than the general population.

Mononucleosis

A. General information.
    1. Mono is usually a self-limited illness caused by the Epstein-Barr virus (EBV).
        a. Member of the herpesvirus family.
        b. Transmitted by oral secretions.
            i. After infection, the patient secretes EBV in the saliva either continuously or intermittently for months.
    2. Peak incidence occurs between 15 and 25 years old.
        a. 1–3% of college students become infected each school year.
        b. Roommates of infected individuals are at no greater risk of contracting mono than the general population.

3. No greater incidence in ice hockey compared to other sports. Discussed here because of return-to-play considerations for contact and collision sport.
B. Pathophysiology.
    1. EBV attacks B-lymphocytes.
        a. Leads to production of IgM antibodies.
        b. Production of autoimmune antibodies also occurs.
            i. Rheumatoid factor.
            ii. Antinuclear antibodies.
        c. T-lymphocyte proliferation.
            i. Lymphoid hyperplasia.
            ii. Leukocytosis.
            iii. Atypical lymphocytes.
    2. Incubation of primary disease is about 30–50 days.
        a. Prodrome.
            i. Headache.
            ii. Malaise.
            iii. Fatigue.
            iv. Myalgias.
        b. Classic signs and symptoms.
            i. Pharyngitis.
            ii. Tonsillar enlargement with or without exudates.
            iii. Posterior palatine petechiae.
            iv. Generalized lymphadenopathy.
                • Tender posterior cervical nodes.
            v. Splenomegaly.
                • Commonly occurs by second week.
                • Only palpable in 20–50% of cases.
                • Best detected by US or CT scan.
                    – Present by US in nearly all patients with mono.
    3. Laboratory tests.
        a. Leukocytosis ($10,000–20,000/mm^3$).
        b. Absolute lymphocytosis (> 50% of total WBC count).
            i. 10–20% atypical lymphocytes.
        c. Thrombocytopenia.
        d. Elevated liver enzymes.
        e. Monospot test positive.
            i. Detects presence of heterophile antibodies.
            ii. Only 60% will have a positive test at 2 weeks.
C. Clinical course.
    1. Generally unremarkable.
    2. Treatment.
        a. Supportive measures to alleviate throat pain, headaches, and myalgias.

    b. Rest.

    c. Corticosteroids may be considered, particularly if any of the following conditions exist:

        i. Hepatitis.

        ii. Myocarditits.

        iii. Neurologic complications.

        iv. Airway obstruction.

3. Athletes may respond differently to EBV infection than nonathletes.

    a. Nonathletes show symptomatic:subclinical cases ratio of 3:1.

    b. Athletes show symptomatic:subclinical cases ratio of 1:3.

    c. Athletes tend to return to training more quickly than nonathletes return to their usual activities.

4. Life-threatening complications.

    a. Airway obstruction.

    b. Splenic rupture.

        i. Occurs in 0.1–0.2% of all cases of mono.

        ii. The mechanism for spontaneous rupture is hypothetical.

            • Lymphocytic infiltration $\rightarrow$ distortion and fragility of normal tissue anatomy including support structures.

               – It is uncertain how long these changes continue.

        iii. Maki and Reich (1982) reviewed 55 patients with splenic rupture and found:

            • All patients suffering splenic rupture had enlarged spleens (2–3 × normal).

            • < 50% of the spleens were palpable.

            • Nearly all splenic ruptures occured between days 4 and 21 of symptomatic illness.

            • There was no correlation between severity of illness and susceptibility to rupture.

            • A large proportion of splenic ruptures were spontaneous.

            • Trauma or significant physical exertion or strain implicated in 50% of cases.

            • 90% occured in males.

            • Few cases were reported in blacks.

            • Leukocytosis ($15,000–30,000/mm^3$) with significant absolute neutrophilia ($> 8,000/mm^3$) in the second and third weeks of illness was noted in over half of the cases.

        iv. Frelinger (1973) reported on 22 cases of traumatic splenic rupture in athletes.

- 17 cases (77%) were related to football participation.
- Only 8 (36%) of the cases were in athletes with confirmed mono infection.
  - **v.** Discussion of the detection and treatment of splenic rupture can be found in Chapter 5, Alpine Skiing.
- **D.** Controversies in mononucleosis management.
  - **1.** To image or not to image.
    - **a.** Pros.
      - **i.** More accurately detect splenomegaly in athletes with mono.
    - **b.** Cons.
      - **i.** Nearly all patients with mono will have splenomegaly on imaging studies despite no clinically palpable spleen.
      - **ii.** Athletes whose spleens are naturally larger than normal parameters may be disqualified from play unnecessarily.
      - **iii.** Once splenomegaly is diagnosed radiographically, documentation of return to normal size is advocated prior to return to contact sports.
        - This could take months, which may unnecessarily disqualify some participants without increasing their risk for rupture.
  - **2.** When to return to sport.
    - **a.** There is no consensus on the appropriate timing of return to sports participation.
      - **i.** Recommendations range from 4 weeks to 6 months.
    - **b.** There is no current study showing an increased incidence of splenic rupture in athletes who resume full activity 4 weeks after infection compared to those who remained activity-free for 6 months.
    - **c.** Two issues are generally agreed upon.
      - **i.** No participation is allowed if the athlete is still showing clinical signs and/or symptoms of acute illness.
      - **ii.** Even if the athlete is feeling well, he/she should be held if the spleen is palpable.
    - **d.** Recommendations.
      - **i.** Athletes diagnosed with mono should be held from sport participation for at least the first 3 weeks of illness.
      - **ii.** Return to light activity after 3–4 weeks if the acute phase of the illness has resolved (i.e., no fever, sore throat, fatigue, myalgias, headache) *and* there is no splenic enlargement.

iii. More vigorous training, contact and collision activities are usually held for at least one more week.
- Slow return to more vigorous and physical play begun at that time.

Exercise-Induced Bronchospasm

See Chapter 2, Pulmonary Physiology.

MUSCULOSKELETAL INJURIES

AC Sprains

A. Mechanism of injury.
  1. Inferiorly directed blow to the top of the shoulder, often with the arm in an adducted position.
     a. Contact with boards/glass.
     b. Contact with opponent.
     c. Contact with ice.
  2. Acromion-clavicle complex shifts inferiorly, and clavicle makes contact with first rib and stops. AC and coracoclavicular ligaments stressed.
B. History.
  1. Pain.
     a. Located directly over AC joint.
     b. Worsened with shoulder motion.
  2. Swelling or gross deformity over the AC region may be present.
  3. Ipsilateral arm paresthesias may be present.
C. Physical examination.
  1. Deformity or swelling may be apparent (Figure 11-2).
     a. May be more easily noted if examiner looks upward at the AC joint from a 10–15° angle.
  2. Tenderness at the AC joint.
     a. Worsened with active and passive motion.
     b. Adduction particularly painful.
  3. Decreased shoulder ROM due to pain.
  4. Neurovascular status usually remains intact.
  5. Positive crossover test.
D. Radiographs should be obtained in all cases of AC sprain.
  1. AP projections parallel to and/or from 10–15° inferior to the joint are recommended (Figure 11-3).

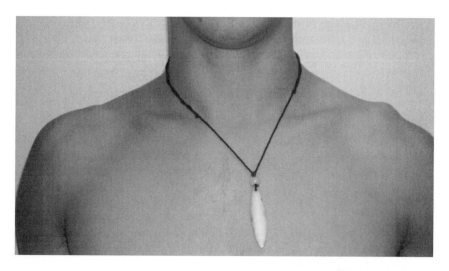

FIGURE 11-2   Gross appearance of a left type III AC separation (nonacute) in a hockey player. Photo courtesy of James L. Moeller, MD.

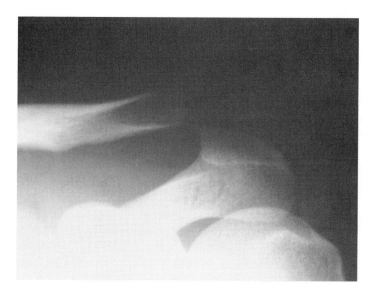

FIGURE 11-3   AP radiograph of a left type III AC separation (radiographs of the patient pictured in Figure 11-2). Image courtesy of James L. Moeller, MD.

      a. Rule out distal clavicle fracture.

      b. Document degree and direction of AC separation.

   2. Weighted images are uncomfortable for the patient and do not tend to change treatment plans, so these are no longer routinely obtained.

   3. Additional diagnostic tests are not usually needed.

E. Classification.

   1. Type I.

      a. Stretch/irritation of AC ligament.

      b. No displacement of clavicle in relationship to acromion.

   2. Type II.

      a. Tear of AC ligament, and coracoclavicular ligaments stretched/ irritated.

      b. Clavicle displaced up to 25% superiorly.

   3. Type III.

      a. Tear of AC and coracoclavicular ligaments.

      b. Clavicle displaced 25–100% superiorly.

   4. Type IV.

      a. Tear of AC and coracoclavicular ligaments.

      b. Deltotrapezial fascia detached.

      c. Clavicle displaced posteriorly. May pierce through trapezius muscle.

   5. Type V.

      a. Tear of AC and coracoclavicular ligaments.

      b. Deltotrapezial fascia detached.

      c. Clavicle displaced 100–300% superiorly.

   6. Type VI.

      a. Tear of AC and coracoclavicular ligaments.

      b. Deltotrapezial fascia detached.

      c. Clavicle displaced inferiorly.

F. Treatment.

   1. Type I and II injuries are treated nonoperatively.

      a. Early treatment.

         i. Sling immobilization.

            • Typically needed for 1–2 weeks.

            • Kenny-Howard slings generally no longer used.

               – May cause skin breakdown over the AC joint.

               – May lead to compression injury to anterior osseous nerve.

         ii. Ice.

         iii. Antiinflammatory medications.

      b. Rehabilitation.

      i. ROM exercises.

      ii. Strengthening exercise.

      iii. Sport-specific training.

   c. Return to play.

      i. Possible in 2–3 weeks in many cases of type I injuries.

      ii. May take 6–8 weeks for type II injuries.

2. Type III injuries.

   a. Initial treatment is controversial with both nonsurgical and surgical treatments being considered.

   b. Nonoperative treatment has been shown to be an excellent option with return of pain-free activities, full motion, and full strength for the majority of patients.

      i. Treatment similar to that listed for type I and II injuries above.

       • Sling immobilization for comfort may be needed for up to 4 weeks.

       • Guarded return to sports can begin over 2–3 months.

   c. Surgical treatment should be strongly considered in certain situations:

      i. Significant nerve or vascular compromise.

      ii. Significant tenting of the skin.

      iii. Chronic pain after nonoperative treatment.

      iv. Cosmetically unacceptable to patient.

   d. Return to contact/collision sports may take 3–5 months.

3. Type IV, V, and VI injuries should all be treated operatively.

Pseudo-Sprain of the AC Joint

A. Seen mainly in younger athletes.

B. Mechanism same as for AC sprain.

C. Pathophysiology.

   1. Distal clavicle surrounded by a thick periosteal tube all the way to AC joint.

      a. Coracoclavicular ligaments tightly bound to inferior border of periosteal tube.

      b. Protects AC joint from injury.

   2. Distal clavicle fractures while the periosteal tube remains intact.

      a. Nondisplaced fractures may be occult, evident only after callous formation takes place.

       i. Nondisplaced injuries often diagnosed as type I sprains.

      b. Displaced fractures heal nicely due to intact periosteal tube.

Clavicle Fracture

A. Mechanism of injury is direct impact to the shoulder.
1. Contact with boards/glass.
2. Contact with opponent.
3. Contact with stick.
4. Contact with ice.
B. Most fractures are in the mid-shaft region.
C. History.
1. Pain in the shoulder region.
   a. Worsened by attempted motion.
2. Gross deformity often noted by the patient.
3. Paresthesias may be present.
D. Physical examination.
1. Gross deformity of the clavicle.
2. Pain on gentle palpation.
3. Decreased ROM.
4. Neurovascular status usually intact.
E. Radiographs are diagnostic (Figure 11-4). It is important to note the following:
1. Displacement.
2. Angulation.
3. Shortening.

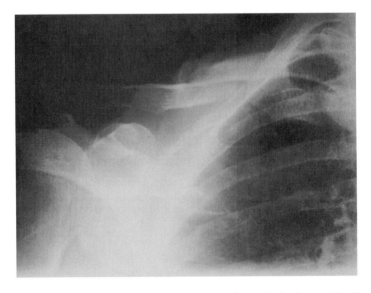

FIGURE 11-4   AP radiograph shows a right mid-shaft clavicle fracture with displacement and shortening. Image courtesy of James L. Moeller, MD.

F. Treatment of mid-shaft fractures.
1. Nonoperative treatment is appropriate for nearly all mid-shaft clavicle fractures, particularly in children.
   a. Patients < 12 years old.
      i. Immobilization.
         - Arm sling.
         - Figure-of-eight sling.
           – May assist with realignment of the more angulated, displaced fractures.
         - Ultimate outcome no different comparing arm sling to figure-of-eight.
      ii. Reduction usually not required, even when large degrees of angulation, displacement are present.
      iii. Clinical healing takes place over 3–6 weeks.
         - Remodeling continues for 6–12 months.
   b. Patients > 12 years old.
      i. Immobilization as above.
      ii. Reduction may be required for gross displacement or severe angulation.
         - Closed manipulation.
         - Conscious sedation or local hematoma block.
      iii. Clinical healing takes place over 6–8 weeks.
2. Operative treatment indications.
   a. Debridement of open fractures (absolute indication).
   b. Fracture associated with neurovascular compromise.
   c. Grossly displaced fracture that cannot be reduced by closed techniques.
   d. Nonunion.

Forearm Fractures

Forearm fractures most commonly occur from receiving a slash to the forearm between the distal end of the elbow pad and proximal extension of the glove.
A. Radiographs are necessary not only for diagnosis but for planning appropriate treatment.
B. Discussion of forearm fractures can be found in Chapter 6, Snowboarding.

Hamate Fracture

A. Though not commonly reported, fractures of the hook of the hamate are most commonly seen in sports that utilize a racquet, club, or stick.

1. Mechanism of injury is repetitive trauma of the stick against the hypothenar eminence. A sudden, single traumatic event may also lead to fracture.
2. Examination reveals tenderness over the hypothenar eminence/hamate bone.
   a. Ulnar nerve symptoms may be present.
   b. Radiographs should be obtained when hamate fracture is suspected.
      i. Carpal tunnel views should be included in the series.
      ii. CT scan may be necessary to make a definitive diagnosis.
3. Treatment.
   a. Nondisplaced fractures can be treated with cast immobilization.
      i. Surgical treatment should be considered if ulnar nerve symptoms exist.
   b. Displaced fractures and nonunion cases are treated surgically.
      i. Excision of the fracture fragment is most commonly performed.
      ii. Operative fixation of the fracture fragment can be attempted but is technically difficult due to the small size of the fracture fragment and tenuous blood supply to this bone.

Forearm Periostitis and Stress Fractures

Forearm periostitis and stress fractures are most commonly described in athletes who use their upper extremities for weight bearing, e.g., gymnasts. Periostitis has been described, however, in throwers and hockey players.
A. The mechanism of ulnar periostitis in hockey players is believed to be resistive forces applied to hand/digit flexors during the slap shot.
   1. Flexor digitorum profundus originates from the proximal ulnar diaphysis.
   2. The at-risk arm is the low arm on the stick (i.e., the left arm in a left-handed player, right arm in the right-handed player).
B. Chief complaint is forearm pain that is worsened with slap shot.
   1. Physical examination may reveal tenderness to palpation of the ulna, but may be unremarkable.
C. Diagnostic tests.
   1. X-rays are typically negative.

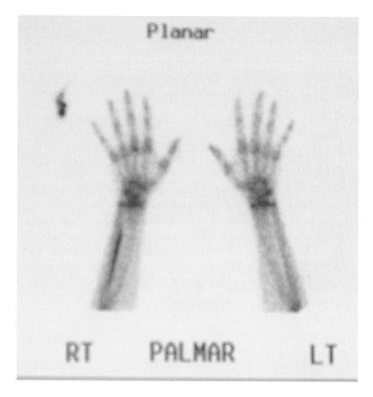

FIGURE 11-5   Radionuclide bone scan image of the forearms reveals diffuse radiotracer uptake in the right ulna, consistent with periostitis. Image courtesy of James L. Moeller, MD.

    2. Bone scan reveals diffuse tracer uptake along the proximal ulnar diaphysis (Figure 11-5).

D. Treatment is removal of the inciting activity, i.e., the slap shot.

    1. Remove player from all hockey activity if pain is present with lower-impact activities such as wrist shot and passing and receiving passes.

    2. Some are able to continue to play by simply eliminating the slap shot and should be allowed to do so as long as they are pain-free.

    3. Once pain-free for 2–4 weeks (the length of time is debatable and not based on any scientific study), reintroduction of the slap shot can be attempted.

E. Misdiagnosis or allowing the player to continue full activity in the face of ulnar periostitis may lead to stress fracture.

Traumatic Olecranon Bursitis

E. Even though the elbow is protected by an elbow pad, many skaters who fall directly onto the tip of the elbow present with pain and localized swelling at the site of impact.

B. For full discussion of traumatic olecranon bursitis, see Chapter 12, Figure Skating.

Groin and Abdominal Muscle Strains

A. Groin (hip adductor and hip flexor) and abdominal muscle strain injuries in elite ice hockey are a significant problem, causing an estimated loss of 25 player games per year at the NHL level.

    1. Injury incidence rose from 12.99 injuries/100 players/year in the 1991–92 season to 19.87 injuries/100 players/year in 1996–97.

    2. Groin strains are more common than abdominal wall strains (3:1).

        a. Hip adductor strains are the most common muscle strains encountered in ice hockey.

B. Most muscle strain injuries are noncontact injuries.

C. More groin and abdominal muscle strains take place during training camp that at other times of the year.

    1. Injuries 5 times more likely during training camp than in the regular season.

    2. Injuries 20 times more likely during training camp than in the postseason.

D. More common in forwards (> 60%) than defensemen and goalies.

E. Abdominal strains lead to greater lost time from practice/play than groin strains.

F. Risk factors: Identification of risk factors can allow for development of prevention programs.

    1. Factors found to increase the risk of groin strains (during training camp) in elite ice hockey include:

        a. < 18 total sport-specific (i.e., skating) training sessions in the off-season.

        b. < 12 sport-specific training sessions in the month prior to the onset of training camp.

        c. Previous injury.

        d. Veterans are more likely to experience injury than rookies.

    2. Low peak adductor torque/strength may be a risk factor for groin strain although this has not been shown to be the case in all studies.

        a. Adductor-to-abductor strength ratio may be a better predictor of groin injury than adductor strength alone.

    i. It has been shown that adductor strength < 80% of abductor strength is associated with a 17 times greater risk of adductor strain.

   b. There is evidence that an adductor-targeted strengthening program may decrease the incidence of adductor strain in an at-risk population.

  3. Total preseason adductor flexibility has not been shown to be a predictor of adductor strain.

Foot Fractures

A. Mechanism of injury is being struck in the foot by a shot puck.
B. The first and fifth metatarsals are the most commonly fractured bones.
C. Radiographs are necessary not only for diagnosis but for planning appropriate treatment.
D. Treatment choices follow standard fracture care guidelines.

Common Peroneal Nerve (CPN) Injury

A. The CPN arises from the dorsal branches of L4 and L5 and the ventral rami of S1 and S2.
  1. Runs obliquely through the lateral portion of the popliteal fossa.
  2. Curves lateral to the fibular neck before dividing into superficial and deep branches.
B. CPN and its branches provide motor and sensory innervation to the lower leg, ankle, and foot.
  1. Motor innervation to ankle dorsiflexors and evertors as well as toe extensors.
  2. Sensory innervation to anterolateral lower leg and dorsum of the foot.
C. Anatomical location of the nerve at the fibular neck places it at risk for injury.
  1. Direct trauma (see further discussion below).
    a. Blunt.
    b. Penetrating.
    c. Hockey shin pad design often leaves the CPN exposed, thereby increasing the risk of injury.
  2. Cryotherapy-induced.
    a. Due to close proximity to the skin surface and a relative lack of fat layer insulation, the CPN is at risk for injury due to ice therapy.

      i. This risk may be increased if the nerve has already been injured by some type of blunt trauma.
- Use caution when applying ice to the lateral knee of an athlete who sustained blunt trauma to the lateral knee area, particularly if signs of CPN injury exist.

      ii. Direct icing over the lateral knee/fibular head region should be of limited duration.

D. CPN injuries in hockey.
1. Lacerations of the CPN from a skate blade have been reported. Nerve lacerations typically lead to significant long-term deficits.
2. Blunt trauma to the CPN from hockey does occur although it has not been widely reported.
   - **a.** Stick trauma (slash) to the area is the most commonly reported mechanism.
   - **b.** Being struck by the puck is the other common mechanism.
   - **c.** Blunt CPN injury is more common during games (80%) than in practice.
   - **d.** Recovery is typically complete, but may take up to six months.
3. Equipment alterations to provide better protection to the CPN have been recommended.

Quadriceps Contusion

A. Mechanism of injury.
1. Direct impact to the anterior thigh musculature causing a crush-type injury.
2. Most common mechanisms are:
   - **a.** Knee versus thigh.
   - **b.** Shoulder versus thigh.

B. History.
1. Acute pain in the anterior thigh.
2. Pain with weight bearing.
3. Decreased range of motion.

C. Physical examination.
1. Thigh may appear grossly normal or may appear swollen.
2. Increased tissue tension noted on palpation in comparison to opposite side.
3. Tender on palpation of the quadriceps musculature.
4. Pain with passive quadriceps stretch.
   - **a.** Aggressive stretching may increase or reestablish bleeding.

D. Diagnostic tests.
1. X-rays are obtained if there is concern of femur fracture.
2. No further tests are necessary for diagnostic purposes.

E. Treatment.
    1. Early treatment.
        a. Stop the bleeding.
            i. Methods in the first 24 hours include:
              • Ice, compression, and elevation.
              • Maintain knee in a flexion position.
            ii. Risk of rebleed is high in the first 7–10 days.
        b. Crutch ambulation.
    2. Treatment after the first 2–3 days.
        a. Active and passive gentle motion exercises.
        b. Stretching.
        c. Massage.
        d. Strength training.
        e. Proprioception exercises.
F. Return to play considered when:
    1. Pain-free through 120° of flexion.
    2. Pain-free with rehabilitation activities as outlined above.
    3. Strength within 90% of uninjured leg.
    4. Additional thigh padding recommended to prevent recurrent injury.
G. Complications.
    1. Myositis ossificans (MO).
        a. Osteoblasts replace fibroblasts in the residual hematoma, causing new bone formation (Figure 11-6).
            i. Begins one week following the injury.
            ii. Radiographic appearance of MO may be present in as early as three weeks.
        b. Signs and symptoms include:
            i. Pain.
            ii. Palpable lump.
            iii. Decreased flexibility.
            iv. Decreased strength.

AXIAL INJURIES

Sportsman's Hernia

A. The very existence of this injury is controversial, due to lack of a clinically palpable hernia.
B. Most commonly encountered in ice hockey and soccer players.
C. Lower abdominal wall, inguinal canal anatomy.

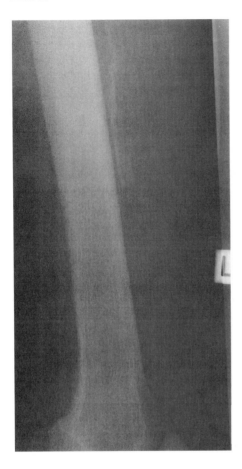

   1. Anterior wall
     a. External oblique aponeurosis.
     b. Internal oblique muscle.
   2. Posterior wall.
     a. Fascia transversalis.
     b. Conjoined tendon.
D. Pathology noted at time of repair of sportsman's hernia is variable depending upon report.
   1. Tear of external oblique aponeurosis is universal to all reports of sportsman's hernia.
   2. Other pathologies reported include:
     a. Conjoined tendon damage.
     b. Fascia transversalis weakness.
     c. Rectus abdominis tears.
     d. Ilioinguinal nerve entrapment.

E. The main complaint of athletes with sportsman's hernia is pain.
  1. Noted in lower abdomen/groin region but may present in hip or scrotum.
    a. Pain is worsened by vigorous activity that requires combinations of hip motion.
    b. Relieved by rest.
  2. Typically unilateral but can be bilateral.
  3. Often present for months prior to initial evaluation.
    a. Many athletes have already tried to treat self for "groin strain."
      i. Avoidance of inciting activity.
      ii. Heat.
      iii. Massage.
      iv. Adductor and hip flexor stretching.
    b. Pain is often reduced during self-rehabilitation but returns upon return to sport activity.
  4. Discomfort may be noted with cough, sneeze, or other activities that cause increased intraabdominal pressure.
F. Physical examination findings are subtle at best and may include:
  1. Discomfort with resisted hip adduction.
  2. Vague discomfort to palpation of inguinal region.
  3. No palpable hernia.
    a. Tender, slightly dilated superficial inguinal ring.
      i. More uncomfortable on the index side.
      ii. Cough impulse may be prominent.
  4. The most important role of the physical examination is to rule out other pathologies.
G. Diagnostic studies are typically negative.
  1. X-rays should be obtained but are typically negative.
  2. Bone scan is helpful to rule out osteitis pubis and pubic ramus stress fracture.
    a. Sportsman's hernia may be present along with these other problems.
  3. CT not typically necessary; should be obtained only if suspicion high for other pathologies.
  4. MRI may be obtained to look for specific soft-tissue pathologies but is usually negative.
    a. Performing the MRI with the patient in a prone position may make a sportsman's hernia easier to identify by increasing the pressure imparted to the anterior abdominal wall.
  5. EMG is considered to rule out nerve entrapment disorders.
    a. Obturator nerve entrapment.
    b. Ilioinguinal nerve entrapment.
  6. Herniography may be positive.

H. Treatment.
    1. Definitive treatment is surgical repair.
    2. Conservative measures should be considered in certain circumstances:
        a. The diagnosis is in question.
        b. Late in the season.
            i. Postoperative recovery (return to play) may take 8–12 weeks.
            ii. Conservative treatment may allow the player to complete the season prior to surgical repair without significantly worsening the condition.
        c. Conservative treatments include:
            i. Relative rest.
            ii. Activity modification.
            iii. Core flexibility and strengthening.
            iv. One of the hallmarks of this process is that despite appropriate conservative treatment, symptoms recur with return to vigorous activity.
    3. 1998 report of sportsman's hernia in 11 NHL players.
        a. Pathology.
            i. Torn external oblique aponeurosis/muscle.
            ii. Ilioinguinal nerve entrapment.
        b. 100% returned to play within 12 weeks after surgical repair.
    4. 2000 report of 157 subjects (recreational to pro athletes).
        a. Pathology.
            i. Torn external oblique aponeurosis.
            ii. Rectus abdominis injury.
               • Thinning (17%).
               • Tear (6%).
               • Hematoma (11%).
        b. 96.8% returned to former level of play after surgical repair.

Spinal Injury

A. Prior to 1980, spinal injuries in ice hockey were seldom reported. The incidence increased through the 1980s and early 1990s.
    1. From 1982 to 1993, reports from Canada, the United States, and Europe showed an average of 16.8 cases of hockey-related spinal injury per year.
        a. Data included fractures and/or dislocations with or without spinal cord or nerve root injury.
        b. Sprains, strains, and whiplash-type injuries and transient neurological injuries without spinal damage were not recorded.

      c. Majority of injured players were male (97.1%).

      d. Mean age of injured players was 20.7 years (median 18 years).

         i. 51.9% age 16–20 years.

         ii. 17.5% age 11–15 years.

      e. 89.1% of cases involved the cervical spine.

         i. C5-C6 was the most common level injured (19%).

         ii. 2.8% thoracic.

         iii. 4.7% thoracolumbar.

         iv. 3.3% lumbosacral.

  2. From 1966 to 1996, the Canadian registry of spinal injuries from ice hockey reported 14 cases per year average (same inclusion criteria as noted above).

      a. 12.75% of cases (31/243) reported prior to 1981.

         i. 38.7% of these injuries were severe (12/31).

      b. Of the 212 cases of injury after 1981, 24% (51/212) were considered severe.

B. Mechanism of injury.

  1. Most commonly a check from behind into the boards.

      a. Neck flexes slightly, creating a segmented column as axial load is applied to the head.

      b. Accounts for 36.6–50% of cases for which mechanism is known.

  2. Other, less common mechanisms of injury include:

      a. Direct contact with another player.

      b. Tripping on ice, sliding headfirst into the boards.

      c. Check or push, not from behind, causing player to slide into boards.

      d. Tripped by an opponent, striking head into the boards.

  3. Overall, contact with the boards accounts for > 70% of the severe spinal injuries.

  4. The vast majority of injuries take place in a game setting.

C. Hockey governing bodies have made an attempt to decrease the incidence of spinal injury. Although the incidence has not changed through the years, the number of severe injuries (permanent neurological injury) has seemingly decreased. Reduction measures have included:

  1. Mandatory helmet use at all levels of play. Facial protection options exist. It has been postulated that use of full facial protection increases the risk of spinal injury due to a false sense of invincibility.

      a. Players wearing full shields have not been shown to have a higher incidence of spinal injury compared to those wearing half-shields.

    b. Full-shield use significantly reduces the risk of ocular injury, facial laceration, and dental trauma.
2. Rule changes making it illegal to check from behind. Strict enforcement of this rule is critical.
3. Educating coaches and players of the dangers of checking from behind.

Immobilization of the C-Spine-Injured Athlete

A. Follow BLS guidelines; ABCs are first priority.
B. Cervical spine immobilization and spine board use are necessary for transport. *The athlete should be boarded with the helmet and shoulder pads intact.*
    1. It has been determined that removal of the hockey helmet for C-spine immobilization leads to a significant increase in sub-axial (C2-C7) cervical lordosis compared to leaving helmet and shoulder pads intact ($p < 0.003$).
        a. The majority of this motion is at the C6-C7 level.
    2. There is a chance for head motion within the helmet after immobilization, but this is not considered to be excessive.
        a. $5.54°$ of motion compared to $4.88°$ of motion in a football helmet ($p > 0.05$).
    3. Hockey face masks can be easily removed or flipped up to allow for airway access.
C. The above recommendations are based on studies of helmeted players. It does not extend to goalies who wear face masks, as the mask itself would have to be removed to allow airway access.

After immobilization, transport to an appropriate medical facility for definitive workup and treatment is necessary.
A. Neurosurgery or orthopedic spine surgery consultation should be obtained immediately if fracture or cord injury is present.

Suggested Readings

Andersen K, Jensen PO, Lauritzen J. Treatment of clavicular fractures: Figure-of-eight bandage versus a simple sling. *Acta Orthop Scand* 1987;58:71–74.

Ardèvol J, Henríquez A. Hook of the hamate nonunion: Suspicion of stress-induced mechanism in a hockey player. *Knee Surg, Sports Traumatol, Arthrosc* 2002;10:61–63.

Arnett MG. Effects of specificity training on the recovery process during inter-mittent activity in ice hockey. *J Strength Cond Res* 1996;10:124.

Aubry M, Cantu R, Dvorak J, et al. Summary and agreement statement of the first international symposium on concussion in sport, Vienna, 2001. *CJSM* 2002;12(1):6–11.

Baker PK, Fagan CD. Determination of a physiological profile for female ice hockey players. *Can J Appl Physiol* 1998;5:476 (Abstract).

Beaulieu S, Leclerc Y. Ulnar periostitis due to stress in hockey players. *AJSM* 2000;28(5):746–47.

Bell G, Game A, Voaklander D, Draper H, Syrotuik D. The relationship between Vo$_2$max, pulmonary function, and oxyhemoglobin saturation in female varsity hockey players. *Can J Appl Physiol* 1999;24:427 (Abstract).

Benson BW, Mohtadi NG, Rose MS, Meeuwisse WH. Head and neck injuries among ice hockey players wearing full face shields vs. half face shields. *JAMA* 1999;282(24):2328–32.

Benson BW, Rose MS, Meeuwisse WH. The impact of face shield use on concussions in ice hockey: A multivariate analysis. *Br J Sports Med* 2002;36:27–32.

Biasca N, Simmen H-P, Bartolozzi AR, Trentz O. Review of typical ice hockey injuries: Survey of the North American NHL and Hockey Canada versus European leagues. *Unfallchirurg* 1995;98:283–88.

Bracko MR. High-performance skating for hockey. *Pulse* 1999;13:13.

Bracko MR. On-ice performance characteristics of elite and non-elite female ice hockey players. *J Strength Cond Res* 2001;15:42.

Bracko MR, Fellingham GW. Comparison of physical performance characteristics of female and male ice hockey players. *Ped Ex Sci* 2001;13:26.

Bracko MR, Geithner CA. Effect of a season of play on young female ice hockey players. *Med Sci Sports Exerc* 2000;32:S216 (Abstract).

Bracko MR, George JD. Prediction of ice skating performance with off-ice testing in women's ice hockey players. *J Strength Cond Res* 2001;15:116.

Bracko MR, Hall LT, Fisher AG, Fellingham GW, Cryer W. Performance skating characteristics of professional ice hockey forwards. *Sports Med Training Rehab* 1998;8:251–63.

Craig EV. Fractures of the clavicle. In: Rockwood CA, Green DP, Bucholz RW, Heckman JD, eds. *Rockwood and Green's Fractures in Adults*. 4th ed. Philadelphia, PA: Lippincott-Raven; 1996.

Dryden DM, Francescutti LH, Rowe BH, et al. Epidemiology of women's recreational ice hockey injuries. *MSSE* 2000;32(8):1378–83.

Echemendia RJ, Putukian M, Mackin RS, et al. Neuropsychological test performance prior to and following sports-related mild traumatic brain injury. *CJSM* 2001;11(1):23–31.

Emery CA, Meeuwisse WH. Risk factors for groin injuries in hockey. *MSSE* 2001;33(9):1423–33.

Emery CA, Meeuwisse WH, Powell JW. Groin and abdominal strain injuries in the National Hockey League. *CJSM* 1999;9(3):151–56.

Frelinger DP. The ruptured spleen in college athletes: A preliminary report. *J Am Coll Health Assoc* 1973;26:216.

Geithner CA, Bracko MR. Somatic profile of female ice hockey players. *Ped Ex Sci* 2001a;13:93 (Abstract).

Geithner CA, Bracko MR. Growth, maturity status, and fitness characteristics of young female ice hockey players. *Ped Ex Sci* 2001b;13:308 (Abstract).

Goodman D, Gaetz M, Meichenbaum D. Concussions in hockey: There is cause for concern. *MSSE* 2001;33(12):2004–9.

Green JP, Grenier SE, McGill SM. Low-back stiffness is altered with warmup and bench rest: Implications for athletes. *Med Sci Sports Exerc* 2002; 34:1076.

Gröger A. Ten years of ice hockey–related injuries in the German Ice Hockey Federation: A ten-year prospective study/523 international games. *Sportverl Sportschad* 2001;15:82–86.

Grossman S, Hines T. National Hockey League players from North America are more violent than those from Europe. *Percept Mot Skills* 1996;83: 589–90.

Hache A. *The Physics of Hockey.* Vancouver, BC: Raincoast Books; 2002.

Kaiser PK, Pineda R 2nd. A study of topical nonsteroidal antiinflammatory drops and no pressure patching in the treatment of corneal abrasions: Corneal Abrasion Patching Study Group. *Ophthalmology* 1997;194(8): 1353–59.

Kirkpatrick HN, Hoh HB, Cook SD. No eye pad for corneal abrasion. *Eye* 1993;7:468–71.

Lacroix VJ, Kinnear DG, Mulder DS, Brown RA. Lower abdominal pain syndrome in National Hockey League players: A report of 11 cases. *Clin J Sport Med* 1998;8(1):5–9.

Lahti H, Sane J, Ylipaavalniemi P. Dental injuries in ice hockey games and training. *MSSE* 2002;34(3):400–2.

LaPrade RF, Burnett QM, Zaraour R, Moss R. The effect of the mandatory use of face masks on facial lacerations and head and neck injuries in ice hockey: A prospective study. *AJSM* 1995;23(6):773–75.

LaPrade RF, Schnetzler KA, Broxterman RJ, et al. Cervical spine alignment in the immobilized ice hockey player: A computed tomographic analysis of the effects of helmet removal. *AJSM* 2000;28(6):800–3.

Lateef F. Commotio cordis: An underappreciated cause of sudden death in athletes. *Sports Med* 2000;30(4):301–8.

Lau S, Berg K, Latin RW, et al. Comparison of active and passive recovery of blood lactate and subsequent performance of repeated work bouts in ice hockey players. *J Strength Cond Res* 2001;15:367.

Leite J. Measuring the effects of lightweight pucks in women's hockey. Canadian Hockey Association. Presentation at Hockey Development Council Meeting, Regina, Canada, May 2001.

Lemos MJ. The evaluation and treatment of the injured acromioclavicular joint in athletes. *AJSM* 1998;26(1):137–44.

Link MS, Maron BJ, VanderBrink BA, et al. Impact directly over the cardiac silhouette is necessary to produce ventricular fibrillation in an experimental model of commotio cordis. *J Am Coll Cardiol* 2001;37(2):649–54.

MacDonald PB, Strange G, Hodgkinson R, Dyck M. Injuries to the peroneal nerve in professional hockey. *CJSM* 2002;12(1):39–40.

Maki DG, Reich RM. Infectious mononucleosis in the athlete: Diagnosis, complications and management. *AJSM* 1982;10(3):163–73.

Maron BJ, Gohman TE, Kyle SB, et al. Clinical profile and spectrum of commotio cordis. *JAMA* 2002;287(9):1142–46.

Maroon JC, Lovell MR, Norwig J, et al. Cerebral concussion in athletes: Evaluation and neuropsychological testing. *Neurosurgery* 2000;47(3): 659–72.

McArdle WD, Katch FI, Katch VI. *Exercise Physiology: Energy, Nutrition, and Human Performance.* Baltimore, MD: Williams & Wilkins; 1996.

Meyers WC, Foley DP, Garrett WE, et al. Management of severe lower abdominal or inguinal pain in high-performance athletes. *AJSM* 2000;28(1):2–8.

Moeller JL, Monroe J, McKeag DB. Cryotherapy-induced common peroneal nerve palsy. *CJSM* 1997;7(3):212–16.

Möhrenschlager M, Seidl HP, Schnopp C, et al. Professional ice hockey players: A high-risk group for fungal infection of the foot? *Dermatology* 2001;203:271.

Mölsä J, Kujala U, Näsman O, et al. Injury profile in ice hockey from the 1970s through the 1990s in Finland. *AJSM* 2000;28(3):322–27.

Mölsä JJ, Tegner Y, Alaranta H, et al. Spinal cord injuries in ice hockey in Finland and Sweden from 1980 to 1996. *Int J Sports Med* 1999;20:64–67.

Napier SM, Baker RS, Sanford DG, Easterbrook M. Eye injuries in athletics and recreation. *Surv Ophthalmol* 1996;41(3):229–44.

Newsome PRH, Tran DC, Cooke MS. The role of the mouthguard in the prevention of sports-related dental injuries: A review. *Int J Pediatr Dent* 2001;11:396–404.

Pashby T. Saving sight in sports. *Can J Ophthalmol* 2000;35(4):181–82.

Roberts WO. Field care of the injured tooth. *Phys Sportsmed* 2000;28(1):101–2.

Roberts WO, Brust JD, Leonard B, Hebert BJ. Fair-play rules and injury reduction in ice hockey. *Arch Pediatr Adolesc Med* 1996;150:140–45.

Rockwood CA, Williams GR, Young DC. Injuries to the acromioclavicular joint. In: Rockwood CA, Green DP, Bucholz RW, Heckman JD, eds. *Rockwood and Green's Fractures in Adults.* 4th ed. Philadelphia, PA: Lippincott-Raven; 1996.

Rundell KW, Jenkinson DM. Exercise-induced bronchospasm in the elite athlete. *Sports Med* 2002;32:583.

Sanders JO, Rockwood CA, Curtis RJ. Fractures and dislocations of the humeral shaft and shoulder. In: Rockwood CA, Wilkins KE, Beaty JH, eds. *Rockwood and Green's Fractures in Children.* 4th ed. Philadelphia, PA: Lippincott-Raven; 1996.

Schlegel TF, Burks RT, Marcus RL, Dunn HK. A prospective evaluation of untreated acute grade III acromioclavicular separations. *AJSM* 2001;29(6):699–703.

Shevell M, Stewart J. Laceration of the common peroneal nerve by a skate blade. *Can Med Assoc J* 1988;139:311–12.

Stuart MJ, Smith A. Injuries in Junior A ice hockey: A three-year prospective study. *AJSM* 1995;23(4):458–61.

Stuart MJ, Smith AM, Malo-Ortiguera SA, et al. A comparison of facial protection and the incidence of head, neck, and facial injuries in Junior A hockey players: A function of individual playing time. *AJSM* 2002;30(1): 39–44.

Stuart MJ, Smith AM, Nieva JJ, Rock MG. Injuries in youth ice hockey: A pilot surveillance strategy. *Mayo Clin Proc* 1995;70:350–56.

Tator CH, Carson JD, Cushman R. Hockey injuries of the spine in Canada, 1966–1996. *CMAJ* 2000;162(6):787–88.

Tator CH, Carson JD, Edmonds VE. New spinal injuries in hockey. *CJSM* 1997;7(1):17–21.

Torok PG, Mader TH. Corneal abrasions: Diagnosis and management. *Am Fam Physician* 1996;53(8):2521–29.

Tyler TF, Nicholas SJ, Campbell RJ, McHugh MP. The association of hip strength and flexibility with the incidence of adductor muscle strains in professional ice hockey players. *AJSM* 2001;29(2):124–28.

Tyler TF, Nicholas SJ, Campbell RJ, et al. The effectiveness of a preseason exercise program to prevent adductor muscle strains in professional ice hockey players. *AJSM* 2002;30(5):680–83.

Viano DC, Bir CA, Cheney BA, Janda DH. Prevention of commotio cordis in baseball: An evaluation of chest protectors. *J Trauma* 2000;49(6):1023–28.

Voaklander DC, Saunders LD, Quinney HA, Macnab RBJ. Epidemiology of recreational and old-timer ice hockey injuries. *CJSM* 1996;60(1):15–21.

Waninger KN, Richards JG, Pan WT, et al. An evaluation of head movement in backboard-immobilized helmeted football, lacrosse, and ice hockey players. *CJSM* 2001;11(2):82–86.

Yap JJL, Curl LA, Kvitne RS, McFarland EG. The value of weighted views of the acromioclavicular joint: Results of a survey. *AJSM* 1999;27(6):806–9.

12

FIGURE SKATING

James L. Moeller
Sami F. Rifat
Ann Snyder

GENERAL INFORMATION

History

A. Origins of the sport as we know it today are linked to the American Jackson Haines in the late 1800s.
    1. Haines introduced dance elements and artistry to what had been a somewhat stiff and rigid sport.
    2. In the beginning, programs consisted primarily of footwork maneuvers, spins, and low-level jumping.

B. Figure skating as an Olympic sport.
    1. Men's singles and pairs competition introduced in 1908 at the London Summer Games.
        a. Did not appear in 1912.
        b. Returned in 1920 at the Antwerp Summer Games.
        c. Moved to Winter Games in 1924 (Chamonix).
    2. Women's singles competition introduced in 1920 at the Antwerp Summer Games.
        a. Moved to Winter Games in 1924 (Chamonix).
    3. Ice dancing competition introduced in 1976 at the Innsbruck Winter Games.

Injury Statistics

A. Incidence of injury in figure skating is approximately 1.4 per 1000 hours of skating, which is relatively low compared to other sports.

B. 56% of the injuries are acute in nature while 44% are chronic or of the overuse variety.

C. Pairs skating has a higher rate of injury than the other skating disciplines.

    1. Lifts and throws predispose the female skater to falls (Figure 12-1).

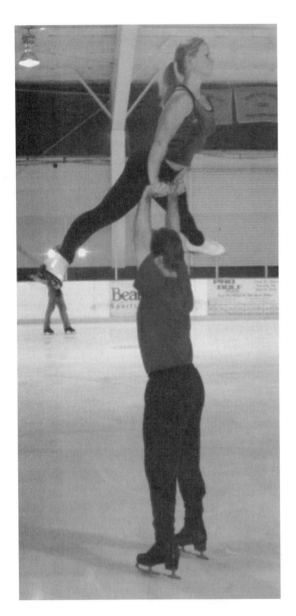

FIGURE 12-1 Pairs team demonstrating a common lift. Photo courtesy of James L. Moeller, MD.

2. May lead to impacts of up to six times body weight.
3. When a pair falls out of a lift, the female skater may fall from heights of over 6 feet.
D. The risk of collision is highest in precision skating.

Competitive Categories

The United States Figure Skating Association (USFSA) has established four distinct disciplines in skating.
A. Singles free skating.
 1. Men and women participate.
 2. Divided into two parts.
  a. Short program (formerly called the original or technical program).
   i. Skaters must execute 8 required elements (Table 12-1).
   ii. Deductions for failures or falls.
  b. Free (long) skate.
   i. No required elements.
   ii. Falling or omitting element(s) counts against skater by reducing overall difficulty.
B. Pairs skating.
 1. Male and female partners perform a short and long program to music as in singles.
 2. Due to the nature of the lifts and throws, this discipline requires a strong male partner and a relatively lightweight female partner.
C. Ice dancing.
 1. Male and female partners perform complex routines to different types of music.
 2. Competition consists of two compulsory dances, an original dance, and a freestyle dance.
 3. Ice dancing is the discipline that remains closest to its original form; however, the physical demands of ice dancing continue to heighten with more innovative and athletic programs.
 4. Ice dancers attempt to demonstrate their full range of technical skills by utilizing changes in position, varied dance holds, and difficult footwork. Contrary to pairs skating, ice dancers utilize small lifts and do not perform jumps.
D. Precision (team) skating.
 1. Large groups (approximately 20) of skaters are on the ice at one time.
 2. The skaters perform synchronized, choreographed, complex movements that involve footwork and intricate close connecting moves.

TABLE 12-1

Required elements of short program.

Men	Women	Pairs
Double or triple Axel	Double Axel	Overhead lift
Triple or quadruple jump preceded by connecting steps	Double or triple jump preceded by connecting steps	Double twist
A combination of a double jump and a triple jump with a triple or quadruple jump	A combination of a double jump and a triple jump or two triple jumps, without intervening steps	Side-by-side double or triple jumps
A flying spin; the flying position must be achieved in the air and the skater must do at least 8 rotations in spinning position	A flying spin; the flying position must be achieved in the air and the skater must do at least 8 rotations in spinning position	Side-by-side spin combinations, with a change of foot, at least one change of position, and at least 5 rotations on each foot
A camel spin or sit spin with a change of foot; at least 6 rotations on each foot	A layback spin; at least 8 rotations in layback position	Pair spin combination with a change of foot and at least one change in position and at least 8 rotations in all
A spin combination with a change of foot and at least two changes of position; the spin must include camel, sit, and upright positions, and there must be at least 6 rotations	A spin combination with a change of foot and at least two changes of position; the spin must include camel, sit, and upright positions, and there must be at least 6 rotations	Death spiral
Step sequence	A spiral step sequence	A step sequence or a spiral step sequence
Another (different) step sequence	Another step sequence	A double or triple throw jump

3. There are no jumps or spins.
4. Precision skating is not an Olympic sport.

Special Considerations and Demographics

A. Many figure skaters begin lessons at a very young age and by age 13 they may be competing at the national or international level. Therefore, the physician caring for figure skating athletes has to be cognizant of several factors including:
1. Growth and development.
2. Nutrition.
3. Social and psychological factors.
4. Pediatric and adolescent medical concerns.
B. Practices typically involve long hours both on and off ice and include not only skating but dance, choreography, and weight training.
C. Ice rink conditions may not be optimal for the health and performance of the skater due to cold temperatures, poor ventilation, and potentially poor air quality.
1. For a complete discussion of cold injury and cold-weather physiology, see Chapters 1 to 3.
2. Carbon monoxide (CO) and nitrogen dioxide (NO_2) exposure produced by the ice-resurfacing machine.
   a. Symptoms of CO poisoning include: headache, nausea, vomiting, weakness, tachypnea, and incoordination.
   b. Symptoms of NO_2 poisoning include: cough, hemoptysis, dyspnea, chest pain, sweating, nausea, dehydration, weakness, and anxiety.

PHYSIOLOGY AND BIOMECHANICS

Skating Techniques

A. Stroking skills.
1. Actions in propulsive muscles include hip extension and abduction, knee extension, and ankle plantar flexion, while stabilization occurs in the trunk and gliding leg.
2. Different ways to traverse the ice surface:
   a. Power stroking: Explosive push off the ice to quickly traverse the ice.
   b. Glides: Traversing the ice via the momentum of a previous stroke—no additional movement may be done on one or both feet.
   c. Sculling: Traversing the ice without lifting either foot.

  B. Stops.

     1. Performed by pressing the skate blade downward against the ice.

     2. May be accomplished single- or double-footed.

     3. Various styles.

       a. T-stop: Back foot placed perpendicular to lead foot.

       b. Snow plow: Skates in chevron position.

       c. Hockey-style stop: Skates are parallel to one another, then suddenly turned perpendicular to direction of motion.

  C. Crossovers—used to go around the corners of an ice rink.

     1. One foot lifted and placed over the other; can be performed with either foot and in either direction.

     2. Actions in propulsive muscles include hip extension and abduction, knee extension, and ankle plantar flexion, while stabilization occurs in the trunk and gliding leg.

  D. Spirals—arms out to the side, trunk bent forward to 90° from the legs, and one leg is lifted behind slowly.

     1. Requiring control, balance, and flexibility.

     2. Stabilization occurs in the trunk and upper and lower extremities.

  E. Turns—performed by both feet and in both directions.

     1. Usually performed to connect skills.

     2. Actions in propulsive muscles include hip extension and abduction, knee extension, and ankle plantar flexion.

  F. Spins.

     1. Rotations over a single spot; spins should be centered and controlled with good velocity.

       a. Stabilization occurs in the trunk, with propulsion occurring with the upper and lower extremities.

       b. Forward spins occur on the back inside edge, while backward spins occur on back outside edge of the opposite foot.

     2. Types of spins.

       a. Upright spins.

         i. Two-footed spin—usually the first spin learned. Head should be up with body erect and arms pulled in across the chest.

         ii. One-footed spin—usually performed on right foot with left foot resting at knee level.

         iii. Forward open spin—similar to one-footed spin, except that the free leg is held out to the side rather than bent, with the foot and knee level.

         iv. Back open spin—similar to forward spin, but performed on the back outside edge of right skate.

      v. Forward scratch spin—similar to one-footed spin, except after a few revolutions the free foot crosses the skating foot and rests on the outside of the skating foot.

      vi. Backward scratch spin—performed on the back outside edge of the right foot, opposite that of the forward scratch spin.

      vii. Cross-foot spin—performed on two feet with the left foot in front of the right foot and the toes pointed toward each other.

  b. Sit spins.

      i. Forward sit spin—a forward shoot-the-duck in a spin.

      ii. Back sit spin—same as forward sit spin, but performed on the opposite foot.

  c. Camel spins—adaptations from the front camel occur in how the skate is grasped and include: catch-foot camel, curly camel, and back camel.

  d. Layback spins (Figure 12-2).

      i. Layback spin—performed on one foot as the body bends back and the arms are gracefully placed overhead.

      ii. Biellmann—a combination of a catch-foot camel and a layback spin as the skater pulls the free foot over his/her head, ending in a near split position on one foot.

  e. Flying spins.

      i. Flying camel—an upward jump from the left outer edge that lands in a back camel spin.

      ii. Flying sit spin—an upward jump from the left outer edge that ends in a sitting position before the body lands and continues the spin.

G. Jumps.

  1. Takeoff and landing generally occur on the strongest leg. Rhythm and timing of all body parts is important.

    a. At takeoff the propulsive actions are hip and knee extension and ankle plantar flexion.

    b. Trunk stability occurs throughout with hip flexion, knee flexion, and ankle dorsiflexion occurring during landing.

    c. Jumps are generally considered to be the most important component of a skating routine.

  2. Types of jumps.

    a. Edge jumps—bunny hops, waltz jump, Axel, Salchow, loop, Walley.

    b. Toe jumps—split, flip, toe loop, Lutz, toe Walley, stag jump.

    c. Jumps that take off and land on same foot—loop, flip, Lutz.

    d. Jumps that change feet—bunny hop, waltz jump, Axel, Salchow, toe loop.

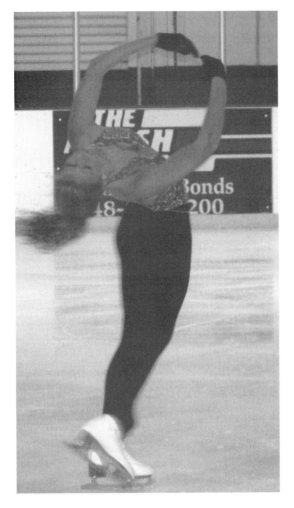

FIGURE 12-2
Position for a layback spin. The extreme spine extension position may put skaters at risk for specific injuries including spondylolysis. Photo courtesy of James L. Moeller, MD.

3. Descriptions of jumps.
   a. Bunny hop—a skip performed on skates.
   b. Waltz jump—a half turn in the air, such that takeoff is from the left outer edge and landing is on the right outer edge.
   c. Salchow—similar to the waltz jump, except that a full revolution occurs and it begins on the back inner edge and ends on the back outer edge.
   d. Loop—begins and ends on the right back outer edge with a full revolution occurring in between.

   e. Walley—begins from the right back inner edge and ends on the right back outer edge with a full revolution occurring in between.
   f. Axel—begins from the right forward outer edge and ends on the right back outer edge with one and a half revolutions occurring in between.
   g. Split—begins from the left back inner edge and ends on the left toe, with one half revolution in the air.
   h. Stag—similar to the split, except that the front leg is bent in a stag position.
   i. Toe loop—begins from the right back outer edge and ends with the right back outer edge with one revolution in between.
   j. Flip—begins from the left back inner edge and ends on the right back outer edge with one revolution in between.
   k. Lutz—similar to the flip, except that it begins from the left back outer edge rather than the left back inner edge.

Physiologic Demands

A. The skating program is performed at an intensity that elicits a heart rate of approximately 92% of maximal values.
B. Greater heart rate observed as skills increase in difficulty.

Characteristics of Elite Figure Skaters

These are averages based on collected data and in no way serve as recommendations or absolutes.
A. Males.
   1. 167–173 cm tall.
   2. 60–66 kg in weight.
   3. 5–9% body fat.
   4. Unremarkable maximal aerobic power ($\approx$ 60 mL/kg/min).
B. Females.
   1. 158–161 cm tall.
   2. 49–51 kg in weight.
   3. 9–12% body fat.
   4. Unremarkable maximal aerobic power ($\approx$ 50 mL/kg/min).

Typical Training Practices of Elite Figure Skaters

A. 30–33 hours/week of training.
   1. Approximately 27 hours/week performing on-ice activities (82%).

   2. Approximately 5.8 hours/week spent completing strength and aerobic activities (17%).

   3. Approximately 0.2 hours/week doing preskating warm-up (1%).

Recommended Exercise and Conditioning Practices

A. On-ice training.

   1. Stress skill work, yet allow sufficient recovery (through use of other training methods) so that highly technical skills can be performed on the ice.

   2. Muscular strength should not be gained primarily on the ice as has been the rule in the past.

   3. Needs to incorporate an appropriate warm-up where low-intensity activity is performed until the body actually becomes warm (usually shown by sweating).

   4. Following on-ice exercise, a cool-down should be performed of low-intensity exercise to facilitate the body returning to homeostasis, especially the flow of the blood.

B. Resistance training.

   1. Muscular strength and power are important to a figure skater as a higher jump may produce greater scores for technical merit.

     a. Significant relationships have been found between maximal knee extension force and jump height for the single and double Axel.

       i. Knee extension accounts for 78% of the variance in the jumps.

     b. Off-ice training has been shown to increase not only muscular strength but also aerobic ability.

   2. Recommended resistance training schedule.

     a. Frequency: 2–3 sessions per week.

     b. Duration: 45–50 minutes per session.

     c. Intensity:

       i. 3 sets of 8–12 repetitions.

       ii. Increase weight when > 12 repetitions can be performed.

       iii. Allow adequate rest between sets (approximately one minute).

     d. Recommended resistance training exercises (with major muscles involved) include:

       i. Hang pull—semimembranosus, semitendinosus, biceps femoris, vastus lateralis, vastus intermedius, vastus medialis, rectus femoris, gluteus maximus, gastrocenemius, soleus, trapezius.

      ii. Back squat—gluteus maximus, semimembranosus, semitendinosus, biceps femoris, vastus lateralis, vastus intermedius, vastus medialis, rectus femoris.

      iii. Bent-knee deadlift—gluteus maximus, semimembranosus, semitendinosus, biceps femoris, vastus lateralis, vastus intermedius, vastus medialis, rectus femoris.

      iv. Calf raise—soleus, gastrocnemius.

      v. Bench press—pectoralis major.

      vi. Push press—gluteus maximus, semimembranosus, semitendinosus, biceps femoris, vastus lateralis, vastus intermedius, rectus femoris, soleus, gastrocnemius, deltoids.

      vii. Bent-over rows—latissumus dorsi, teres major, middle trapezius, rhomboids.

      viii. Push-ups—pectoralis major, deltoids, triceps.

      ix. Abdominal crunches—rectus abdominis.

      x. Ankle rocker balances—gastrocnemius, soleus, tibialis.

C. Flexibility.
  1. Injury prevention.
    a. In an uninjured population, stretching activities have not been proven effective in reducing injuries.
  2. Required for performance of spirals and split jumps.
  3. Warm-up prior to performing stretching exercises; perform after skating or other exercise.
  4. Perform static stretches and hold each stretch for 15–30 seconds.
  5. Stretch all muscle groups used in skating and off-ice training.

D. Off-ice specific training.
  1. Many of the on-ice skills can be performed off-ice.
    a. Off-ice jump training can teach body awareness, coordination, and overall body control.
    b. Balance training can strengthen the muscles of the lower extremity while also enhancing motor ability and total body control.
    c. Sport cords can be used for off-ice training of jumps and spins.

E. Plyometric exercises.
  1. Used to train the nervous system to perform a forceful and/or quick muscular contraction.
  2. Exercises include:
    a. Jumping drills (from boxes or weighted ropes).
    b. Use of weighted belts or vests during normal activities.
    c. Medicine ball.
  3. Plyometric exercises result in eccentric contractions that can cause soreness and microscopic damage to the muscle.

    a. Should be performed in supervised setting when first trying these exercises (athletic trainer, physical therapist, certified personal trainer).

    b. Should only be performed by advanced athletes with sufficient recovery allowed following the exercise.

F. Cross-training.

    1. Aerobic ability, while not primarily used during the skating programs, is important so that training for the skating programs can be performed.

    2. Cross-training activities can enhance aerobic ability and give the athlete another type of activity to perform to alleviate boredom and reduce the risk of injuries. Common cross-training exercises include:

    a. Jogging.

    b. Cycling.

    c. In-line skating.

    d. Climbing events (upper body).

    e. Yoga and/or martial arts for flexibility.

G. Periodization.

    1. Training programs should be tailored to lead to the greatest performances at the top-level competitions.

    2. The yearly training program (macrocycle) should be broken into four mesocycles.

    a. Off-season.

       i. High volume.

       ii. Low intensity.

       iii. Activities:

- Off-ice aerobic training.
- Resistance training.
- On-ice stroking skills.

    b. Preseason.

       i. Volume decreases.

       ii. Intensity increases.

       iii. Activities:

- Continue off-ice aerobic training.
- Continue resistance training.
- More on-ice skill training including spins, jumps, and turns now that the skater is physiologically strong enough to perform them.

    c. Competition season.

       i. Volume decreases to its lowest level.

       ii. Intensity is at its highest.

- Practices may simulate competition.
- Competitions taking place.

    d. Recovery.
      i. Active rest.
      ii. Minimal on-ice activities.
      iii. Low-intensity cross-training exercises performed.
  3. The length of the different mesocycles will depend on the athlete, but the recovery mesocycle should be at least one month long.
    a. Each mesocycle can be further broken down into microcycles (typically a one-week block).
      i. Within each meso- and microcycle variations must occur in intensity and duration of the exercise (including recovery time).
      ii. Recovery days and weeks have to occur throughout the micro- and mesocycles in order for the body to adapt to the stresses placed upon it, allowing for athlete performance to be enhanced maximally.

Nutrition

A. Both male and female skaters have been observed to consume only about 80% of the calories that a typical sedentary person would consume.
  1. Regardless of mesocycle.
  2. Breakfast found to be a very low-carbohydrate meal with most skaters not consuming sufficient macro- or micronutrients.
B. Prolonged training on a daily basis depletes the body of glycogen stores.
  1. Figure skaters should follow the food pyramid and consume approximately 60% of their calories as carbohydrates.
  2. Consumption of approximately 300 kcals of carbohydrates within two hours post-exercise has been shown to enhance muscle glycogen resynthesis and is therefore recommended for figure skaters.
C. Fluids.
  1. Should be consumed every 20–30 minutes during training.
  2. Should be made available at all exercise and competition sites.
  3. Optimal fluid source.
    a. Plain water is an excellent fluid choice, especially for shorter-duration exercise sessions.
    b. A fluid source with up to 6% carbohydrate should be considered for longer-duration activity sessions.
  4. Monitoring of body weight before and after practice sessions can be used to detect weight loss due to dehydration.
  5. Any weight lost during the exercise session should be replenished with fluids prior to the next exercise session.

MEDICAL ISSUES

Eating Disorders

Figure skating is a unique winter sport in that it is judged not only on athletic ability but on aesthetic quality as well. This fact increases the potential for eating disorders among figure skating athletes.

A. Anorexia nervosa (AN).
  1. The prevalence of AN is about 1% in the adolescent and young adult female population; however, the prevalence of disordered eating is higher in figure skating athletes.
  2. Diagnostic criteria for AN:
    a. Refusal to maintain body weight at or above a minimally normal weight for age and height (85% of expected weight).
    b. Intense fear of gaining weight or becoming fat, even though the patient is underweight.
    c. Altered body image.
    d. Amenorrhea in post-menarchal females.
B. Bulimia nervosa (BN).
  1. Prevalence in the general population is 1–3%; however, as in the case of AN, the incidence of BN in young female and male skaters is difficult to determine.
  2. Diagnostic criteria.
    a. Recurrent episodes of binge eating characterized by eating a larger than "normal" amount of food in a discrete period of time and a sense of lack of control over eating during the episodes.
    b. Recurrent inappropriate compensatory behavior in order to prevent weight gain (e.g., self-induced vomiting, laxative use, etc.).
    c. The above activities occur, on average, at least twice weekly for three months.
    d. Self-evaluation is unduly influenced by body shape and weight.
    e. The disturbance does not occur exclusively during episodes of AN.
  3. Characteristics of athletes at risk for eating disorders.
    a. Participation in a subjectively judged sport.
    b. Perfectionist.
    c. Overachiever.
      i. A "minor" comment from a coach or parent (e.g., "that dress looks a little tight") may cause a young skater to experience feelings of self-doubt and fear of losing acceptance in the sport because his/her weight is outside of an acceptable range.

4. Treatment.
   a. AN and BN should be considered potentially life-threatening conditions. Treatment needs to be started immediately and aggressively.
   b. Nutritional and overall health assessment should be performed.
   c. Behavioral therapy and nutritional interventions should be initiated as part of a multidisciplinary approach to treatment.

Menstrual Irregularities

A. Young female athletes commonly experience menstrual irregularities. Menstrual abnormalities may be seen as an isolated entity or may be associated with eating disorders and osteoporosis.
   1. Amenorrheic athletes have a decreased leutinizing hormone (LH) surge at mid-cycle due to decreases in gonadotropin-releasing hormone (GnRH) pulse generation in the hypothalamus.
   2. Peripheral aromatization of dihydroepiandrosterone is decreased compared to the nonathletic population.
B. Delayed onset of menses (primary amenorrhea) is frequently seen in young female figure skaters.
   1. Primary amenorrhea is defined as failure of onset of menses by the age of 16 years.
      a. Menarche is often delayed in athletes but the reason(s) for this have not fully been determined.
         i. May be due in part to decreased body weight and/or decreased body fat percentage noted in many young female skaters.
   2. Secondary amenorrhea is the cessation of previously established menses. This is very common in athletes, especially as frequency, intensity, and duration of participation increases.
      a. Secondary amenorrhea in an athlete that corresponds to training increases is often assumed to be "athletic amenorrhea."
         i. If spontaneous return of menses occurs with decreases in training, no further workup is considered necessary.
C. Workup of menstrual irregularities begins with a detailed medical and menstrual history.
D. Physical examination should include sexual maturity staging and a thorough genitourinary examination.

1. Secondary sex characteristics may or may not be present.
   a. If secondary sex characteristics are present, consider an anovulatory process such as polycystic ovary disease.
   b. If secondary sex characteristics are absent, gonadal dysgenesis, adrenal enzyme, and hypothalamic-pituitary disorders should be considered.
E. Laboratory evaluation.
   1. Rule out pregnancy either with urine or serum pregnancy test.
   2. Thyroid-stimulating hormone and prolactin levels are drawn as part of the initial workup to rule out thyroid disease and hyperprolactinemia.
   3. Follicle-stimulating hormone and LH hormone levels can be considered but are often obtained, if necessary, at a later stage in the workup.
F. Progestin challenge test.
   1. Medroxyprogesterone 10 mg administered daily for five days.
      a. Withdrawal bleeding occurring 2–5 days later indicates adequate levels of circulating estrogen and no outflow obstruction.
      b. No withdrawal bleeding indicates inadequate estrogen levels or outflow track obstruction.
         i. At this time, FSH and LH should be obtained if not done previously.
            • Premature ovarian failure is associated with increased FSH and LH levels.
            • Hypothalamic or pituitary dysfunction is associated with normal or decreased FSH and LH levels.
G. Treatment.
   1. Anovulatory, normal estrogen level patients are treated with progesterone to stimulate withdrawal bleeding.
      a. Hormone administration to cause menstruation every 3 months is considered adequate.
   2. Low-estrogen, amenorrheic patients need to be treated with estrogens and progesterone. This is usually accomplished in the form of an oral contraceptive pill (OCP).
   3. Patients with athletic amenorrhea may require OCP treatment if their training and amenorrhea last longer than three months. Other components of treatment may include:
      a. Decrease in training regimen (most athletes are not willing to change their training).
      b. Increase in body weight and/or body fat (most athletes are not willing to try this treatment idea either).

    c. Dietary changes.
      i. Increase total caloric intake.
      ii. Increase protein intake.
      iii. Maintain adequate calcium intake (1500 mg per day) to guard against bone mineral loss that may accompany a hypoestrogen state.

Female Athlete Triad

A. The triad consists of:
    1. Disordered eating.
      a. AN.
      b. BN.
    2. Menstrual irregularities.
      a. Oligomenorrhea.
      b. Amenorrhea.
    3. Osteoporosis.
      a. Develops secondary to:
        i. Hypoestrogen state.
        ii. Poor nutritional status.
      b. True osteoporosis is relatively rare; osteopenia is much more common and is now commonly recognized as the third arm of this triad.
B. Incidence of the triad is difficult to assess.
    1. Believed to be higher in judged sports.
      a. Figure skating.
      b. Gymnastics.
      c. Diving.
    2. May go undetected for a prolonged period of time.
      a. Athletes rarely present to sports doctors for evaluation of eating disorder or menstrual irregularities.
      b. Primary care providers often see young patients for menstrual irregularities but may be unaware of the female athlete triad.
C. Clinical suspicion needs to be high when a female athlete presents with an overuse bone injury such as periostitis or stress fracture.
    1. History should include:
      a. Location and timing of pain.
      b. Training information.
        i. Recent changes.
        ii. Frequency.
        iii. Intensity.
        iv. Duration.

    c. Dietary information.

    d. Menstrual history.

  2. If suspicion of female athlete triad exists, additional testing should be considered.

    a. Bone densitometry.

    b. Blood laboratories to evaluate the hypothalamic-pituitary-gonadal axis (see Menstrual Irregularities, E).

    c. 3- or 5-day dietary log.

D. Treatment is multifaceted including behavioral, nutritional, and medical interventions.

Concussion

A. Mild traumatic brain injury typically occurs due to direct head trauma. In figure skating, this is usually due to striking the head against the ice during a fall.

  1. A hard fall onto the buttocks may transmit significant enough force along the spinal column to the head, causing concussion.

  2. For a full discussion of concussion, see Chapter 11, Ice Hockey.

Exercise-Induced Bronchospasm

See Chapter 2, Pulmonary Physiology.

TRAUMATIC MUSCULOSKELETAL INJURIES

General

The great majority of acute injuries in figure skating occur as a result of falls. The majority of injuries involve the lower extremities though upper extremity and head injuries may occur as well.

Wrist Injuries

A. Wrist fractures are not uncommon and are typically due to falling onto an outstretched arm. Special attention must be paid to the scaphoid bone of the wrist.

  1. Scaphoid fractures are notorious for their occult nature (not readily seen on initial radiographs) and poor healing (especially proximal pole and displaced injuries).

  2. Suspicion of scaphoid fracture should prompt immobilization even if radiographs are negative.

  3. For a full discussion on scaphoid fractures, see Chapter 13, Speed Skating.

Olecranon Injuries

A. These injuries typically occur due to a fall directly onto a flexed elbow and may range in severity from a simple contusion to traumatic olecranon bursitis and even fracture.

  1. Any skater who falls directly onto the elbow and has pain on palpation should be considered to have a fracture until proven otherwise.

    a. A more indirect type of insult may result in fracture, such as when violent triceps muscle contraction is imparted on a partially flexed elbow.

    b. In light of these mechanisms of injury, it is prudent to obtain radiographs prior to any vigorous examination or intervention.

B. Olecranon fractures.

  1. Pain after either direct or indirect trauma is the main complaint.

    a. Joint effusion is present in the majority of cases.

    b. There may be a palpable deformity or sulcus.

    c. Motion is typically limited but the patient should be able to extend the elbow against gravity if the triceps attachment is intact.

    d. Always be sure to document neurovascular status as ulnar nerve and vascular injury may occur due to the trauma.

  2. Diagnostic tests.

    a. Radiographs should be obtained.

      i. AP and true lateral projections should adequately reveal the fracture (Figure 12-3).

      ii. Oblique projections may be included but may not show the true extent of the injury.

    b. Additional diagnostic studies are not typically necessary.

  3. Treatment.

    a. Nondisplaced fractures may be treated in a conservative manner with long-arm cast with the elbow at 45–90° of flexion for up to three weeks.

      i. A fracture is considered nondisplaced in the following circumstances:

        • < 2 mm displacement that does not increase with elbow flexion to 90°.

        • Patient is able to extend elbow actively against gravity, showing that the triceps mechanism is intact.

      ii. Repeat X-rays should be obtained 5–7 days post-injury to ensure that no displacement has occurred.

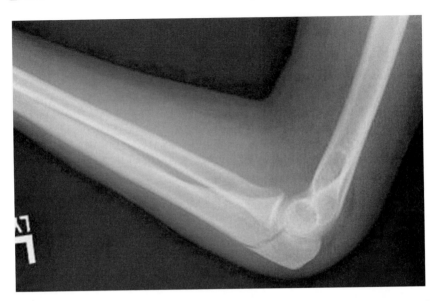

FIGURE 12-3   Lateral elbow radiograph reveals a minimally displaced olecranon fracture. Careful evaluation also reveals the presence an anterior fat pad. Image courtesy of James L. Moeller, MD.

    iii. Even though the fracture won't be completely healed for 6–8 weeks, most are stable in 3 weeks. The cast is removed and gentle range of motion activities are initiated to avoid excessive stiffness and potential long-term motion loss. Once bony union has occurred, more aggressive therapy can be initiated.

  b. All displaced fractures should be treated by an orthopedic surgeon.

    i. Although nonoperative treatment is an option, it is fraught with potential complications. Therefore, ORIF and excision of the fracture fragment are the most common methods of treatment.

C. Traumatic olecranon bursitis.

  1. Many skaters who fall directly onto the tip of the elbow present with pain and localized swelling at the site of impact. The swollen area is discrete and fluctuant and is consistent with olecranon bursitis.

    a. Elbow motion should be full although there may be some discomfort due to the trauma.

    b. Neurovascular examination should be normal.

    c. Radiographs show no evidence of fracture.

2. Treatment is conservative and may initially consist of the very simple regimen of compression wrap, ice, antiinflammatory medications, and activity modification to avoid recurrent injury.
3. Many physicians aspirate the bursa on the initial evaluation as an adjunct to the initial treatment outlined above.
    a. The aspirate will be bloody but should not appear infected.
        i. If the aspirate appears infected, fluid analysis with culture and sensitivity testing should be done.
        ii. It is prudent to start antibiotic treatment empirically while awaiting for culture results.
        iii. If infection is present, open drainage should be considered.
    b. The physician should visually examine the aspirate to look for fat droplets that may indicate an occult fracture.
        i. If fat droplets are present, one must assume that an open fracture situation is present and the patient should be started on antibiotics along with the general treatment.
    c. Corticosteroid injection after aspiration in the acute traumatic setting is controversial.

Hip Apophyseal Injuries

Hip apophyseal injuries may be acute or chronic in nature.
A. Acute injuries occur due to a sudden, violent muscle contraction that may avulse the apophysis from its normal position.
B. Chronic injuries are due to consistent, repetitive action of the abdominal, pelvic, and thigh musculature on their attachment sites (see Table 12-2).
C. Hip apophyseal avulsion injuries.
    1. History.
        a. Pain is the chief complaint.
            i. Location: Depends on apophysis involved.
                • Ischial tuberosity avulsion causes buttock or hamstring pain.
                • ASIS and AIIS avulsions cause anterior hip pain.
                • Iliac crest avulsions cause lateral and anterolateral pain.
                • Lesser trochanter avulsion causes groin pain.
            ii. Onset is usually sudden, most commonly associated with jumps.
            iii. Provoked by activities, relieved by rest.

TABLE 12-2

Hip apophyses and muscular attachment.

Apophysis	Muscle	Lower Extremity Position at Time of Injury
Anterior inferior iliac spine	Rectus femoris	Hip in extension, knee in flexion
Anterior superior iliac spine	Sartorius	Hip in extension, knee in flexion
Iliac crest	Abdominal obliques	Trunk rotation
Ischial tuberosity	Hamstrings	Hip in flexion, knee in extension
Lesser trochanter	Iliopsoas	Hip in extension, knee in flexion

2. Physical examination findings may include:
   a. Antalgic gait.
   b. Swelling (more easily noted with injury to the ASIS).
   c. Tenderness to direct palpation over the apophysis.
   d. Pain and weakness on testing of the appropriate muscle group (strength often limited by discomfort).
   e. Neurovascular status remains intact.
3. Diagnostic tests.
   a. Radiographs should be obtained with comparison views of the opposite apophysis.
   b. Displacement of the apophysis compared to the opposite side in the above clinical setting is diagnostic for an acute avulsion fracture (Figure 12-4).
4. Treatment.
   a. Brief period of non-weight-bearing may be necessary.
      i. Non-weight-bearing may be needed as long as two weeks.
      ii. The patient should be encouraged to advance to partial weight-bearing status, then full weight bearing as tolerated. This may take many weeks to achieve.
   b. Ice.
   c. Analgesic medications.
      i. Acetaminophen.
      ii. NSAIDs.
   d. Rehabilitation begins as pain decreases.

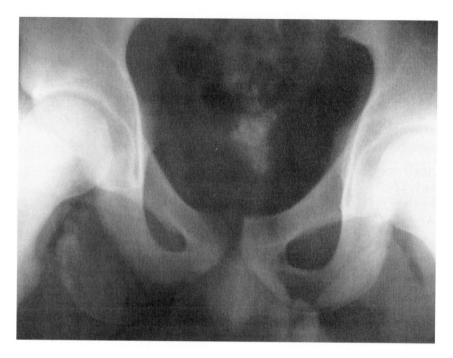

FIGURE 12-4 AP radiograph of the pelvis reveals an avulsion fracture of the right ischial tuberosity. Image courtesy of Sami F. Rifat, MD.

 i. Strengthening.
 ii. Flexibility.
 iii. Balance and coordination training.
 iv. Advancement of activities should proceed in a pain-free manner.
 v. Some migration of the avulsed apophysis may occur during treatment, but this does not appear to adversely affect long-term hip motion or function either for normal daily or sports activities.
 5. Full return to sport may take months.
 6. Surgical treatment may be required.
 a. Wide (> 2cm) displacement.
 b. Prolonged pain despite appropriate nonoperative management.
D. Apophysitis.
 1. Presents as insidious onset anterior hip pain.
 2. Pain is typically less severe than that encountered in avulsion fractures.

3. Radiographs show no apparent differences between the injured and noninjured side.
4. Treatment follows a similar course as outlined for avulsion fracture, though the patient is usually able to progress through rehabilitation and back to full activities in a shorter length of time.

Ankle Sprains

Ankle sprains, though very common in other sports, are not particularly common in figure skating due to the relative protection afforded by the skating boot.

A. For a full discussion of ankle sprains, see Chapter 6, Snowboarding.

OVERUSE MUSCULOSKELETAL INJURIES

The majority of lower extremity injuries encountered in figure skating are of the overuse variety.

Back Pain

A. In adults, most back pain complaints are due to either muscular strain or disc pathology. Empiric treatment can often be initiated safely. If symptoms fail to improve, then a more specific diagnostic workup is initiated.

B. Back pain in a child or adolescent should prompt early, aggressive workup to identify an underlying cause prior to the initiation of significant therapeutic interventions.

1. Most competitive figure skaters are in the adolescent and young adult age groups and the threshold for evaluation should be low.

Spondylolysis

A. The most common cause of low back pain in active adolescents who seek medical attention for their pain.

1. More likely to occur in males.
2. Spondylolisthesis (bilateral spondylolysis that results in anterior/ posterior slippage of the adjacent vertebral segments) is more common in females.

B. It is felt that repetitive hyperextension activities put the posterior elements of the spinal column at risk for injury in young athletes and are the primary cause of this injury.

    1. Landing multiple jumps.

    2. Layback spins.

    3. Lifts in pairs skating put the back at risk by increasing the axial load to the male partner's spine due to holding the female partner overhead. Increased low back lordosis may occur during this maneuver as well.

C. Primary care physicians who do not regularly treat spondylolysis should strongly consider referring these patients to a sports medicine physician.

D. History.

    1. Pain.

        a. Can be unilateral or bilateral.

        b. Usually does not radiate.

        c. Worsened by extension activities, relieved (at least partially) by rest.

    2. Radicular symptoms usually absent.

    3. Bowel/bladder control issues absent.

    4. Not associated with fever, sweats, chills, or unexplained weight loss.

    5. Onset is usually insidious although some patients will report a traumatic event.

    6. There may be a family history of this problem.

E. Physical examination.

    1. Tenderness.

        a. Usually present on palpation in the paravertebral muscle areas.

        b. Worsened by motion, particularly hyperextension.

            i. One-leg standing hyperextension test (stork test) is likely the most sensitive and specific clinical test.

    2. Other components of the examination are usually normal.

F. Diagnostic tests.

    1. Plain X-rays. Should be obtained when spondylolysis suspected. X-rays, however, do not fully confirm the diagnosis of active stress lesions.

        a. AP view (Figure 12-5a).

            i. Lucencies consistent with spondylolysis can be seen.

            ii. Spina bifida occulta (a risk factor for the development of this condition) can be seen (Figure 12-6).

        b. Lateral view.

            i. Lucencies consistent with spondylolysis can be seen.

            ii. Spondylolisthesis can be easily identified.

        c. Oblique views (Figure 12-5b); once considered the most important view of the X-ray series for the diagnosis of spondylolysis.

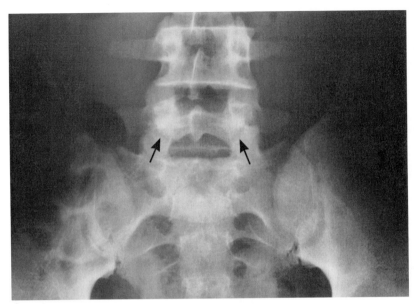

A

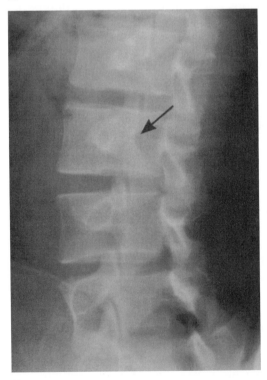

B

FIGURE   12·5
Spondylolysis: a) AP radiograph of the lumbar spine
shows bilateral pars interarticularis defects at the L5
level; b) oblique radiograph
of the lumbar spine shows a
fracture through the pars
interarticularis region of L3
(the neck of the "Scotty
Dog"). The age and metabolic activity cannot be determined by the appearance of
either X-ray. Images courtesy
of James L. Moeller, MD.

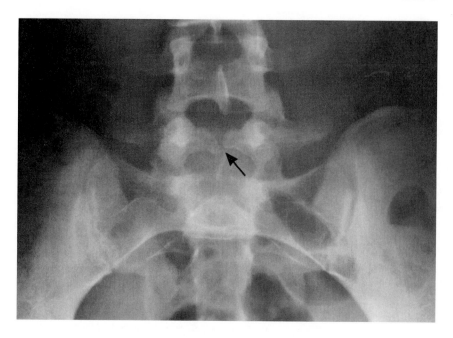

FIGURE 12-6 AP radiograph of the lumbar spine showing spina bifida occulta (SBO). The presence of SBO has been associated with spondylolysis. Image courtesy of James L. Moeller, MD.

     i. Best view to see the pars interarticularis.
      • "Scotty Dog" view.
     ii. Lucencies or frank fractures through the pars region can be seen.
  2. Radionucleotide bone scan (Figure 12-7).
    a. Very sensitive tool for indicating metabolic activity of bone.
    b. Many feel that a positive bone scan and SPECT images confirm the diagnosis of active spondylolysis.
  3. Computerized tomography (CT) scan.
    a. More specific than bone scan.
    b. May provide additional information regarding the state of healing.
  4. Magnetic resonance imaging (MRI).
    a. Excellent tool for looking at soft tissues of the spine.
    b. The role of MRI in the diagnosis of spondylolysis is evolving.
G. Treatment.
  1. Conservative management is the mainstay of early treatment.

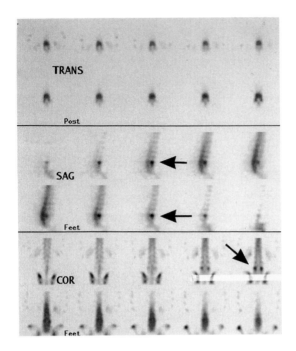

FIGURE 12-7
Radionucleotide bone scan SPECT images show increased uptake in the bilateral pars interarticularis regions indicating active stress fractures. Image courtesy of James L. Moeller, MD.

    a. Restrict the athlete's activity from competition, practice, and training that involves hyperextension of the lower back and movement that provokes symptoms.
    b. Ice and/or heat may provide comfort and can be used alone or in a contrast pattern.
    c. Acetaminophen or NSAIDs can be used to alleviate the discomfort.
    d. Rehabilitation program can be initiated early with special care to avoid hyperextension activities.
        i. Lower extremity flexibility.
        ii. Abdominal strengthening and trunk stabilization program.
    e. Thoracolumbarsacral orthosis can be added if these initial measures are unsuccessful.
        i. Bracing should be used in conjunction with the rehabilitation regimen outlined above.
  2. Return to activities: Following successful rehabilitation of spondylolysis, activities should be introduced at a very low intensity with a slow progression to full activity.

Spondylolisthesis

A. Presents with clinical symptoms similar to spondylolysis.

TABLE 12-3

Grading system for spondylolisthesis.

Grade	Amount of Displacement
I	1–25%
II	26–50%
III	51–75%
IV	76–100%
V (Spondyloptosis)	>100%

B. Lateral radiograph used to determine the degree of anterior/posterior displacement of adjacent vertebral bodies. The amount of slippage can be reported as a percentage or grade (see Table 12-3).
   1. For purposes of follow-up, it may be best to express the degree of spondylolisthesis as a percentage because a significant change in status may not be reflected as a change in grade (e.g., a patient with a 27% slip advances to a 45% slip but is still a grade II).
C. Progression of spondylolisthesis should be monitored closely during an adolescent's maximum linear growth stage due to the increased risk of vertebral body displacement during this period.
D. Treatment and activity recommendations.
   1. Many patients with a grade I injury are asymptomatic and can compete normally without symptoms or long-term problems.
   2. Larger degrees of displacement or rapid increases may require a thoracolumbarsacral orthosis.
   3. Surgical intervention may be necessary if the degree of displacement increases or neurological compromise develops.

Osteochondritis Dissecans (OCD)

A. General considerations.
   1. Most agree that OCD results from cumulative stress causing subchondral stress fractures.
   2. The subchondral injury causes vascular compromise leading to the common finding of bony injury covered by intact articular cartilage.
   3. Incidence.
      a. 18/100,000 females.
      b. 29/100,000 males.

B. History.
    1. Insidious onset of pain in the knee.
        a. Typically described as medial pain but may be global.
        b. Worsened with activities, relieved by rest.
    2. Swelling may be noted.
    3. Grinding or clicking may be described.
    4. Catching or locking may be described.
C. Physical examination.
    1. Limp may be noted.
    2. Effusion may be present.
    3. Tender to palpation of the involved femoral condyle.
    4. Flexion/circumduction may cause discomfort.
        a. Can be mistaken for a meniscus tear.
D. Diagnostic tests.
    1. X-rays should be obtained.
        a. AP, lateral, and sunrise views make up a typical radiographic knee series but OCD is not always evident on these views.
        b. If OCD suspected, adding a notch view to the standard series can be very helpful, bringing the weight-bearing surfaces of the femur into better view (Figure 12-8).
    2. MRI is now the standard diagnostic test utilized in staging OCD lesions and the authors recommend that MRI be obtained in all cases (Figure 12-9).
E. Treatment.
    1. Nonoperative.
        a. Can be attempted in cases of stable OCD lesions.
        b. Goal: Lesion healing before physis closure.
            i. Healing can occur in up to 50% of patients over a 10–18 month period.

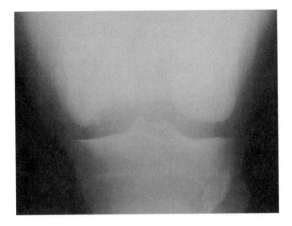

FIGURE 12·8
Notch radiograph of the knee reveals OCD lesion of the medial femoral condyle. Image courtesy of James L. Moeller, MD.

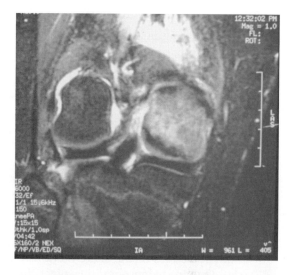

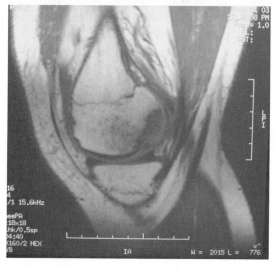

FIGURE 12-9 MRI scan of the knee (same patient as in Figure 12-8) reveals OCD lesion and bone edema of the medial femoral condyle. Images courtesy of James L. Moeller, MD.

    c. A course of non-weight-bearing is commonly advised.

    d. Controversy over early immobilization exists.

    e. Serial radiographs should be obtained to document progression of healing.

  2. Operative.

    a. Surgical intervention recommended when:

      i. Lesion is unstable.

      ii. Closed physes or patient nearing age of physis closure.

      iii. Failure of conservative treatment.

    b. Surgical approach (ORIF, graft, drilling) depends on the size, fragmentation, and stability of the lesion.

Fibular Stress Fractures

A. Lower leg stress fractures are very common in sport, but most involve the tibia. In figure skating, however, primary care physicians need to be cognizant of the possibility of fibular stress fractures.

    1. Most of these injuries occur in the area of the fibula that corresponds to the top of the skating boot. The compressive force of the skating boot at this location is believed to play a role in the development of fibular stress fractures.

    2. Figure skaters take off and land from jumps while leaning on either the inside or outside of the foot (known as inside and outside edges of the skate blade).

        a. Outside edge activities place increased stress on the peroneal musculature and fibula and contribute to the risk of fibular stress fracture.

    3. Other potential risk factors for development of fibular stress fractures in skaters include:

        a. Poor diet (primarily poor calcium and vitamin D intake).

        b. Abnormal foot mechanics.

        c. Poor jumping/landing mechanics.

        d. Muscle imbalances.

        e. The boot itself may fit poorly, may be too stiff, or may not be supportive enough.

        f. Menstrual irregularities (see Medical Issues, Menstrual Irregularities).

B. History.

    1. The athlete typically presents with lateral lower leg pain that is worsened by activity and relieved by rest.

        a. In more severe cases, routine daily activities may cause discomfort.

    2. The onset of pain is usually insidious; however, some skaters may relate the onset of pain to a specific fall or other trauma.

    3. The patient may report soft-tissue swelling with this type of injury but less often reports ecchymosis, erythema, and paresthesias or other evidence of neurovascular compromise.

C. Examination.

    1. Palpation reveals tenderness along the fibula, which may mimic isolated peroneal muscle/tendon tenderness.

    2. Significant swelling along the surface of the fibula increases the likelihood that a stress fracture is present.

3. Muscle strength testing against resistance may provoke tenderness in the affected area; however, a positive finding in this component of the physical exam may not be helpful in differentiating between a stress fracture of the fibula and simple soft-tissue injuries to muscle and tendons in the lower leg.
4. Increased pain due to vibratory stimulus (tuning fork testing) should increase suspicion of this problem.
D. Differential diagnosis.
  1. Muscle strain.
  2. Tendinopathy.
  3. Peroneal nerve entrapment.
  4. Chronic exertional compartment syndrome.
E. Diagnostic testing.
  1. Radiographs should always be obtained when fibular pain is present.
    a. Periosteal thickening, periosteal elevation, or the presence of a cortical lucency are all positive radiographic findings that are consistent with a stress fracture (Figure 12-10).
    b. Negative radiographs do not rule out the presence of stress fracture.
  2. Bone scan should be obtained if clinical findings are consistent with stress fracture in spite of normal X-rays.
    a. A definitive diagnosis confirming the presence or absence of a stress fracture of the fibula is very important because the treatment for stress fracture is drastically different from the treatment of muscle strains and tendinopathies.

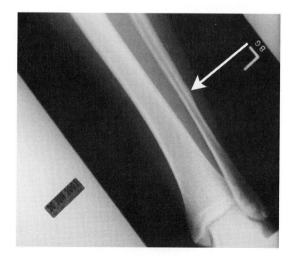

FIGURE 12-10 AP radiograph of the tibia/fibula shows cortical thickening and irregularity at the level of the top of the skating boot in a figure skater with lateral lower leg pain indicating fibula stress fracture. X-rays are often negative in this condition and if so, a follow-up bone scan should be considered. Image courtesy of James L. Moeller, MD.

F. Treatment.
1. Address factors that may play a role in the development of this lesion and remove the athlete from activities that result in high stress to the injured bone.
    a. If the patient has pain with routine activity, non-weight-bearing or partial weight bearing may be of benefit.
    b. Crutches should be weaned as soon as pain permits because weight bearing stimulates bone metabolism.
    c. During the rest period, the athlete should be encouraged to remain as physically active as possible by engaging in activities that do not cause pain to the injured area.
        i. This continuing physical activity should be performed to prevent deconditioning both from a muscular and cardiovascular standpoint.
        ii. Activities may include bicycling, swimming, water running, and some resistance training.
2. Progress the athlete to more vigorous physical activity when the signs and symptoms of the stress fracture have resolved and when the athlete is able to perform routine activities of daily living in a pain-free manner.
    a. Activities should start at low intensity with slow progression back to full activity.
3. When treated inappropriately, the young athlete may experience an adverse outcome (e.g., progression to a completed fibular fracture).

Foot and Ankle Tendinopathy

Tendinitis, or perhaps more appropriately tendinosis, is a very common overuse injury in figure skaters.
A. Although much of the power for skating and jumping is generated from the hip, gluteal, and thigh musculature, the foot and ankle plantar flexors also play a large role in speed development and fine control of jumping and landing. For this reason, the muscles and tendons involved in foot and ankle plantar flexion are exposed to a high degree of eccentric activity and a high risk of injury.
1. Foot and ankle plantar flexor muscles include:
    a. The gastrocnemius and soleus muscles in the superficial posterior compartment. Together these muscles become the Achilles tendon.
    b. The tibialis posterior, flexor hallucis, and flexor digitorum muscles/tendons on the medial side of the ankle (deep posterior muscle compartment).
    c. The peroneus longus and brevis muscles/tendons on the lateral side of the ankle (lateral compartment).

B. Skaters present with pain in the lower leg, usually around the ankle, that is worsened by activity and relieved by rest.

1. The pain usually starts insidiously and is not related to any specific fall or other trauma.
2. Localized swelling may be reported.

C. The main physical examination finding is tenderness to palpation of the tendon along with increased tenderness on resisted muscle testing.

1. Some mild swelling may be noted by the examiner.
2. The ankle is nontender to careful palpation of bony prominences and ligamentous regions.
   a. If bony tenderness is present at the tendon insertion site, stress injury to the bone must be considered as part of the differential diagnosis.
3. Joint motion is full and generally nontender.
4. The ankle is ligamentously stable.
5. Neurovascular status is intact.

D. Radiographs are not necessary for the diagnosis of tendinopathy, but should be considered if bony or joint pathology is being considered as a cause of the skater's pain.

E. Many muscle and tendon injuries can be treated aggressively with rehabilitation while the athlete continues to skate at a decreased level of intensity.

1. Pain, swelling, and inflammation can be treated with a combination of activity modification, compression, elevation, ice, and NSAID use.
2. Muscle stretching and strength and endurance training are initiated as soon as pain permits.
3. Balance and proprioception training is another important component to the rehabilitation program. These activities should be initiated once motion is full and mostly pain-free.
4. Activities should be performed below the soreness threshold (**REST** = **R**esume **E**xercise below the **S**oreness **T**hreshold) throughout the rehabilitation process.
5. In more severe cases, electrical stimulation and ultrasound may be of benefit. In cases in which the signs and symptoms of injury are severe or more refractive to the above interventions, iontophoresis or phonophoresis may prove helpful.
6. Extracorporeal shock wave treatment may also be considered.

Malleolar Bursitis

A. An interesting entity peculiar to skating athletes. Bursae do not typically develop over the malleoli; however, adventitial bursae

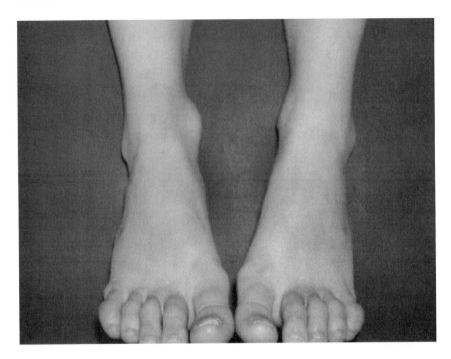

FIGURE 12-11   Medial malleolar bursitis of the right ankle in a figure skater. Photo courtesy of James L. Moeller, MD.

may develop in this region if the ankle is exposed to consistent stress and frictional forces (Figure 12-11).

1. This bursa can grow large enough to cause improper fit of the skating boot, which worsens the friction and creates a vicious inflammatory cycle.
2. Many skaters present due to the swelling rather than pain.

B. There typically is no history of trauma to the affected area and no significant history of pain.

C. Fluctuant swelling is located directly over the malleolus.
1. The bursa is usually painless on palpation.
2. Redness or heat should raise the suspicion of infection.

D. Radiographs are of limited value in making an accurate diagnosis.

E. Treatment: Malleolar bursitis typically does not respond well to simple, conservative measures.
1. Boot stretching may be helpful in order to allow proper fit of the skate, but this may not entirely solve the problem.
2. Aspiration of the bursal fluid may be both diagnostic and therapeutic.

    a. A large-gauge needle is used to aspirate the thick, gelatinous fluid. The viscosity of the fluid may make it difficult or impossible to aspirate through a small-bore needle.

      i. If there are no clinical signs of infection and the bursal fluid appears clear, a small amount of corticosteroid can be injected into the bursal sac in an attempt to decrease inflammation within the bursa.

      ii. If infection is suspected (redness, warmth, fever, cloudy appearing fluid, etc.), corticosteroid should not be used.

        • The bursal fluid should be sent to the laboratory for culture and the patient should be started on empiric antibiotic therapy.

    b. A pressure wrap should be applied.

3. Ice and NSAIDs can be used to lessen the chance of fluid reaccumulation.

4. Aperture pad for return to skating.

5. Even with appropriate interventions, the risk of fluid reaccumulation is high and surgical excision of the bursa may be required.

Suggested Readings

Brown TD, Varney TE, Micheli LJ. Malleolar bursitis in figure skaters: Indications for operative and nonoperative treatment. *AJSM* 2000;28(1): 109–11.

Cahill BR. Osteochondritis dissecans of the knee: Treatment of juvenile and adult forms. *J Am Acad Orthop Surg* 1995;3:237–47.

Congeni J, McCulloch J, Swanson K. Lumbar spondylolysis: A study of natural progression in athletes. *Am J Sports Med* 1997;25(2):248–53.

Davison KK, Earnest MB, Birch LL. Participation in aesthetic sports and girls' weight concerns at ages 5 and 7 years. *Int J Eat Disord* 2002 Apr;31(3): 312–17.

Dutton JAE, Hughes SPF, Peters AM. SPECT in the management of patients with back pain and spondylolysis. *Clin Nucl Med* 2000;25(2):93–96.

Eating disorders. In: *Diagnostic and Statistical Manual of Mental Disorders*. 4th ed. Washington, DC: American Psychiatric Association; 1994:539–50.

Kazis K, Iglesias E. The female athlete triad. *Adolesc Med* 2003 Feb; 14(1):87–95.

Khan KM, Liu-Ambrose T, Sran MM, et al. New criteria for female athlete triad syndrome? As osteoporosis is rare, should osteopenia be among the criteria for defining the female athlete triad syndrome? *BJSM* 2002;36(1): 10–13.

Micheli LJ, Wood R. Back pain in young athletes: Significant differences from adults in causes and patterns. *Arch Pediatr Adolesc Med* 1995;149:15–18.

Moeller JL. Pelvic and hip apophyseal avulsion injuries in young athletes. *Curr Sports Med Rep* 2003;2(2):110–15.

Oleson CV, Busconi BD, Baran DT. Bone density in competitive figure skaters. *Arch Phys Med Rehabil* 2002;83(1):122–28.

Pecina M, Bojanic I, Dubravcic S. Stress fractures in figure skaters. *AJSM* 1990;18(3):277–79.

Poe CM. *Conditioning for Figure Skating.* Chicago, IL: Contemporary Books; 2002.

Rossi F, Dragoni S. Acute avulsion fractures of the pelvis in adolescent competitive athletes: Prevalence, location, and sports distribution of 203 cases collected. *Skeletal Radiol* 2001;30:127–31.

Sabatini S. The female athlete triad. *Am J Med Sci* 2001;322(4):193–95.

Sherman WM. Carbohydrate feedings before and after exercise. In: Lamb DR, Williams MH, eds. *Ergogenics: Enhancement of Performance in Exercise and Sport, Perspectives in Exercise Science and Medicine.* Vol 4. Indianapolis, IN: W. C. Brown and Benchmark Publishers; 1991:1.

Shulman C. *The Complete Book of Figure Skating.* Champaign, IL: Human Kinetics; 2002.

Snyder AC, Foster C. Physiology and nutrition of skating. In: Lamb DR, Knuttgen HG, Murray R, eds. *Physiology and Nutrition for Competitive Sport, Perspectives in Exercise Science and Sports Medicine.* Vol 7. Carmel, IN: Cooper Publishing Group; 1994:181.

13

SPEED SKATING

James L. Moeller
Eric A. Heiden
Carl Foster
Jos J. deKoning

GENERAL INFORMATION

Types

There are two types of competitive speed skating: long track and short track.

A. Long track.
   1. 400-m oval.
      a. Two lanes.
   2. Two racers skate at a time.
      a. Lane crossovers occur on back stretch.
      b. Pack-style racing was popular early in the sport and was even used in the Olympic Games as late as the 1932 Lake Placid Games.
   3. Equipment.
      a. Skates.
         i. Klapskate.
            • Used at higher levels of competition.
            • Front skate post is hinged, rear post free to open to allow for increased blade contact with ice surface during push-off.
         ii. Standard skate.
            • Front and rear posts fixed.
         iii. Blade bending.
            • More common practice in short track.

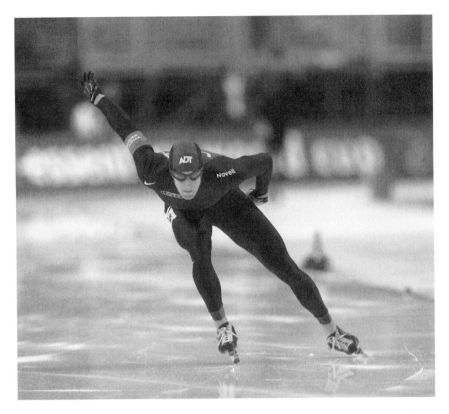

FIGURE 13-1   Long-track speed skater in aerodynamic skin suit. Photo courtesy of U.S. Speedskating.

- Bending full length of blade has not been proven to be advantageous for long-track skaters.
    - Sacrifices speed in the straight portions of the track.
    - Sprint distance skaters (500 m, 1000 m, and 1500 m) are now experimenting with bending the front of the blade only.
  b. Skating suit.
    i. Aerodynamic design and materials utilized (Figure 13-1).
      - Some manufacturers use six different materials in each suit.
        - Each material specific to the aerodynamic need of the different body areas.
      - Wind tunnel testing utilized to maximize aerodynamic benefit.

      ii. It is estimated that some suits may improve a skater's speed by ~ 0.25 seconds per lap in the longer races.
- Men may benefit more than women.
  - Perhaps due to a greater aerodynamic disadvantage to start with.
- Studies are ongoing.

  4. Racing distances (M = men's, L = ladies').
    a. M/L 500 m.
    b. M/L 1000 m.
    c. M/L 1500 m.
    d. L 3000 m.
    e. M/L 5000 m.
    f. M 10,000 m.

B. Short track.
  1. 111.12-m track.
    a. No distinct lanes.
  2. Pack-style racing, up to 6 racers per heat (Figure 13-2).
  3. Equipment.
    a. Skates.

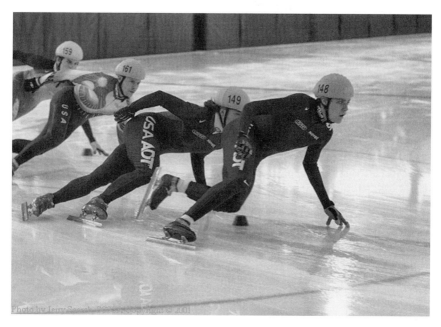

FIGURE 13-2 Short-track speed skaters. Note the pack-style racing, multiple racers, and special equipment including helmets, neck guards, and cut-resistant gloves. Photo courtesy of Jerry Search.

      i. Front and rear posts fixed to boot.
      ii. Boot custom molded, reinforced to withstand high centrifugal forces encountered in turns.
      iii. Blades offset to allow for greater lean in the turns.
- Right skate blade set to medial portion of boot.
- Left skate blade set to lateral portion of boot.

      iv. Many skaters bend the skate blades into a curved shape (concave left) to assist in holding the turns at high speeds.
- Advantageous in short track because the percentage of time spent cornering is high.

  b. Skating suit.
      i. Shin guards and knee pads often incorporated into suit.
  c. Helmet.
  d. Cut-proof gloves.
  e. Neck guard.

4. Distances.
  a. Individual races.
      i. M/L 500 m (4.5 laps).
      ii. M/L 1000 m (9 laps).
      iii. M/L 1500 m (13.5 laps).
      iv. M/L 3000 m (27 laps).
  b. Relay (4-person team) races.
      i. L 3000 m (27 laps).
      ii. M 5000 m (45 laps).

Evolution of the Skate

A. Thirteenth century: Skates fashioned from the long bones of large animals, strapped to the shoe.
B. Fourteenth century: Man-made, wood runners strapped to the shoes took the place of animal bones.
C. 1400: Metal runners added to the bottom of the wood component of the blade.
D. 1572: All-iron skate introduced.
E. 1850: All-steel skate introduced.
F. 1995: Introduction of Klapskate.

History of Long Track

A. Competition.
  1. 1763: World's first organized speed skating race.
    a. Held on the Fens in England.
    b. Distance covered: just over 24 km.

    2. 1863: First modern speed skating competition was held in Norway.

    3. 1889: First World Championships (men only) were held in Amsterdam, Netherlands.

    4. 1936: First World Championships for ladies were held in Stockholm, Sweden.

B. 1892: International Skating Union established.

C. Olympic Games history.

    1. 1924: Speed skating appeared in the first Olympic Winter Games in Chamonix, France (men only).

    2. 1932: Women's speed skating introduced as an Olympic exhibition sport in Lake Placid, NY.

    3. 1960: Women's speed skating an official medal sport at Squaw Valley, CA.

History of Short Track

A. Originated in Canada and the United States in 1905.

    1. Became part of the ISU in 1967.

B. Competition.

    1. First known competition took place in 1909.

    2. International competitions began in the 1970s.

    3. 1976: First ISU-sanctioned competition.

    4. 1981: First World Championships held at Meudon-la-Forêt, France.

C. Olympic Games history.

    1. 1988: Introduced as a demonstration sport at Calgary, Canada.

    2. 1992: Full medal sport at Albertville, France.

Injury Statistics

A. There are no major published reports on the incidence of specific injuries encountered in speed skating.

PHYSIOLOGY AND BIOMECHANICS

Nature of the Sport

A. Speed skating is an energy-demand or power-balance sport.

B. In long track, and in part in short track, competitive results are defined by the average velocity the athlete can achieve.

    1. The athlete with the greatest average velocity has the smallest time and becomes the winner.

    2. The ability to record a high average velocity depends on the balance between the power generated by the athlete's muscles and the power lost to the environment.

C. Power production is attributable to:

    1. Aerobic power output, reflected by:

        a. Vo_2 max.

        b. Threshold of sustainable aerobic power.

            i. Blood lactate threshold.

            ii. Ventilatory threshold.

    2. Anaerobic power output, reflected by:

        a. Peak anaerobic power output.

        b. Anaerobic capacity.

    3. Efficiency of the transfer of power to the ice.

        a. Klapskate technology has allowed for more efficient transfer of power to the ice.

D. Power losses are attributable to:

    1. Air friction.

        a. Larger source of power loss compared to ice friction.

        b. Main factors:

            i. Air density.

- Lower at higher altitudes.
  - Not surprisingly, most world records in long track have occurred at higher-altitude ovals (Table 13-1).
- Local barometric pressure is an important factor.

            ii. Net air movement in the oval.

- A following wind is beneficial.
- Skaters warming up on the inner lane can create a biased airflow; therefore, there are rules regarding the number of skaters who may skate in that lane at any one time during competition.

            iii. Frontal surface area of the skater, perhaps the largest factor in creating air resistance, dependent upon:

- Size of the skater.
- Skating position.
  - As the pre-extension knee angle and trunk angle decrease, the effective frontal area decreases.

            iv. Air resistance qualities of the skating suit.

- Loose-fitting, thick suits increase air resistance.
- Form-fitting suits decrease resistance.
- Texture of the material is important.
  - Some textures act like the dimpling of a golf ball, changing the airflow characteristics over the skater's body.
  - Different textures used over different body areas.

TABLE 13-1

World record performances during speed skating. World records in track and field and in cycling are appended below the table for reference. The location where the world record was recorded is noted after the time.

Distance (meters)	Men	Women
500	34.32 SLC	37.22 Calgary
1000	1:07.18 SLC	1:13.83 SLC
1500	1:43.95 SLC	1:54.02 SLC
3000	3:42.75* Calgary	3:57.70 SLC
5000	6:14.66 SLC	6:46.91 SLC
10,000	12:59.92 SLC	14:22.60* Calgary
1-hour	41,040 m	34,507 m

*Not a normally contested event in senior competition.

Running (men/women): 800 m = 1:41.11/1:53.28; 1500 m = 3:26.00/3:50.46; 3000 m = 7:20.67/8:06.11; 5000 m = 12:39.36/14:28.09; 10,000 m = 26:22.75/29:31.78; 1-hour = 21,101m/18,340m.

Cycling (men/women): 500 m = */34.01; 1000 m = 58.88/*; 3000 m = */3:39.82; 4000 m = 4:11.11/*; 1-hour = 49,441/45,094.

    2. Ice friction.
       a. Depends mainly on temperature of ice.
       b. Remarkably similar at all of the major competitive ovals in the world.

Velocity Profile

A. In most events, there is a tendency to slow throughout the latter half of the event (Figure 13-3).
    1. This pacing pattern also common in cycling events of comparable duration.
    2. Reflects that:
       a. Velocity at the end of the race is wasted kinetic energy.
       b. In both skating and cycling, velocity will remain quite high even if power output goes to zero.
B. At any given competitive distance, cycling is ~ 10% faster than skating (and skating is about twice as fast as running) (Table 13-1). The speed differences between skating and cycling are attributable to:

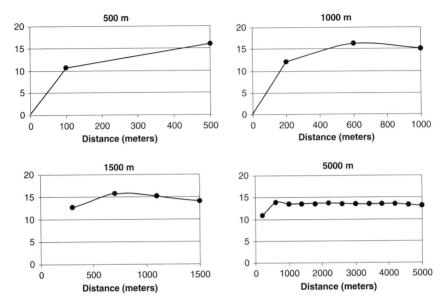

FIGURE 13-3 Pattern of velocity during the gold-medal performance during the four shortest men's events of the 2002 Olympic Winter Games in Salt Lake City. Note that there is a tendency to slow during the latter part of all of the longer events. High-resolution data that is not yet published also indicates there is a tendency to slow during the last part of the 500-m event. This data reflects the reality that velocity at the end of a race is essentially wasted kinetic energy. Given that these were the best performances in each event, the athlete obviously found the best trade-off between not wasting kinetic energy and risking a competitively meaningful slowdown at the end of the race.

    1. Slightly higher aerobic power can be generated during cycling.
       a. Related to the restriction of muscle blood flow during skating, which is the central unique physiological fact of speed skating (see further discussion under The Stance).
    2. Slightly higher efficiency during cycling compared to skating.
  C. Power outputs requiring Vo_2 max can be sustained for about 6–7 minutes.
    1. Power output during skating exceeds that attributable to aerobic metabolism in all but the 10,000 m.
    2. In correspondence with this, during standard laboratory testing, the power output during cycling in elite male and female skaters in relation to duration decreases in a regular fashion. (Figure 13-4).

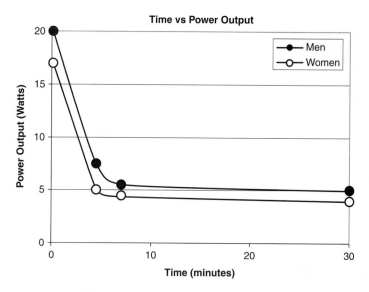

FIGURE 13-4   Time versus power output (watts/kg) relationship based on laboratory tests using cycle ergometry in elite speed skaters. In our experience almost all skaters successful in international competition will be above the gender-specific curve. Given that most athletes can sustain a work intensity associated with Vo_2 max for 6–7 minutes, and that most speed skating events are performed at intensities exceeding Vo_2 max, the importance of anaerobic energetic resources should be evident.

  3. Time-dependent sustainable power outputs represent the summation of aerobic and anaerobic metabolic contributions.

The Stance

The first rule of skating is to sit deeper (Figure 13-5).
A. The smaller the pre-extension knee angle and the lower the trunk angle, the smaller the effective frontal area presented to the wind.
  1. Minimizes power losses to air friction.
  2. 10° reduction in pre-extension knee angle will result in ~ 7-second (~ 3%) improvement in performance in the 3000 m.
  3. 5° reduction in trunk angle will result in ~ 12-second (~ 5%) improvement in performance.
B. Sitting deeper is not easy.
  1. The very high muscle forces required to achieve a low pre-extension knee angle probably contribute to a reduction in muscle blood flow.
    a. Leads to reduction in aerobic metabolism.

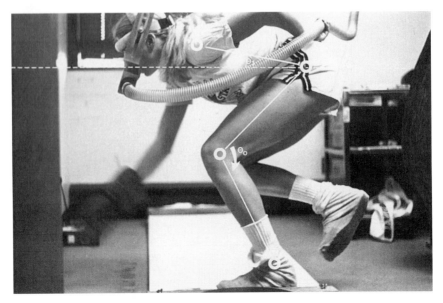

FIGURE 13-5 The first rule of skating is to sit low, to present a small frontal area to the wind. Biomechanically, this is defined by the pre-extension knee angle and the angle of the trunk with the horizontal. Even small improvements in the ability to achieve and maintain an idealized skating position have very large implications for performance.

2. A very low trunk angle can potentially interfere with ventilation during skating and presents a significant challenge to the musculature of the lower back.
3. Early data, based on simulated competitions on the slideboard (as depicted in the figure), suggests that one of the major adaptations to training is the ability to sit deeper and to maintain this position throughout the event.

The Skating Push-Off

A. Skating is dominated by a very long gliding phase which, although not productive of power output, is very fatiguing.
B. Power production comes from the push-off, which is very short but extremely powerful.
C. The characteristics of the push-off are very similar to a jump from one leg, though from a starting position which is far too low for effective jumping.
1. One of the unique muscular adaptations observed in speed skaters is the ability to generate high values of torque at the very beginning of the range of motion.

D. The duty cycle in skating (gliding + push-off) is very long, exceeding 50%, while the tempo (~ 80 push-offs/min) is relatively slow.
  1. Duty cycle in cycling ~ 30%, tempo 180–200 strokes/min.
  2. Duty cycle in running ~ 10%.
E. The interval between push-offs is comparatively longer during skating than during cycling.

Pattern of Power Output during Competition

A. Pacing strategy is largely determined by how the athlete chooses to use anaerobic energy reserves. Power outputs that cannot be provided for by aerobic metabolism must rely on anaerobic sources.
  1. At the start of exercise, aerobic metabolism increases rapidly.
  2. Because of the short duration of most speed skating events, the power output exceeds that provided by Vo_2 max.
B. There is evidence that there is a maximal amount of anaerobic work that can be done by a given athlete.
  1. Anaerobic energy sources involve:
    a. Depletion of intramuscular phosphagens.
    b. Ability to accumulate metabolites, principally lactic acid, without causing a change in pH that is limiting to muscular contraction.
C. Given that the anaerobic capacity is a fixed quantity, the athlete's strategy for expending this reserve dictates the pattern of how races are completed.
  1. The data for the pattern of power output during speed skating competitons is limited, and still quite preliminary.
  2. More extensive data collected during cycle time trials in the laboratory has allowed us to make some reasonable approximations of how aerobic and anaerobic energetic resources are used during the course of competition. (Figure 13-6).
    a. The common denominator seems to be a powerful start for the first few seconds, followed by a proportional utilization of anaerobic resources, so this energy system is exhausted very close to the finish line.
    b. Longer events: The athletes seem to retain some anaerobic energy reserves to allow for a "finishing kick."
    c. Middle distance events: Appears that the athlete is trying to bring the anaerobic energy reserves to zero as close to the finish line as possible.
    d. In speed skating and other air-resisted sports in which it is possible to glide at high speed even with no power output, the athlete has to balance the factor that velocity at the finish line is essentially wasted kinetic energy that might have profitably been used to get to the line sooner.

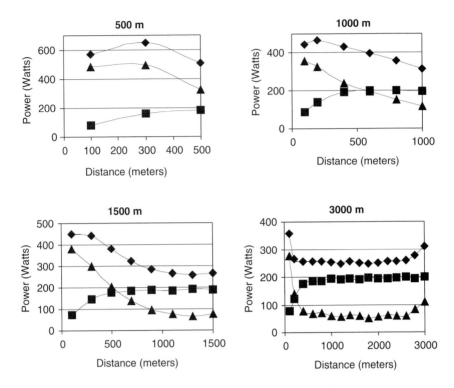

FIGURE 13-6 Pattern of power output during simulated competitions on the cycle in events representative of common speed skating events. The total power output (diamonds) generally declines after an early period of very high power output. In the longer events, there is an increase in power output associated with a finishing "kick." The power output attributable to aerobic metabolism (squares) increases rapidly to a constant value, which is maintained throughout the remainder of the event. The power output attributable to anaerobic sources (triangles) is very high at the beginning of the event, and then decreases to very low values at the end of the event. In the longer events, the increase in power output associated with the "kick" appears to be attributable to anaerobic sources. Recent evidence suggests that the pattern of power output during speed skating is very similar to these simulations performed during cycling.

Limitation of Skeletal Muscle Blood Flow

A. The fairly high muscle forces required to allow the athlete to sit in the characteristic deep sitting posture of the speed skater may compress the small arterioles in the hip and knee extensors to the point that blood flow is limited.

1. Evidence for this is provided:
   a. By the lower Vo_2 max during low-position skating compared to a higher position.
   b. By a lower stroke volume and cardiac output and a higher systemic vascular resistance during skating (Figure 13-7).
   c. By the more rapid accumulation of lactate, particularly in the low position (Figure 13-8).
   d. By greater O_2 desaturation in the knee extensors, particularly in the low position (Figure 13-9).
      i. More pronounced when the weight is supported on one leg as compared to two legs (i.e., higher intramuscular forces).

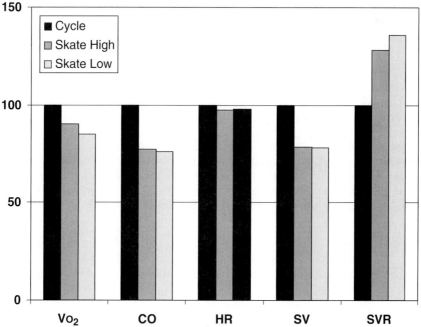

FIGURE 13-7 Hemodynamic responses during maximal exertion during cycling, skating in a high position typical of in-line racing, and skating in a low position typical of metric-style speed skating. The values are normalized to the values observed during cycling. The pattern of responses is consistent with a reduction of muscle blood flow secondary to increases in afterload, attributable to crimping of the small arterioles by the high muscular forces during speed skating.

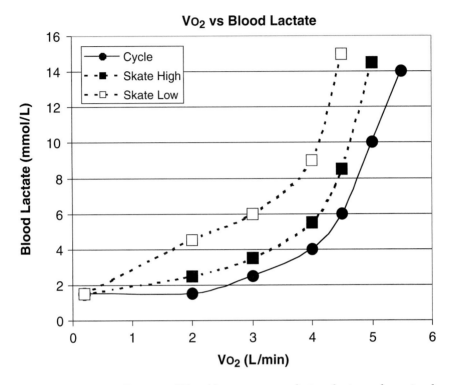

FIGURE 13-8   Pattern of blood lactate accumulation during submaximal and maximal cycling and skating in a high position typical of in-line racing and a low position typical of metric-style speed skating. Note that blood lactate accumulates much more rapidly during skating, especially in the low position, consistent with the hypothesis of a restricted muscle blood flow during skating.

    2. As much as this loss of power production from aerobic metabolism is a hindrance to performance, it is more than balanced by the reductions in power losses to air friction.

Anaerobic Metabolism

A. Markers of anaerobic metabolism are rather robust in speed skaters.

    1. Measures of anaerobic cycling performance in elite speed skaters are as high in speed skaters as in any group of athletes (regardless of measurement technique).

        a. Peak value.

        b. Average over 30 seconds.

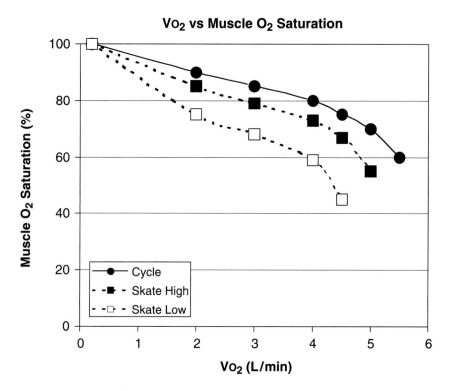

FIGURE 13-9 Pattern of muscle O_2 saturation during submaximal and maximal cycling and speed skating in the high position typical of in-line racing and in a low position typical of metric-style racing. The pattern of responses is consistent with the hypothesis that muscle blood flow is limited during skating, particularly by the high muscle forces typical of the low position, leading to a relative tissue O_2 desaturation.

    2. Postcompetition blood lactate accumulation is as great in skaters as in any group of athletes (Figure 13-10a).
        a. Isolated postcompetition (long track) blood lactate concentrations of 27 mmol/L have been observed.
        b. Following a short-track relay race (e.g., repetitive skating efforts with a very short rest) we have observed 30 mmol/L.
        c. To our knowledge, these are the highest blood lactate concentrations observed in humans.
  B. The rate of lactate accumulation is much more rapid during skating than during similar distance time trials on the cycle (Figure 13-10b).

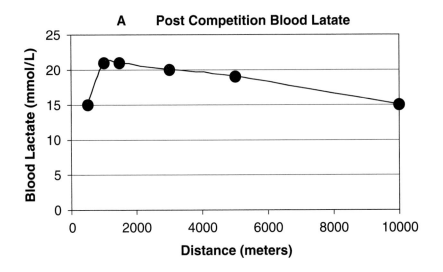

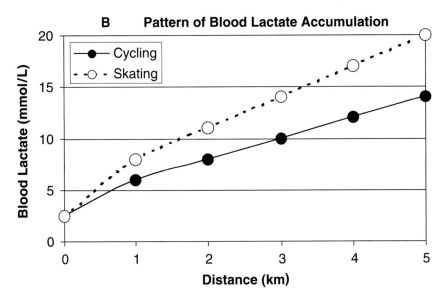

FIGURE 13-10   a) Magnitude of post-exercise blood lactate accumulation following competitions of different distances. This magnitude of blood lactate accumulation is among the highest observed in humans following athletic competitions. b) Pattern of blood lactate accumulation in relation to the proportion of a 5-km competition completed for both cycling and skating.

The Bottom Line

A. Speed skating is a unique sport, depending on the balance of power output and power losses to define the achievable velocity, which dictates the competitive result.
B. Because of the need to achieve a low body position to minimize frictional power losses to air resistance, the physiology of speed skating is uniquely constrained.
  1. Represents an example whereby the biomechanics of the sport dictate that suboptimal physiological conditions are better for the overall competitive result.
  a. Very low skating position.
    i. Allows minimization of power losses to air friction.
    ii. Requires very high intramuscular forces which crimp the smaller arterioles.
      • Limits power production from aerobic sources.
      • Causes a very large reliance on anaerobic power production.
C. Whether from training or selection, speed skaters seem to have some of the largest values for various markers of anaerobic energy supply among athletes.

LONG-TRACK SPEED SKATING INJURIES

Overuse

Most injuries in long-track skating are of the overuse variety.

Back Pain

A. Common complaint in long-track skaters, due in part to the body position required for efficient skating.
  1. Low trunk flexion angle needed to reduce frontal surface area puts a great deal of stress on spinal support musculature.
B. Pain tends to be mechanical in nature, most commonly from lumbar muscle strain, although disc pathology may occur.
C. History.
  1. Pain, typically in low back region without radiation.
  2. May worsen with prolonged activity; however, shorter-duration activity may partially relieve discomfort.
  3. Onset is usually insidious with gradual worsening over time.
  4. Mechanism of injury is usually atraumatic but may be related to a fall or other trauma.

   5. Associated signs/symptoms usually absent.
      a. Radiation of pain into lower extremities.
      b. Numbness, weakness in lower extremities.
      c. Bowel/bladder dysfunction.
      d. Fevers, sweats, chills.
      e. Unexplained weight loss.
D. Physical examination findings may be limited.
   1. Tenderness on palpation may or may not be elicited.
   2. Range of spine motion may be decreased or painful.
      a. Be sure to evaluate hip ROM.
   3. Strength, sensation, and reflexes typically full and intact.
   4. Special tests are typically negative.
      a. Straight leg raise.
      b. Faber's test.
      c. Stork test.
E. Diagnostic tests.
   1. Radiographs.
      a. Consider early in adolescent population.
      b. Obtain in adults when "red flag" signs are present. If no red flags, then consider if:
         i. Pain present for 4–6 weeks despite conservative treatment.
         ii. Pain worsens or red flags develop during initial treatment.
         iii. Pain is chronic on initial presentation.
   2. MRI.
      a. Very helpful if disc pathology suspected.
      b. Typically not necessary early in the treatment course.
   3. Bone scan.
      a. Excellent sensitivity for bony injury, lacks specificity.
      b. Consider if suspicion of spondylolysis high.
      c. Consider if suspicion of occult fracture high.
   4. CT scan.
      a. Can be used to look for disc pathology but generally more helpful due to its specificity for bony injury.
F. Findings from experience with elite speed skaters with back pain (unreported data collected 1995–97):
   1. Decreased hamstring flexibility.
   2. Decreased adductor flexibility of the left leg compared to right.
      a. On turns, the left leg holds the line of the turn as the right leg crosses over.
   3. Weak abdominal musculature.
   4. Majority of skaters had resolution of back pain symptoms when the above mechanical issues were addressed.

Patellofemoral Knee Pain

A. Perhaps the most common cause of anterior knee pain.
1. Overuse injury.
2. May occur at any age or level of competition.
B. Caused by unbalanced friction between the undersurface of the patella and the trochlea of the femur.
1. Subchondral bony injury.
2. Articular cartilage injury.
3. Synovial injury.
C. Biomechanics.
1. Resultant forces of the patella against the femur dependent upon:
   a. Quadriceps forces.
   b. Patellar tendon forces.
   c. Knee flexion angle.
      i. The greater the angle, the greater the resultant force for any given quadriceps/patella force.
2. Quadriceps activation leads to knee extension and lateral patellar motion/tilt.
   a. Vector forces of vastus lateralis, vastus intermedius, and rectus femoris move the patella laterally.
   b. Vastus medialis is the only quadriceps muscle that imparts a medially directed vector force.
3. The optimal "sit deeper" skating position (Figure 13-11) demands greater knee flexion angles and quadriceps and patellar forces, thereby increasing patellofemoral joint forces.
D. Intrinsic risk factors: Through prospective study, the following were found to be positive risk factors for the development of patellofemoral pain:
1. Decreased quadriceps flexibility.
2. Altered (faster) VMO muscle reflex response time.
3. Decreased explosive strength (measured with vertical jump).
4. Hypermobile patella.
5. Other possible, though not proven, risk factors include:
   a. Increased Q-angle.
   b. Hindfoot pronation/pes planus.
E. History.
1. Knee pain.
   a. Location.
      i. Anterior.
      ii. Peripatellar.
      iii. Nonradiating.
   b. Insidious onset with gradual worsening.

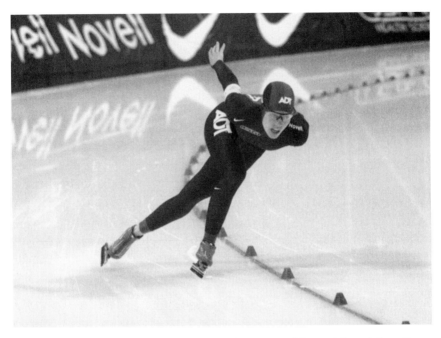

FIGURE 13-11 Long-track speed skater in a "deep sit" position. Deep knee flexion angles along with high quadriceps and patellar tendon forces lead to high patellofemoral joint forces. Photo courtesy of U.S. Speedskating.

    c. Provocative activities.
        i. Ascending/descending stairs.
        ii. Rising from a seated position (theater sign).
        iii. Deep knee bend/squat position (i.e., effective skating position).
  2. Negatives.
    a. Swelling is uncommon.
    b. No locking.
    c. No instability.
F. Physical examination.
  1. Positive findings.
    a. Peripatellar tenderness.
    b. Patellar facet tenderness.
    c. Subpatellar crepitus.
    d. Positive grind test.
        i. Compress patella against the femur and have patient activate quadriceps.
        ii. Pain with this maneuver is a positive test.

   2. Negative findings.
   - **a.** No effusion.
   - **b.** No ligamentous laxity.
   - **c.** Negative meniscus tests.
     - **i.** McMurray's.
     - **ii.** Apley's compression/distraction test.
     - **iii.** Flexion/circumduction test.

G. Diagnostic tests.
   1. X-rays often negative but may show:
   - **a.** Lateral patellar tilt.
   - **b.** Patellofemoral arthrosis.
   - **c.** Loose bodies.

   2. Other diagnostic tests not usually needed.

H. Treatment.
   1. Mainstay of treatment is vastus medialis obliquus (VMO) strengthening.
   - **a.** Isolated contraction of the VMO during quad exercises does not take place.
   - **b.** Open chain exercise programs (home program and formal physical therapy) have been shown to be effective in decreasing patellofemoral pain in adults and adolescents. Examples of open chain exercises include:
     - **i.** Isometric, maximal quad contraction with knee in full extension.
     - **ii.** Straight leg raise from supine position.
     - **iii.** Leg adduction from the lateral decubitus position.
   - **c.** Closed chain exercise may be slightly more effective than open chain exercises. Examples include:
     - **i.** Seated leg press.
     - **ii.** One-third knee bends.
       - One leg.
       - Two-legged.

   2. Patellar taping.
   - **a.** Can decrease patellofemoral pain symptoms.
   - **b.** Effects on the VMO may or may not be of benefit.
     - **i.** May alter the temporal characteristics of VMO firing in a positive manner.
     - **ii.** Decreases the relative activity of the VMO in comparison to the vastus lateralis.

   3. Patellar stabilizer knee sleeves.
   - **a.** May reduce pain in some patients, but not consistently successful.
   - **b.** Do not correct patellar tracking patterns based on kinematic MRI studies.

   c. Simple elastic sleeves have been shown to be at least as effective (if not more) in controlling pain compared to certain knee sleeves with silicone patellar rings.

4. Ice as needed.
5. Medications as needed.
   a. Acetaminophen.
   b. NSAIDs.
   c. Narcotic analgesics rarely required.
6. Activity modification.
   a. Difficult to modify skating position as this will negatively affect performance.
   b. Skaters do a great deal of cross-training (in-line skating, cycling, weight training) and it may be easier to modify these activities.
      i. Avoid high-impact, deep knee bend positions.
        • In-line skate in a more upright position.
        • Elevate bike seat.
        • Avoid deep squat and leg press weight training.
      ii. Avoid hill training and/or stair running.
7. Address other mechanical issues.
   a. If hindfoot valgus and/or pes planus present, custom orthotics for shoes and skates can be considered.
      i. In elite skaters, skates are often custom-molded.
   b. Blade position may need to be altered to reduce pain.
8. Surgical treatment.
   a. Typically reserved for patients who fail 6–12 months of adequate attempts at nonsurgical treatment.
   b. Various procedures available.
      i. Lateral release.
      ii. Tibial tubercle transfer.
      iii. Debridement of the patellofemoral joint.

Hip Flexor Strain

A. Common injury in both long- and short-track speed skating.
B. Muscles involved in hip flexion.
   1. Sartorius.
   2. Quadriceps.
   3. Iliopsoas.
C. Mechanism of injury is eccentric loading of the hip flexor muscles.
   1. Hip flexors at greatest eccentric load at the end of the push-off.
      a. Muscles act as decelerators to hip extension.
      b. Simultaneous production of flexion forces to return leg to proper position for glide.

2. Pre-Klapskate era.
    a. Toe of skate would often drag into ice.
        i. Toe digs into ice during push-off: Skater flexes hip and knee prematurely in order to lift blade off ice, creating eccentric forces.
        ii. If toe dragged during hip flexion, resistive forces (and therefore eccentric forces) increase.
3. Klapskate era.
    a. Incidence of hip flexor strain felt to be the same as in the pre-Klapskate era.
    b. The Klapskate mechanism allows for the full blade to maintain contact with the ice throughout the push-off stroke (Figure 13-12).

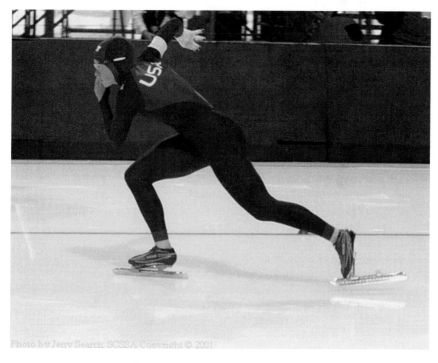

Photo by Jerry Search. SCSSA Copyright © 2001

FIGURE 13-12 Klapskate technology allows the skate blade to stay in contact with the ice throughout the push-off, allowing for more efficient transfer of power to the ice. Greater hip extension can be achieved during the skating stroke in Klapskates compared to conventional skates, potentially creating increased eccentric forces on the hip flexor musculature. Photo courtesy of Jerry Search.

    i. Toe does not dig into ice during push-off.

    ii. Greater hip extension achieved; this may add to the eccentric load of the hip flexors.

    iii. The toe may still drag on ice during active hip flexion as noted above.

D. History.

  1. Pain.

    a. Onset: May be acute or insidious.

    b. Location: Anterior hip region.

    c. Provocative activities.

      i. Fast skating.

      ii. Running (sprints).

      iii. Stretching anterior hip.

    d. Palliative activities.

      i. Relative rest.

      ii. Ice or heat.

  2. Weakness may or may not be present, but exercise performance is often hindered.

E. Physical examination.

  1. Positive findings.

    a. Tender over hip flexor musculature.

    b. Pain with passive hip flexor stretch.

    c. Pain with resisted hip flexion.

    d. Weakness may or may not be present; strength assessment hindered by pain.

  2. Negative findings.

    a. Swelling and bruising rare unless injury is acute.

    b. Neurovascular status intact.

    c. Passive hip motion is nontender (except extension).

    d. Nontender on bony palpation.

F. Differential diagnosis.

  1. Abdominal wall strain.

  2. Hernia.

    a. Inguinal.

    b. Sportsman's: See Chapter 11, Ice Hockey.

  3. Osteitis pubis: Consider if running is major component of cross-training.

  4. Femoral neck stress fracture: Consider if running is major component of cross-training.

  5. Apophysitis or apophyseal avulsion fracture.

G. Diagnostic tests are not generally needed to make hip flexor strain diagnosis.

  1. X-rays should be obtained in skeletally immature athletes who present with hip pain or when:

      a. The diagnosis is in question.

      b. Other pathologies need to be ruled out.

H. Treatment.

   1. Acute injury.

      a. Control pain and inflammation.

         i. Ice initially; heat can be added in after 48–72 hours.

         ii. NSAIDs or other analgesics.

            • Due to risk of increased bleeding after acute injury, acetaminophen should be considered in the first 24–48 hours.

         iii. Relative rest. May require a short period of rest from skating altogether.

      b. ROME.

         i. Active ROM.

         ii. Passive stretching.

      c. Strength training.

      d. Balance/proprioception training.

      e. Sport-specific activities.

   2. Chronic or overuse injury.

      a. Inflammation probably limited if present at all. NSAIDs can be used for analgesic effect.

      b. Treatment follows same progression as with acute injury.

         i. Usually able to continue activity during rehabilitation at a lower intensity.

Apophyseal Avulsion Fractures and Apophysitis

A. Apophyseal avulsion fractures.

   1. Most commonly seen in the adolescent age group.

   2. Anterior superior iliac spine (ASIS) and anterior inferior iliac spine (AIIS) injuries can mimic hip flexor strains.

      a. ASIS is origin of sartorius.

      b. AIIS is origin of straight head of rectus femoris.

   3. Avulsion fractures present as acute onset of anterior hip pain.

      a. Most likely to occur during the running phase of the start.

   4. For full discussion of hip apophyseal avulsion fractures and apophysitis, see Chapter 12, Figure Skating.

Patellar Tendinitis and Tendinosis

A. Mechanism of injury.

   1. Overloading of the patellar tendon leading to tissue changes and discomfort.

      a. May be due to multiple "physiologic" loads.

      b. May be due to fewer "supraphysiologic" loads.

    2. Inflammation present early in the process; typically resolves within one month even if symptoms persist.

    3. Later in process, changes in the tendon matrix develop, including microtears.

B. History.
  1. Pain.
    a. Onset: Insidious.
    b. Location: Anterior knee.
      i. Inferior pole of patella.
      ii. Mid-substance patellar tendon.
    c. Provocative activities.
      i. Deep squat activities.
        • Skating position.
      ii. Running, jumping.
  2. Negatives.
    a. No swelling.
    b. No instability.
    c. No locking.

C. Physical examination.
  1. Positives.
    a. Tender at inferior patellar pole and/or patellar tendon.
    b. Tender resisted knee extension.
      i. Strength full unless limited by pain.
  2. Negatives.
    a. No effusion.
    b. No ligamentous laxity.
    c. Negative meniscus tests.
    d. Negative grind test.

D. Differential diagnosis.
  1. Skeletally mature athletes.
    a. Patellofemoral knee pain.
    b. Infrapatellar bursitis.
    c. Meniscus injury.
  2. Skeletally immature athletes.
    a. Patellofemoral knee pain.
    b. Osgood-Schlatter.
    c. Sindig-Larsen-Johansson.
    d. Osteochondritis dessicans (OCD).
      i. For complete discussion of OCD, see Chapter 12, Figure Skating.

E. Diagnostic tests.
  1. Not needed to make this diagnosis.
  2. Utilized when diagnosis in question or to rule out other pathologies.

      a. If obtained, X-rays should include AP, lateral, and sunrise views.
        i. Include notch view if OCD considered.
        ii. Comparison views of contralateral knee helpful in skeletally immature skaters.

F. Treatment.
   1. Conservative treatment is usually effective though may take a number of months.
      a. Activity modification to reduce discomfort.
      b. Stretching exercises.
        i. Quadriceps.
        ii. Hamstrings.
      c. Eccentric loading program (e.g., drop squats).
        i. Controlled eccentric load to tendon.
        ii. Stimulates neovascularization.
        iii. Helps reestablish normal collagen matrix of the tendon.
        iv. May be uncomfortable to perform in early stages.
      d. Ice application.
      e. Analgesic medications.
        i. Inflammation may be minimal or even absent; therefore NSAIDs are used primarily for analgesic effect.
        ii. Acetaminophen.
      f. Bracing.
        i. Patellar knee sleeve with superior buttress.
        ii. Patellar tendon strap.
      g. Cross-friction massage.
      h. Extracorporeal shock wave therapy.
   2. Surgical treatment may be necessary in recalcitrant cases.

Chronic Exertional Compartment Syndrome (CECS)

A. An infrequently diagnosed cause of lower leg pain in athletes.
B. Four compartments in the lower leg; any or all may develop pathologic elevated intercompartmental pressures during exercise.
   1. Anterior compartment.
      a. Muscles.
        i. Tibialis anterior.
        ii. Extensor hallucis longus.
        iii. Extensor digitorum longus.
      b. Neurovascular structures.
        i. Anterior tibial artery and vein.
        ii. Deep peroneal nerve.
      c. Most common compartment involved in CECS.

2. Deep posterior compartment.
    a. Muscles.
        i. Tibialis posterior.
        ii. Flexor hallucis longus.
        iii. Flexor digitorum longus.
    b. Neurovascular structures.
        i. Peroneal artery and vein.
        ii. Posterior tibial artery and vein.
        iii. Tibial nerve.
3. Lateral compartment.
    a. Muscles.
        i. Peroneus longus.
        ii. Peroneus brevis.
    b. Neurovascular structures.
        i. Superficial peroneal nerve.
4. Superficial posterior compartment.
    a. Muscles.
        i. Gastrocnemius.
        ii. Soleus.
    b. Neurovascular structures.
        i. Medial sural cutaneous nerve.
C. History.
    1. Pain.
        a. Location: Lower leg.
        b. Onset: Insidious, gradual worsening with continued activities.
        c. Relieved by rest.
        d. Swelling may be noted occasionally.
    2. Late symptoms.
        a. Numbness of lower leg and foot.
        b. Weakness of lower leg.
            i. Foot drop.
            ii. Steppage gait.
D. Physical examination.
    1. Exam is often normal.
        a. Most patients present to office after a period of rest.
        b. May be beneficial to have athlete exercise prior to evaluation.
    2. Positives.
        a. Tender to palpation of anterior lower leg.
            i. Anterior muscle compartment.
            ii. Medial edge of tibia.
        b. Other areas of the lower leg may be tender depending on compartments involved.
        c. Discomfort with passive stretching of involved compartments.

    d. Discomfort with resisted strength testing.
      i. Strength usually full.
      ii. Weakness may be noted in some cases, particularly if the athlete exercises just prior to examination.
  3. Negatives.
    a. Sensation usually intact.
      i. Sensation may be decreased late in the disease process.
    b. Pulses intact.
    c. Reflexes intact.
E. Differential diagnosis.
  1. Bone pain.
    a. Periostitis.
    b. Stress fracture.
    c. Tumor.
  2. Nerve pain.
    a. Peroneal nerve entrapment.
    b. Other peroneal nerve injury.
      i. Direct trauma.
      ii. Cryotherapy induced.
    c. Radicular pain.
  3. Vascular.
    a. Claudication/PVD.
    b. DVT.
    c. Embolism.
  4. Muscular pain.
    a. Strain.
    b. Contusion.
    c. Primary muscular disease.
    d. Muscle herniation.
F. Diagnostic testing (all typically negative in CECS).
  1. Radiographs.
    a. AP and lateral tibia/fibula views should be obtained early in workup.
    b. Signs of stress fracture include:
      i. Cortical thickening.
      ii. Periosteal elevation.
      iii. "Dreaded black line."
        • Indicates anterior cortex stress fracture.
  2. Bone scan.
    a. Diffuse, linear uptake indicative of periostitis.
    b. Fusiform uptake indicative of stress fracture.
  3. Ultrasound.
    a. Noninvasive test of choice to rule out vascular pathology.
    b. Excellent choice to evaluate for muscle herniation.

4. MRI.
   a. Excellent choice to evaluate for muscle herniation.
5. EMG/NCV.
   a. Test of choice to evaluate for radiculopathy and peripheral neuropathy.
   b. Typically negative in CECS, but may turn positive late in process.
6. Compartment pressure measurement.
   a. "Gold standard" test for CECS.
   b. Compartment pressures measured pre-exercise (baseline) and at timed intervals after exercise challenge (athlete exercises to pain).
   c. Positive pressures.
      i. Opening pressure $\geq$ 15 mm Hg.
      ii. 1-minute post-exercise $\geq$ 30 mm Hg.
      iii. 5-minutes post-exercise $\geq$ 20 mm Hg.

G. Treatment.
   1. Conservative treatments are generally not effective in competitive athletes. Conservative therapies include:
      a. Remove athlete from inciting activities.
      b. Massage.
      c. Ice.
      d. NSAIDs.
      e. Support.
         i. Shin splint tape.
         ii. Compressive wrap.
         iii. Lower leg splint.
      f. Pain almost always fully returns when athlete returns to activities.
   2. Fasciotomy is definitive treatment.

SHORT-TRACK SPEED SKATING

Medical Issues

A. Concussion.
   1. Although possible in long track, concussion is much more common in short track.
      a. Higher rate of falls.
      b. Contact with boards at high rate of speed is the primary mechanism of injury.
         i. Boards are padded.
         ii. Striking head against ice is another common mechanism.

     c. Hard-shell helmet use mandatory.
  2. For full discussion of concussion, see Chapter 11, Ice Hockey.
B. Laceration.
  1. Primarily due to contact with skate blade.
     a. Lacerations tend to be clean.
     b. Tend to be linear.
  2. Can occur to any part of the body.
     a. Most commonly encountered on the extremities.
     b. Cut-resistant gloves are required equipment.
     c. Neck guard is required equipment.
  3. Update tetanus immunization if appropriate.
  4. For discussion of preparation and closure options, see Chapter 11, Ice Hockey.
  5. Most athletes are able to resume competition immediately following wound closure.
  6. Sutures should be removed in 7–10 days in most cases.
C. Exercise-induced bronchospasm—see Chapter 2, Pulmonary Physiology.

Musculoskeletal Injuries

A. AC sprains and clavicle fractures.
  1. Mechanism of injury is direct trauma to the superior aspect of the shoulder.
     a. Contact with boards.
     b. Contact with ice.
  2. For full discussion of AC sprains and clavicle fractures, see Chapter 11, Ice Hockey.
B. Scaphoid fracture.
  1. Mechanism of injury.
     a. Fall to ice on outstretched hand.
     b. Using arms to brace for impact with the boards.
  2. History.
     a. Pain.
        i. Radial aspect of wrist.
        ii. Worse with motion.
     b. Other signs/symptoms that may be present:
        i. Swelling: Usually only present with fracture/dislocations.
        ii. Gross deformity (usually more indicative of distal radius fracture).
        iii. Paresthesias.
  3. Physical examination.
     a. Tenderness over scaphoid tubercle.
     b. Tenderness in anatomical snuff-box.

     c. Tender passive ROM.

     d. Document neurovascular status.

4. Radiographs should be obtained in all cases of suspected scaphoid injury.

     a. Views.

         i. AP view (Figure 13-13).

         ii. Lateral view.

         iii. Ulnar deviation or scaphoid views.

     b. Radiographs often negative shortly after injury.

         i. Should be repeated in two weeks if initially negative but suspicion remains high.

5. Other diagnostic tests may be obtained if repeat X-rays are negative or definitive diagnosis needed sooner than the planned two-week follow-up.

     a. Radionuclide bone scan. Becomes positive within 2–3 days of the injury.

     b. CT scan.

     c. MRI scan.

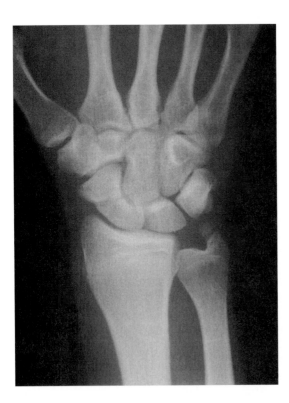

FIGURE 13-13 AP radiograph of the wrist shows a nondisplaced fracture of the waist of the scaphoid. Image courtesy of James L. Moeller, MD.

6. Treatment of scaphoid fracture.
  a. Treatment of fracture is initiated if suspicion of scaphoid fracture is high even if X-rays are initially negative.
    i. Repeat X-rays at follow-up visit.
    ii. May discontinue immobilization if exam and X-rays are negative at follow-up unless suspicion remains high.
  b. Nondisplaced fractures are treated with cast immobilization.
    i. Long-arm versus short-arm thumb spica casting is controversial.
      • Studies have shown decreased time to union and reduced rates of delayed union and nonunion with a long-arm thumb spica cast.
      • Union rates of up to 95% with short-arm casting have been reported.
      • Combination of long-arm and short-arm casting may be most appropriate.
        – Long-arm cast for initial 6 weeks.
        – Short-arm cast from 6 weeks until radiographic healing present.
  c. Healing rates and average healing time depend on location of the fracture due to the blood supply to the different regions of the scaphoid.
    i. Distal pole fractures.
      • Healing rate: Close to 100%.
      • Average time: 10–12 weeks.
    ii. Waist fractures.
      • Healing rate: 80–90%.
      • Average time: 10–12 weeks.
    iii. Proximal pole fractures:
      • Healing rate: 60–70%.
      • Average time: 12–20 weeks.
  d. Poor outcome (nonunion, malunion) more likely to occur if:
    i. Diagnosis is delayed.
    ii. Appropriate treatment delayed.
    iii. Proximal pole fracture.
  e. Although usually treated with surgical fixation, displaced fractures ($\geq$ 1mm) can be treated with closed immobilization.
    i. Surgical options include:
      • Closed reduction and percutaneous pin fixation.
      • Open reduction and fixation.
        – Pin fixation.
        – Compression screw fixation.

7. Return to activities.
   a. Cast immobilization.
      i. Safe to start skating once immobilized.
      ii. Full training and competition may need to be delayed until full healing occurs.
         • Long-arm cast on left arm would not allow skater to make appropriate hand contact on turns.
         • Cast may not allow athlete to wear appropriate equipment (cut-resistant gloves) for full training or competition.
         • Cast may put other competitors at risk for injury and therefore may be cause for disqualification from competitive events.
   b. Surgical fixation.
      i. In contact sport athletes, return to activity 5.8 to 8 weeks after ORIF with a Herbert screw has been reported.
      ii. There is no data currently available regarding return to competition after ORIF of scaphoid fracture in short-track speed skaters.
   C. Discussion of distal radius and forearm fractures can be found in Chapter 6, Snowboarding.
   D. Lower extremity muscle strains.
      1. Very common problem in short-track speed skating.
      2. Discussion of lower extremity muscle strains can be found in multiple areas throughout this book.
         a. Hip flexor strain: See Long-Track Speed Skating Injuries.
         b. Quadriceps strain: See Chapter 14, Sliding Sports.
         c. Hamstring strain: See Chapter 14, Sliding Sports.

Suggested Readings

Abramowitz AJ, Schepsis AA. Chronic exertional compartment syndrome of the lower leg. *Orthop Rev* 1994;23(3):219–25.

Arroll B, Ellis-Pegler E, Edwards A, Sutcliffe G. Patellofemoral pain syndrome: A critical review of the clinical trials on nonoperative therapy. *AJSM* 1997;25(2):207–12.

Cook JL, Khan KM. What is the most appropriate treatment for patellar tendinopathy? *Br J Sports Med* 2001;35(5):291–94.

Cooney WP, Linscheid RL, Dobyns JH. Fractures and dislocations of the wrist. In: Rockwood CA, Green DP, Bucholz RW, Heckman JD, eds. *Rockwood and Green's Fractures in Adults.* 4th ed. Philadelphia, PA: Lippincott-Raven; 1996.

Cowan SM, Bennell KL, Hodges PW. Therapeutic patellar taping changes the timing of vasti muscle activation in people with patellofemoral pain syndrome. *Clin J Sport Med* 2002;12(6):339–47.

deKoning JJ, deGroot G, van Ingen Schenau GJ. A power equation for the sprint in speed skating. *J Biomech* 1992;25:573.

deKoning JJ, Foster C, Bobbert MF, et al. Aerobic and anaerobic kinetics during speed skating competition. Experimental test of some assumptions in the power balance model of skating. *J Appl Physiol* (in press).

deKoning JJ, van Ingen Schenau GJ. Performance determining factors in speed skating. In: Zatsiorsky VM, ed. *Olympic Encyclopedia of Sports Medicine and Science: Biomechanics in Sport—The Scientific Basis of Performance*. Oxford, UK: Blackwell Scientific; 2000:232.

Finestone A, Radin EL, Lev B, et al. Treatment of overuse patellofemoral pain: Prospective randomized controlled clinical trial in a military setting. *Clin Orthop* 1993;293:208–10.

Foster C, Brucker L, Zeman J, et al. Effect of competitive distance on utilization of the anaerobic capacity. *Med Sci Sports Exerc* 2002;34:S134.

Foster C, deKoning JJ. Physiological perspectives in speed skating, In: Gemser H, deKoning JJ, van Ingen Schenau GJ, eds. *Handbook of Competitive Speed Skating*. Leeuwarden, NL: Eisma Publishers bv; 1999:117.

Foster C, deKoning JJ, Hettinga F, et al. Pattern of energy expenditure during simulated competition. *Med Sci Sports Exerc* 2003;35(5):826–31.

Foster C, deKoning JJ, Rundell KW, et al. Physiology of speed skating. In: Garrett WE, Kirkendall DT, eds. *Exercise and Sports Science*. Philadelphia, PA: Lippincott, Williams and Wilkins; 2000:885.

Foster C, Rundell KW, Snyder AC, et al. Evidence for restricted muscle blood flow during speed skating. *Med Sci Sports Exerc* 1999;31:1433.

Gastin PB. Quantitation of anaerobic capacity. *Scand J Med Sci Sports* 1994;4: 91.

Gellman H, Caputo RJ, Carter V, et al. Comparison of short and long thumb-spica casts for nondisplaced fractures of the carpal scaphoid. *JBJS*(A) 1989;71:354–57.

Houdijk H, deKoning JJ, deGroot G, et al. Push-off mechanics in speed skating with conventional and Klapskates. *Med Sci Sports Exerc* 2000;32:635.

Howard JL, Mohtadi NG, Wiley JP. Evaluation of outcomes in patients following surgical treatment of chronic exertional compartment syndrome in the leg. *CJSM* 2000;10(3):176–84.

Khan KM, Cook JL, Bonar F, et al. Histopathology of common tendinopathies: Update and implications for clinical management. *Sports Med* 1999;27(6):393–408.

Moeller JL. Pelvic and hip apophyseal avulsion injuries in young athletes. *Curr Sports Med Rep* 2003;2(2):110–15.

Montgomery S, Haak M. Management of lumbar injuries in athletes. *Sports Med* 1999;27(2):135–41.

Nadler SF, Malanga GA, DePrince M, et al. The relationship between lower extremity injury, low back pain, and hip muscle strength in male and female collegiate athletes. *CJSM* 2000;10(2):89–97.

Ng GY, Cheng JM. The effects of patellar taping on pain and neuromuscular performance in subjects with patellofemoral pain syndrome. *Clin Rehabil* 2002;16(8):821–27.

O'Neill DB, Micheli LJ, Warner JP. Patellofemoral stress: A prospective analysis of exercise treatment in adolescents and adults. *AJSM* 1992;20(2): 151–56.

Pedowitz RA, Hargens AR, Mubarak SJ, Gershuni DH. Modified criteria for the objective diagnosis of chronic compartment syndrome of the leg. *AJSM* 1990;18(1):35–40.

Powers CM, Shellock FG, Beering TV, et al. Effect of bracing on patellar kinematics in patients with patellofemoral joint pain. *Med Sci Sports Exerc* 1999;31(12):1714–20.

Rajalla GM, Neumann DA, Foster C, et al. Quadriceps muscle performance in male speed skaters. *J Strength Cond Res* 1994;8:48.

Rettig AC, Kollias SC. Internal fixation of acute stable scaphoid fractures in the athlete. *AJSM* 1996;24(2):182–86.

Rettig AC, Weidenbener EJ, Gloyeske R. Alternative management of mid-third scaphoid fractures in the athlete. *AJSM* 1994;22(5):711–14.

Rundell KW, Nioka S, Chance B. Hemoglobin/myoglobin desaturation during speed skating. *Med Sci Sports Exerc* 1997;29:248.

Trainor TJ, Wiesel SW. Epidemiology of back pain in the athlete. *Clin Sports Med* 2002;21(1):93–103.

van Ingen Schenau GJ, deGroot G, Scheurs AW, et al. A new skate allowing powerful plantar flexions improves performance. *Med Sci Sports Exerc* 1996;28:531.

van Ingen Schenau GJ, deKoning JJ. Biomechanics of speed skating. In: Gemser H, deKoning JJ, van Ingen Schenau GJ, eds. *Handbook of Competitive Speed Skating.* Leeuwarden, NL: Eisma Publishers bv; 1999:41.

Witvrouw E, Lysens R, Bellemans J, et al. Intrinsic risk factors for the development of anterior knee pain in an athletic population: A two-year prospective study. *AJSM* 2000;28(4):480–89.

14

SLIDING SPORTS

Bradford A. Stephens
Eugene Byrne

BOBSLED

General Information

A. Description.
   1. Winter team sliding sport on artificial ice track.
   2. Bobsled teams.
      1. Two-man team.
         a. Pilot.
         b. Brakeman.
      2. Four-man team.
         a. Pilot.
         b. Two pushers.
         c. Brakeman.
B. Sled.
   1. Cockpit.
      a. Four-man sled.
         i. Length: 3.8 m (maximum).
         ii. Width: 0.67 m.
         iii. Weight: 630 kg (maximum).
            • Weight includes crew.
            • Weight bars may be added to achieve maximum weight.
      b. Two-man sled.
         i. Length: 2.7 m (maximum).
         ii. Width: 0.67 m.
         iii. Weight: 390 kg (maximum).

- Weight includes crew.
- Weight bars may be added to achieve maximum weight.

2. Runners.
   a. Each sled has two sets of paired runner blades.
   b. Bottoms of runners are made of steel.
   c. Runners are carefully smoothed for speed and sharpened for control.
   d. Front runners can be turned for steering.
3. Steering.
   a. Pilot steers by pulling cords attached to the front runners.
   b. Driver seeks the "perfect line" which gives the most speed and shortest distance.
      i. Driver must apply very small changes to runners to stay on-line.
4. Braking.
   a. Two sharpened rods are connected to handles at the rear of the sled.
   b. Brakeman pulls up forcibly on handles to rotate the brake down into the ice.
   c. Out-run is long and uphill.

C. Equipment.
   1. Skin-tight Lycra suit.
   2. Fiberglass helmet with full face shield.
   3. Spiked shoes.
      a. Spikes located under the ball of the foot.
      b. Spikes may not exceed 4 mm in length.
      c. Top of spike may not exceed 1 mm in width.

D. Track.
   1. All bobsled tracks are now combined with luge tracks (see description of luge track in Luge, Description, 4a–c).

E. Race.
   1. First segment is 15 m.
      a. Athletes initiate pushing the sled.
      b. They accelerate the sled as rapidly as possible in this segment.
      c. At the 15-m mark a timing eye starts timing for the race.
   2. Second segment is a 15-m downslope that starts at the 15-m mark.
      a. Athletes accelerate the sled to their maximum running speed and then enter sled.
         i. Usually at the 30–40-m mark.
         ii. All athletes must be in the sled by the 50-m mark.
   3. Stopping.

      a. After finish, the brakeman applies the brakes with as much force as possible.

      b. Sled enters an upgrade, which helps with stopping.

  4. Duration: 2–3 minutes.

      a. World Cup races are a combination of two runs.

      b. Olympic races are a combination of four runs.

      c. Races are timed to one one-thousandth of a second.

      d. After the race the sled and the athletes are weighed together and the runner temperature is measured.

F. Critical factors for maximum performance.

  1. Start.

  2. Driving technique.

  3. Conditioning.

  4. Equipment.

G. History of bobsled.

  1. 1877—Steering mechanism was placed on toboggans in Davos, Switzerland.

  2. 1884—First competition held.

      a. Racers rode from St. Moritz to Celerina.

  3. 1897—First World's "Bobsleigh" Club was founded in St. Moritz.

      a. Bobsled name comes from the "bobbing" maneuver used by crews to try to increase their speed on straightaways.

      b. Early sleds were made of wood, were flat, and had steering wheels to control runners.

  4. 1914—Bobsled races were taking place on natural ice courses.

  5. 1924—First winter Olympics in Chamonix, France, had a four-man bobsled event.

  6. 1932—Two-man event (men only) added at the Lake Placid, NY, Olympic Games.

  7. National bobsled powers.

      a. American-built steel sleds and athletes were very successful through the 1950s.

      b. Switzerland and Germany have been most successful since that time.

  8. 2002—Women's bobsled (two-woman) added at the Salt Lake City, Utah, Olympic Games.

Biomechanics and Physiology

A. The start is the most important part of the race.

  1. Every 0.01 second gained at the start will turn into a 0.03-second advantage at the finish.

2. The start is an explosive rapid movement by the athletes similar to a track start.
   a. The need to apply maximum power to push the heavy sled and to accelerate as rapidly as possible creates large stresses.
   b. The start is an anaerobic event.
3. Phases of the start.
   a. First phase.
      i. Athletes lean into the sled for 1 to 2 seconds to start the sled sliding.
   b. Second phase.
      i. Athletes drop into a starting position similar to a track athlete and initiate an explosive running start.
   c. Third phase.
      i. As athletes reach maximum running speed, they enter the sled.
      ii. The entry must be done in an accelerating fashion.
      iii. Order of entry in a four-man sled.
         • The driver enters first.
         • The two pushers enter after this, with the slower runner entering first.
         • Finally, the brakeman enters.
            – He must be the fastest of all four team members.
B. The slide.
   1. The pushers and brakeman sit with their legs extended, torsos bent forward at the waist as far as possible.
      a. They should "sink" into as relaxed a position as possible.
      b. They do not attempt to move to either side to help with steering.
   2. The driver bends partially forward, keeping his/her head up, and steers with cords.
C. The finish.
   1. The brakeman must pull up on the brake handles with maximum power. This is done by a combination of:
      a. Forced back extension.
      b. Knee extension.
      c. Arm flexion.
D. Training.
   1. Designed to improve conditioning, speed, and power.
      a. Conditioning—running, mostly sprint work.
      b. Power—developed through Olympic lifts and squats.
      c. Speed—developed in sprint work.
   2. Training facilities (North America).

     a. Wheeled push track in Lake Placid, NY.

     b. Indoor ice start track in Calgary, Alberta, Canada.

E. Team selection (USA) for pusher and brakeman positions is based on six tests.

    1. Sprint speed.

       a. 30-m sprint.

       b. 50-m sprint.

    2. 30-m fly.

    3. Vertical jump.

    4. Consecutive hops.

    5. Back squat.

    6. Power clean.

Musculoskeletal Injuries

A. Mechanism of injury.

    1. Repetitive, overuse injuries.

       a. Off-track injuries related to strength training.

       b. Occasional injuries due to lifting heavy sled.

       c. On-track overuse injuries caused by stress of the start sprint.

          i. Hamstring strains.

          ii. Low back strain.

          iii. Hip flexor strain.

    2. Acute trauma from crashes.

       a. High-speed (80-mph) injuries.

          i. The sled tips over and athletes attempt to stay in sled.

            • Helmets strike ice, causing concussions and cervical strains.

            • Shoulders strike ice, causing burns.

          ii. Athletes thrown from sled continue to slide all the way to the bottom of the run.

            • Multiple injuries can occur from striking the ice or track lips.

B. Very little data exists regarding injury statistics in the sport of bobsled. The following data has been generated from injury surveys and training room injury reports from the U.S. bobsled team for the 2002–2003 season. Actual numbers of runs are not available, so incidence rates cannot be calculated.

    1. Total injuries, 32.

       a. Mechanism.

          i. Crashes, 10.

          ii. Noncontact, 22.

2. Anatomic areas affected and injury type.
   a. Head, 12.5% (4/32).
      i. Concussion, 2.
         • For discussion of concussion management, see Chapter 11, Ice Hockey.
      ii. Laceration, 1.
         • For discussion of laceration repair options, see Chapter 11, Ice Hockey.
      iii. TMJ, 1.
   b. Neck, 18.75% (6/32).
      i. Muscle strain, 6.
      ii. Cervical strain is discussed in the Luge section of this chapter.
   c. Back/trunk, 25% (8/32).
      i. Lumbar strain, 4.
         • Discussed in Chapter 13, Speed Skating.
      ii. Rib contusion, 2.
      iii. Sacroiliac joint sprain, 1.
         • Sacroiliitis is discussed in Chapter 9, Cross-Country Skiing.
      iv. Abdominal strain, 1.
         • Discussed in Chapter 11, Ice Hockey.
   d. Shoulder, 9.375% (3/32).
      i. Contusion, 3.
   e. Elbow, 3.125% (1/32).
      i. Contusion, 1.
      ii. Discussion of olecranon injuries (fracture and traumatic bursitis) can be found in Chapter 12, Figure Skating.
   f. Hip, 18.75% (6/32).
      i. Hamstring strain, 4.
         • Discussion of hamstring strain can be found in the Skeleton section of this chapter.
      ii. Adductor strain, 1.
         • See Chapter 11, Ice Hockey.
      iii. Hip flexor strain, 1.
         • See Chapter 13, Speed Skating.
   g. Knee, 9.375% (3/32).
      i. Contusion, 1.
      ii. Tendinitis, 1.
      iii. Iliotibial band syndrome, 1.
         • See Chapter 9, Cross-Country Skiing.
   h. Ankle, 3.125% (1/32).
      i. Peroneal strain, 1.
         • Discussed in Chapter 9, Cross-Country Skiing.

3. Injury severity.
    a. Majority of injuries are relatively minor and result in very little time lost from training or competition.
        i. 97% (31/32) of injuries resulted in 0–5 days lost.
        ii. 6–14 days: 0%.
        iii. > 14 days: 3% (1/32).

Conclusion

A. Bobsled is a very popular, exciting, high-speed sport.
B. Bobsled is relatively safe with a few major injuries.
C. There are few highly-trained competitors worldwide in the sport.
D. Most injuries are mild to moderate.

LUGE

General Information

A. Description.
    1. Winter sliding sport on artificial ice track.
    2. The sled.
        a. Two runner blades.
            i. Bottoms of the runners are made of steel.
            ii. Smoothed for speed and sharpened for steering.
            iii. Front of runners is turned up into Kufens used for steering.
            iv. Runners must not be 5° warmer or colder than control blade.
        b. Pod on which the athlete lies.
        c. Two undivided bridges connecting the pod to the runners.
        d. No brakes.
            i. The athlete must sit up, put feet down, and pull up front of sled to stop.
        e. Sled weight.
            i. 23–25 kg (50.6–55 lbs) singles.
            ii. 25–30 kg (55–66 lbs) doubles.
    3. Equipment (Figure 14-1).
        a. Athlete wears skin-tight Lycra-type suit.
        b. Fiberglass (Kevlar) helmet with full face shield.
        c. Leather gloves with spikes on fingertips or knuckles.
        d. Tight booties on feet.
        e. May wear a weight vest to make up for lighter body weight.
        f. A neck strap to prevent neck extension can be worn.

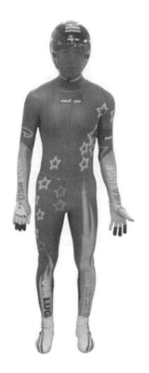

FIGURE 14-1 Front view of a luge athlete. Note the helmet with full face shield, skin-tight Lycra bodysuit, boot covers, and spiked gloves. Photo courtesy of Daniel Smith, ATC, USA Luge.

      i. A single strap from the chin strap of the helmet is connected to a loop around each thigh.
   g. May wear elbow, ankle, and/or forearm protection of molded plastic (orthoplast).
 4. The track.
   a. Artificial iced track.
      i. Men: approximately 1500 m.
     ii. Women and doubles: approximately 1300 m.
   b. Start area.
      i. Approximate 90-m drop for men.
     ii. 60-m drop for women.
        • Women and doubles start lower on the track than men.
   c. Turns.
      i. Usually 15 to 20 turns.
     ii. Include simple, S-shaped and Kreisel (360°).
    iii. Lips are now placed on turns to prevent sleds and athlete from leaving the track.
 5. Races.
   a. Speeds reach an excess of 90 mph.
   b. G-force loads of 4 to 5 have been measured.

    c. Races run as singles for men and women and doubles for men.

    d. Duration: 2 to 3 minutes.

        i. Combined time over four runs.

    e. Races are timed to one one-thousandth of a second.

    f. Critical factors for maximum performance.

        i. Start.

        ii. Sliding technique.

        iii. Conditioning.

        vi. Equipment.

    g. At the end of a race the sled weight, athlete weight, and runner temperature are checked.

B. History.

    1. Sled racing is one of the oldest winter sports.

        a. Believed that the Vikings used two-runner sleds as early as 800 AD.

        b. First chronicled in Norway and the Alps in the 1400s.

    2. "Luge" comes from the French word for sled (called "rodel" in German).

    3. 1883—First international luge race took place in Davos, Switzerland.

        a. 21 athletes from 7 countries participated.

        b. 4-km race; winning time was 9 minutes, 15 seconds.

    4. 1914—First European Championships took place in what is now the Czech Republic.

    5. 1953—Federation Internationale de Luge de Course, the sport's international governing body, formed.

    6. 1955—First World Championships on an artificial track took place in Oslo, Norway.

    7. 1964—Introduced as an Olympic sport at Innsbruck games.

    8. 1979—First North American track built for the 1980 Lake Placid Olympics.

    9. New combined bobsled and luge tracks built recently:

        a. Calgary, Alberta, Canada—1986.

        b. Nagano, Japan—1996.

        c. Salt Lake City, Utah—1997.

        d. Lake Placid, NY—2002.

Biomechanics

A. Start: Most critical part of the overall run.

    1. Explosive, rapid movement.

    2. High stress on wrists, shoulders, and back.

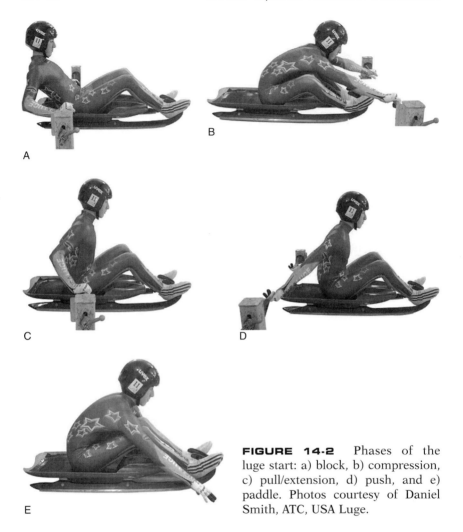

A

B

C

D

E

FIGURE 14-2 Phases of the luge start: a) block, b) compression, c) pull/extension, d) push, and e) paddle. Photos courtesy of Daniel Smith, ATC, USA Luge.

3. There are six basic parts of the start.
   a. Block: Slide sled forward (Figure 14-2a).
      i. Wrists, shoulders, and back in extension.
      ii. Abdominal contraction.
   b. Compression: Forced, fast backward movement of sled (Figure 14-2b).
      i. Upper body compresses down between the knees.
      ii. Elicit stretching effect of muscles.
      iii. Maximal back flexion.
      iv. Shoulder forward flexion.

    c. Pull: Start sled forward (Figure 14-2c).
        i. Natural bounce effect from compression.
        ii. Back extension and shoulder flexion initiated.
    d. Extension: After sled starts its first movement (Figure 14-2c).
        i. Upper and lower back extension.
        ii. Back should stay straight.
        iii. Hip extension and slight straightening of the legs.
    e. Push: Starts as body moves past the start handles (Figure 14-2d).
        i. Torso should stay erect and forward.
        ii. Shoulders go into extension.
    f. Paddle: Continues to propel sled forward (Figure 14-2e).
        i. Spikes on glove fingertips or knuckles used.
        ii. Abdominal muscles tight.
        iii. Back straight, head up, looking down the track.
        iv. Wrist, fingers, and elbows are solid and tight.
        v. Generally 3–4 paddles.
B. Slide: Athlete must be very relaxed and hold body in best aerodynamic position (Figure 14-3).
    1. Ankles and feet are maximally flexed.
    2. Knees are slightly flexed and hips are extended.
    3. Arms are at the side holding handles on inside edge of sled at thigh level.
    4. Neck slightly flexed at approximately 5° to allow vision down the track.
        a. High G-forces of 4–5 force neck into extension.
            i. High stresses on cervical muscles, ligaments, and joints.

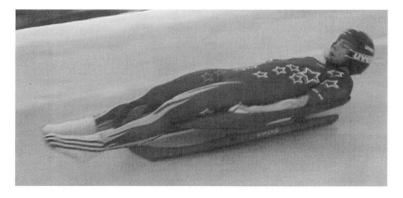

FIGURE 14-3 Aerodynamic sliding position. Photo courtesy of Daniel Smith, ATC, USA Luge.

   b. Athlete can "lose" neck into hyperextension and not be able
      to correct.
      i. Some athletes use the neck strap to prevent this from
         happening.
   5. Abdominal musculature contracted.
   6. Torso, arms, and legs relaxed to allow smooth glide.
C. Steer.
   1. Gentle and subtle pressures used to avoid oversteering.
   2. Pressure on Kufens by the leg on the outside of the turn.
   3. Shoulder on the inside of the turn applies pressure.
   4. Neck rotates to face into the turn.
D. Stopping.
   1. Tracks end with a long, straight uphill with cushioned pads at
      the end.
   2. Athlete sits up, puts feet down, and lifts up on the Kufens.
   3. Requires good leg, arm, and back strength.

Training

A. General aerobic and anaerobic fitness training start early in the
   spring.
B. Flexibility and agility work with alternative training.
C. Base strengthening of legs, neck, and abdominal muscles continually worked on.
   1. Core strengthening.
      a. Dead lifts.
      b. Rows.
      c. Arm extensions.
   2. Speed and power strengthening.
      a. Olympic-style lifts and explosive extensions and pulls.
         i. Power cleans.
         ii. Clean and jerk.
         iii. Snatch lifts.
         iv. Plyometrics.
         v. Explosive extensions and pulls.
D. Start technique continually practiced at the indoor start facilities.

Mechanisms of Injury

A. Repetitive, overuse injuries.
   1. Off-track injuries are most commonly due to strength training.
   2. On-track overuse injuries are due to repetitive practice runs,
      rough ice, and high G-loads.

      a. Cervical strains.

      b. Low back strains.

B. Acute trauma.

    1. High speed (80 mph) results in high-energy injuries.

      a. Strike the lips on track edges.

        i. Direct blows to feet.

        ii. Twisting injuries to ankles.

        iii. Hands protected within sled pod.

      b. Athlete thrown from sled in crash or rollover.

        i. Once thrown, athlete and sled do not stop.

        ii. If you crash at the top of the track you will slide on your own to the bottom.

          • Abrasions and burns from the ice are common.

          • Emergency personnel are stationed at the lowest section of the track.

        iii. Direct blow to the head causes concussions. For discussion of concussion, see Chapter 11, Ice Hockey.

      c. Athlete trying to prevent a crash.

        i. Puts feet down, injuring foot or ankle.

        ii. Puts arm out, injuring hand, wrist, or elbow.

      d. Athlete rarely thrown from track in modern tracks.

        i. If ejected from track, high-energy multiple trauma.

Injuries

A. Incidence.

    1. 1043 athletes suffered 407 injuries on 57,244 runs.

    2. 407 injuries/57,244 runs = 7 injuries/1000 runs.

    3. Risk of injury: 0.39/person/yr.

    4. Risk of injury causing >1 lost day of practice: 0.04/person/year.

B. Male/female comparison.

    1. Athlete gender.

      a. Male: 75% (782/1043).

      b. Female: 25% (261/1043).

    2. Percentage of total injuries.

      a. Male: 69% (281/407).

      b. Female: 31% (126/407).

    3. Major injuries.

      a. Male: 3% (12/407).

      b. Female: 0.8% (3/407).

    4. Conclusions.

      a. Males have slightly less frequent but more severe injuries. Reasons for this may include:

        i. Higher start on the track.

        ii. Higher speeds reached.

        iii. Larger body mass.

C. Crashes were the major cause of injury and account for:
1. 64% of all injuries (260/407).
2. 91% of moderate and major injuries.
3. 70% of contusions.

D. Injury sites.
1. Upper extremity: 51%.
2. Lower extremity: 30%.
3. Torso: 19%.

E. Injury severity.
1. Most injuries minor.
2. Time loss due to injury.
   - **a.** 67% of injuries resulted in no loss of training or competition time.
   - **b.** 22%: 1 day lost.
   - **c.** 9%: 2–7 days lost.
   - **d.** 2%: > 7 days lost.
3. Moderate and major injuries do occur.
   - **a.** Head is the greatest site of moderate/major injury.
   - **b.** Helmets have been greatly improved since the time of the survey cited above.
   - **c.** Concussions 13% of major injuries. For full discussion of concussions, see Chapter 11, Ice Hockey.
     - **i.** 71% caused by crashes.

F. Injury types.
1. Contusions.
   - **a.** Location.

i. Hand:	16%.
ii. Knee:	10%.
iii. Leg:	10%.
iv. Foot:	10%.
v. Shoulder:	10%.

   - **b.** Severity.

i. Mild:	93%.
ii. Moderate:	5%.
iii. Major:	2%.

2. Strains.
   - **a.** Location.

i. Neck:	45%.
ii. Back:	21%.

   - **b.** Severity.

       i. Mild: 96%.

       ii. Moderate: 4%.

3. Lacerations.

   a. Location.

       i. Elbow: 25%.

       ii. Face: 25%.

          • All on chin.

       iii. Hand: 19%.

   b. Severity.

       i. Mild: 81%.

       ii. Moderate: 19%.

4. Sprains.

   a. Location.

       i. Ankle: 50%.

          • Primarily anterior talofibular ligament.

       ii. Knee:

          • Primarily the medial collateral ligament.

       iii. Fingers/interphalangeal joints.

   b. Severity.

       i. Mild: 79%.

       ii. Moderate: 21%.

5. Fractures.

   a. Location.

       i. Foot: 21%.

          • Calcaneus.

          • Fifth metatarsal.

          • First toe.

       ii. Hand: 14%.

       iii. Ankle: 14%.

       iv. Ribs: 14%.

   b. Severity.

       i. Mild: 71%.

       ii. Moderate and major: 29%.

G. Specific injuries.

  1. Neck sprain is the most commonly encountered injury.

    a. General information.

       i. Due to high forces (> 5000 N) pushing neck into extension in curves.

       ii. Trapezius is primary muscle group involved (70% of cases).

       iii. 13% are crash-related.

       iv. Most are mild (96%) in severity.

    b. History.

     i. Posterior neck pain.
- May develop acutely or insidiously.

     ii. Neurological symptoms usually absent.

  c. Physical examination.

     i. Tenderness to palpation of the trapezius and paracervical musculature.

     ii. Range of motion may be limited.

     iii. Neurological evaluation is normal including Spurling's test.

  d. Diagnostic tests.

     i. Radiographs should be obtained if neck pain is acute in onset or due to a crash.

     ii. Radiographs are not routinely necessary if the pain is insidious in onset.

     iii. Other tests not necessary.

  e. Treatment.

     i. Relative rest.
- Cervical strains typically result in limited time lost from training.

     ii. Ice and heat can both be helpful.

     iii. Analgesics or NSAIDs.

     iv. Massage.

     v. Range of motion and stretching exercises.

     vi. Strengthening.

2. Hand contusions.

  a. General information.

     i. Make up 74% of hand injuries.

     ii. Mechanisms.
- Crashes.
- Paddling on starts.

     iii. 98% are mild in nature.

  b. Radiographs are often obtained to rule out fracture.

  c. Do not result in time loss in most cases.

  d. Additional padding of the gloves may reduce pain and prevent further injury.

3. Back injuries.

  a. Majority are mild.

  b. Types.

     i. Strains (64%).
- May be acute or repetitive use in nature.
- Primarily due to starts.

     ii. Contusions (33%).
- Due to crashes.

4. Ankle sprains.
   a. Crashes are the most common mechanism.
   b. 50% of ankle injuries are sprains.
      i. Lateral ligaments most commonly injured.
         • Anterior talofibular ligament.
         • For sliding and steering, ankles are in a slight plantar flexed, inverted position.
      ii. For full discussion of ankle sprains, see Chapter 6, Snowboarding.
   c. Because no significant weight bearing is needed to start, slide, or stop, training can continue during rehabilitation.
      i. Precautions should be taken to avoid further injury in case of another crash.
5. Foot fractures.
   a. Mechanism of injury is crashing into the edges of the ice track.
   b. History.
      i. Athlete presents with pain in the foot after a crash.
      ii. Pain with weight bearing.
      iii. Swelling may be noted by the athlete.
   c. Physical examination.
      i. Limp.
      ii. Foot edema.
      iii. Tender to bony palpation of the foot.
      iv. Neurovascular status intact.
   d. Diagnostic tests.
      i. Radiographs should be obtained.
      ii. A minimum of two views is necessary.
   e. Treatment.
      i. Cast immobilization is considered (though not absolutely necessary) in most cases of foot fracture.
      ii. In cases of nondisplaced metatarsal and phalanx fracture, simple foot support is often adequate for healing.
         • Postoperative shoe.
         • Range of motion walking boot.
      iii. Surgical fixation of acute fractures of the base of the fifth metatarsal should be considered if the fracture is through the vascular watershed area.

Conclusions

A. Luge is an exciting, high-speed, and relatively safe winter sport.
B. There are relatively few high-level, well-trained competitors.

C. Most injuries are caused by crashes.

   1. Low incidence of moderate and major injuries.

SKELETON

General

A. History.

   1. World's first sliding sport, also known as tobogganing.

   a. First toboggan track from Davos to Klosters in Switzerland, 1882.

   b. Skeleton was practiced only in Switzerland until 1905.

   2. The name "skeleton."

   a. Believed to be after an English sled in 1892 of Mr. Child, which looked like a skeleton.

   b. Another theory is that "skele" is an anglicization of the Norwegian word for toboggan.

   3. 1926—Declared an Olympic sport.

   4. 1928—Appeared in Olympic games in St. Moritz.

   a. Jennison Heaton (USA) won the first Olympic gold medal and John Heaton (USA) won the silver medal.

   b. Did not return as an Olympic sport until St. Moritz games of 1948.

   i. Nino Bibbia (ITA) won gold while John Heaton won the silver medal again.

   c. Skeleton did not appear in the Olympics again until 2002.

   5. 1970s—Sport gains increasing popularity in Europe.

   6. 2002—Skeleton returns as an Olympic sport at the Salt Lake City games.

   a. Men's and women's events held.

   i. Tristan Gale (USA) won gold medal in first ever women's Olympic skeleton competition.

   ii. Jim Shea Jr. (USA) wins gold medal in men's competition.

B. Equipment.

   1. Helmet.

   a. All athletes must wear a helmet at all times to protect face from the ice surface, which is 2 inches away.

   b. Helmet must have a chin guard.

   c. Face visor must be shatter- and splinter-proof.

   2. Suit.

   a. Skin-tight rubber suit increases aerodynamics.

   b. Short sleeves and short trousers are not allowed.

3. Shoes.
  a. Spiked.
    i. Maximum of 8 spikes per shoe.
    ii. Maximum spike length is 7 mm.
  b. Enhance traction when sprinting on the ice track.
4. Sled.
  a. Body.
    i. Made of steel and fiberglass.
    ii. Dimensions:
      • Length is from 80 to 120 cm.
      • Height is 8 to 20 cm.
      • Width is 34 to 38 cm.
  b. Runners.
    i. Two runners composed of steel with at least 50% iron.
    ii. Runners are 25 mm wide and 45 cm long.
    iii. Width between runners is 34–38 cm.
    iv. Runners must be within 4°C of the reference runner during competitions.
      • Reference runner is left to cool in the open air at the track for one hour prior to racing.
      • No heating or "juicing" of the runners is allowed.
  c. Weight.
    i. Men's, 43 kg.
      • Maximum weight of sled and driver must not exceed 115 kg.
      • Missing weight may be attached to sled as ballast.
      • No ballast allowed on the athlete.
    ii. Women's, 35 kg.
      • Maximum weight of sled and driver must not exceed 92 kg.
      • Missing weight may be attached to sled as ballast.
      • No ballast allowed on the athlete.
  d. No devices are allowed to assist with steering or braking.
  e. Elbow padding is allowed but not required.
5. Track.
  a. Same track as for bobsled.
  b. 1200–1300 m in length.
    i. 1200 m must be sloping downhill.
    ii. No centrifugal force in excess of 5G is allowed.
    iii. Centrifugal force of 4G is allowed for only 4 seconds.
  c. Deceleration stretch at end to allow the sled to stop without brakes.
  d. Speeds as high as 70 to 80 mph are reached.

    e. Times are measured to one one-hundredth of a second.
       i. Competition determined by combined times of two runs.
       ii. World record times are difficult to determine due to the individual nature of each track.

Biomechanics

A. The start.
   1. Athlete sprints on ice track for 50 m.
     a. Both hands in contact with sled throughout the sprint.
       i. Hips and low back in extreme flexion.
       ii. Neck often held in neutral.
   2. At end of start track, the athlete lunges onto the sled.
     a. Weight of body supported by upper extremities until torso makes contact with sled.
       i. Neck, back, and hips move into an extended position.
     b. Once on the sled, the athlete is in prone position.
       i. Head first.
       ii. Neck extended.
       iii. Arms at sides.
B. Steering.
   1. Accomplished by shifting of body weight.
   2. No other devices allowed to assist with steering.
C. Stopping.
   1. There are no brakes.
   2. The uphill, deceleration stretch of track slows the sled.
     a. End of deceleration stretch is padded.

Injury Data

The information presented here is based on two years of injury data collection from the U.S. National Team.

A. 54 total injuries requiring attention by USOC athletic trainer.
   1. Actual number of runs was not monitored; therefore injury incidence cannot be calculated.
B. 57.4% of the total injuries occurred in males, 42.6% in females.
C. Mechanism of injury.
   1. Contact injuries 72% (39/54).
     a. Wall (30%).
     b. Contact with sled (24%).
     c. Fall off sled (24%).
     d. Crash (19%).
     e. Flipped sled (3%).
   2. Noncontact injuries 28% (15/54).

D. Injury types.
   1. Contusion (45%). Main mechanisms are:
      a. Mounting the sled after sprinting.
      b. Contact with track walls.
      c. Falling off sled.
   2. Sprain/strain (26%).
   3. Concussion (9%).
   4. Facial laceration (6%).
   5. Facial fracture (4%).
   6. Burn/abrasion (4%).
   7. Other (6%).
E. Injury location (Table 14-1).
   1. Thigh (27%).
      a. Hamstring strains account for 53% of the thigh injuries.
         i. Equal distribution between males and females.
      b. Majority of thigh injuries were strains, due to the intense short-distance sprinting needed to accelerate the sled.
   2. Head (20%).
      a. Head at risk for injury due to head-first position coupled with high speed of travel.
      b. Concussion was the most common injury to the head, accounting for 45% of all injuries to this region.
         i. Grade I (mild) concussion, 40%.
         ii. Grade II (moderate), 60%.

TABLE 14-1

Skeleton luge injury sites.

Body Site	Percentage of Total Injuries
Thigh	27
Head	20
Ankle/lower leg	11
Shoulder	9
Neck	7
Elbow	6
Hand	6
Chest	4
Hip	4
Foot	4
Knee	2

c. Higher percentage of concussion in males.

    d. For full discussion of concussion, see Chapter 11, Ice Hockey.

  3. Ankle/lower leg (11%).

  4. Shoulder (9%).

  5. Neck (7%).

    a. Higher percentage of neck injuries in females.

  6. Elbow (6%).

  7. Hand (6%).

  8. Chest (4%).

  9. Hip (4%).

 10. Foot (4%).

 11. Knee (2%).

F. Injury severity.

  1. The majority of injuries led to a loss of 1–7 days of practice/competition.

  2. Only 2% required > 7 days loss of practice/competition.

  3. The remaining injuries led to no lost time from sport.

Specific Injuries

A. Hamstring injuries.

  1. Mechanism of injury. Acute injuries tend to occur at two specific times:

    a. While sprinting during the 50-m start.

    b. While lunging onto the sled.

      i. The athlete accelerates prior to leaping onto the sled.

  2. Risk factors.

    a. Muscular fatigue limits muscle ability to absorb energy.

    b. Hamstring tightness.

      i. Stretching led to a 12% decrease in hamstring strains in military population.

    c. Prior hamstring injury is the largest risk factor for future hamstring injury.

      i. Risk particularly worse if previous injury not rehabilitated properly.

    d. Hamstring to quadriceps (H/Q) strength imbalance.

      i. H/Q ratio of at least 0.55 shown to decrease recurrent hamstring strain in Division I football players.

  3. History.

    a. Sensation of a "pop" or tear in the posterior thigh.

    b. Pain in the posterior thigh.

    c. Difficulty with running due to pain or tightness in posterior thigh.

    d. Many note that before the acute injury, they felt a tightness or impending "pull" that developed into recurring tightness and difficulty with running.

4. Physical examination.

    a. Limp may be noted.

    b. Edema and ecchymosis may be present.

    c. Tenderness to palpation of the hamstring musculature.

    d. Palpable muscle defect may be present.

    e. Decreased flexibility.

    f. Reduced strength.

5. Diagnostic tests.

    a. Plain radiographs.

        i. Important in skeletally immature athletes to look for avulsion fracture of ischial tuberosity.

        ii. Usually negative.

    b. MRI.

        i. Generally not needed for diagnosis and treatment.

        ii. If obtained, can define level and severity of injury.

           • May be helpful for prognosis and to approximate return to play for the elite-level athlete.

6. Injury classification.

    a. First-degree strain: mild pain with minimal disruption of musculotendinous unit.

    b. Second-degree strain: moderate pain with partial disruption of musculotendinous unit.

    c. Third-degree strain: severe pain with complete disruption of musculotendinous unit or a proximal avulsion.

7. Treatment.

    a. Grade I, II, and mid-substance Grade III strains.

        i. RICE.

        ii. NSAIDs.

        iii. Gentle stretching.

           • Avoid ballistic stretching.

           • Avoid painful stretching.

        iv. Gradual introduction of progressive resistance exercises.

        v. Gradual resumption of running activities.

    b. Grade III/complete avulsion of proximal attachment.

        i. Surgical repair recently recommended.

           • Five-year follow-up of acute repairs showed full hip and knee ROM and strength.

        ii. Nonoperative treatment for these injuries often led to less than optimal outcomes.

           • 83% report chronic pulling/cramping in posterior thigh.

           • 42% unable to run or perform sports that require agility.

8. Return to competitive sports may take several days to several weeks depending on grade of strain but should be delayed until the following goals are met:
   a. Full hip and knee ROM.
   b. Full hip extension and knee flexion strength.
   c. Able to run without pain in posterior thigh.
   d. H/Q ratio ≥ 0.6.

B. Quadriceps strain.
   1. Acute injury to the quadriceps musculature.
   2. Very similar to hamstring strain in regard to mechanism, history, physical examination, classification, and treatment.
      a. Occurs during the sprint phase of the start when the quadriceps is eccentrically loaded.
   3. Recurrence is common, particularly if the athlete is returned to sport before the injury is completely rehabilitated.

Suggested Readings

Cummings RS Jr, Shurland AT, Prodoehl JA, et al. Injuries in the sport of luge: Epidemiology and analysis. *AJSM* 1997;25(4):508–13.

Garrett WE Jr. Muscle strain injuries: Clinical and basic aspects. *MSSE* 1990;22(4):436–43.

Hartig DE, Henderson JM. Increasing hamstring flexibility decreases lower extremity overuse injuries in military basic trainees. *AJSM* 1999;27(2): 172–76.

Heiser TM, Weber J, Sullivan G, et al. Prophylaxis and management of hamstring muscle injuries in intercollegiate football players. *AJSM* 1984;12(5): 368–70.

Sallay PI, Friedman RL, Coogan PG, Garrett WE. Hamstring muscle injuries among water skiers: Functional outcome and prevention. *AJSM* 1996;24(2): 130–36.

15

CURLING

Sami F. Rifat

GENERAL CONSIDERATIONS

History

A. Name derived from the "curl" as the stones slide down the ice.

B. Probably originated in the 1500s on the frozen ponds and lakes of northern Europe, although similar games may have been played by prehistoric peoples.

C. The modern game was refined in Scotland in the 1600s and by the nineteenth century they had formalized rules and equipment.

D. In 1832 the first curling club was established in the United States.

E. Curling debuted as a medal sport in the 1998 Winter Olympics.

F. Approximately 1.5 million people curl worldwide.

The Game

A. The object of the game is for two teams of four players each to slide a 42-pound granite stone or rock down a 130-foot long by 15-foot wide sheet of ice.

B. The stones are "delivered" toward a 12-foot-wide target. After 16 rocks have been delivered, the score is determined. Teams score one point for each rock closest to the center of the target.

C. The ice in front of the rock is brushed to polish and heat the surface of the ice to keep the rock moving. This "sweeping" technique makes the rocks travel farther and straighter.

Common Injuries

A. Hand problems.
B. Ligament sprains.
C. Muscle strains.
D. Contusions.
E. Blisters and calluses.

MEDICAL ISSUES

There are no specific medical issues associated with curling. However, concerns regarding air quality are similar to those of the other indoor ice sports.

TRAUMATIC INJURIES

Groin Injuries

A. Groin injuries in curling may occur during the stretch phase of the delivery or the push phase while sweeping if the trailing leg is overextended.
B. These injuries are more common among users of the push-type broom.
C. Groin injuries are discussed further in Chapter 11, Ice Hockey.

Knee Contusions and Prepatellar Bursitis (Curler's Knee)

A. Curler's knee refers to soft tissue and bony contusion of the patella as the result of a fall onto the ice or improper technique. Repetitive trauma to the prepatellar bursa may also develop.
B. Most contusions can be treated with relative rest, ice, and analgesics. Prepatellar bursitis may be treated initially with ice, anti-inflammatory medications, rest (avoidance of trauma or repetitive knee flexion), and compression with an elastic wrap. If symptoms persist or if the bursa is so enlarged that it has become painful, it may be aspirated. If signs of infection (redness, local warmth, fever) are present, the aspirate should be sent for culture. Corticosteroid injection should not be used if infection is suspected and generally should be used with caution because of the risk of creating a fistulous tract in the relatively thin overlying skin.
C. The athlete may return to activity as symptoms allow.
D. Correction of improper technique and use of knee pads can help prevent this condition.

Lumbar Back Strains

A. Injury to the low back can occur as a result of improper sweeping technique or moving the stone incorrectly. The stone should be slid and not lifted. Lifting the stone at the beginning of play may cause injury.

B. The diagnosis and management of lumbar strains are discussed in Chapter 10, Biathlon.

OVERUSE INJURIES

DeQuervain's Tenosynovitis

A. DeQuervain's tenosynovitis is a stenosing tenosynovitis of the first dorsal compartment.

B. The injury affects the abductor pollicis longus and extensor pollicis brevis tendons (Figure 15-1) which abduct and extend the thumb at the MCP joint.

C. The injury occurs as a result of overuse, usually from delivery of the stone.

D. Diagnosis.

    1. The patient usually complains of radial wrist pain and occasional swelling. There is often difficulty abducting the thumb and with ulnar deviation of the wrist.

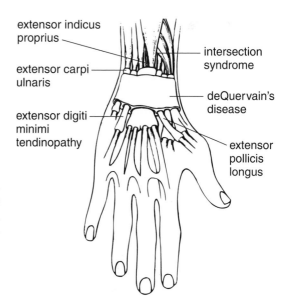

FIGURE 15-1 Dorsal surface anatomy of the wrist and hand. Reprinted with permission from Brukner P, Khan K. *Clinical Sports Medicine*, rev. 2nd ed. New York: McGraw-Hill; 2002, p. 304.

2. On examination swelling may be present and there is tenderness proximal to the radial styloid. Finkelstein test is positive. This test is performed by asking the patient to tuck the thumb inside the other fingers while the examiner passively ulnarly deviates the wrist. Radiographs are usually not necessary unless there is a history of trauma or the examiner is trying to rule out other sources of radial wrist pain.

E. Treatment.
1. Treatment of DeQuervain's tenosynovitis follows basic principles. The patient should avoid aggravating activity and, if still painful, a thumb spica splint is indicated. Ice and analgesic medications may also be helpful. Physical therapy is useful in those individuals with more severe symptoms.
2. Corticosteroid injection of the first dorsal compartment is often helpful in those who do not respond to more conservative measures.
3. Surgical release of the first dorsal compartment may be required if all else fails.

Intersection Syndrome

Intersection syndrome is a tenosynovitis or "friction" tendonitis between the first and second dorsal compartments of the wrist and distal forearm.

A. It is believed to occur as a result of repetitive movement of the wrist, particularly grasping and wringing.
B. These repetitive movements cause the muscle bellies of the extensor pollicis brevis and abductor pollicis longus to irritate the wrist extensor tendons of the second compartment as they cross over them at the dorsal radial distal forearm.
C. Diagnosis.
1. Individuals usually complain of distal forearm pain aggravated by active movement.
2. On examination there is point tenderness on the dorsal radial aspect of the forearm approximately 2 to 3 fingerbreadths proximal to the wrist (Figure 15-1). There is often palpable crepitance with passive or active motion.
D. Treatment of intersection syndrome involves relative rest, ice, and analgesic medication. A thumb spica splint may be helpful. Physical therapy is sometimes necessary. Injection may be useful in refractory cases.

Calluses

Calluses occur at the interface between the skin and an article of equipment or clothing. Most commonly seen on the hands and feet as a compensatory or protective response of the skin. In curlers, calluses often develop on the palms of the hands from gripping the broom handle.

A. Calluses appear as a thickened, hypertrophied stratum corneum over areas of bony prominence.

B. Treatment is often unnecessary unless the callus is painful or to prevent underlying blister formation. Usually the callus can be pared down with a pumice stone or file. Soaking can soften harder calluses prior to paring.

Blisters

Blisters can occur underneath calluses as a result of increased shearing forces. In curlers, these tender, fluid-filled vesicles most often form on the hands due to forces produced by gripping the broom handle.

A. The blister roof should be allowed to remain intact. The fluid may be drained every 12 hours for the first 24 hours. If the epidermal covering has been removed, a hydrocolloid gel (Duoderm) may be applied for 5 to 7 days.

B. Prevention is really the best treatment. Calluses should be pared and the athlete should wear properly fitting shoes and equipment.

APPENDIX

SUGGESTED DOSAGES FOR CORTICOSTEROID AND ANESTHETIC INJECTION BY SITE

Site	Needle	Syringe	Triamcinolone 20 mg/mL	Lidocaine*	Bupivacaine
Shoulder					
Subacromial	1.5 in. 25 g	5–10 mL	1–2 mL	2 mL	2-4 mL
Biceps	1.5 in. 25 g	5 mL	1 mL	1 mL	1 mL
Knee					
Intra-articular					
Anesthetic	1.5 in. 25 g	3 mL	—	2 mL	—
Injection	1.5 in. 18–21 g	10 mL	2–4 mL	2–4 mL	2–4 mL
Aspiration	1.5 in. 18 g	30–60 mL	—	—	—
Pes anserine	1.5 in. 25 g	5 mL	1 mL	1 mL	1 mL
Prepatellar bursa					
Anesthetic	1.5 in. 25 g	3 mL	—	2 mL	—
Aspiration	1–1.5 in. 18 g	10–60 mL	—	—	—
Injection	1.5 in. 18–21 g	5 mL	1–2 mL	1 mL	1 mL
Iliotibial band	1.5 in. 25 g	5 mL	1–2 mL	1 mL	1 mL
Hand and Wrist					
DeQuervain's	1–1.5 in. 25 g	3 mL	0.5 mL	1 mL (2%)	—
Dorsal ganglion					
Anesthetic	1 in. 25 g	3 mL	—	2 mL	—
Aspiration	1 in. 18 g	10 mL	—	—	—
Injection	1 in. 22–25 g	3 mL	1 mL	—	—

continued

(Continued)

Site	Needle	Syringe	Triamcinolone 20 mg/mL	Lidocaine*	Bupivacaine
Elbow					
Lateral epicondyle	1–1.5 in. 25 g	5 mL	1 mL	2 mL	2 mL
Olecranon bursa					
Anesthetic	1.5 in. 25 g	3 mL	—	2 mL	—
Aspiration	1–1.5 in. 18 g	10–60 mL	—	—	—
Injection	1.5 in. 18–21 g	3 mL	1 mL	1 mL	1 mL
Greater Trochanteric Bursa	1.5–2 in. 22–25 g	10 mL	2 mL	2 mL	2–6 mL
Plantar Fascia	1.5 in. 25 g	5 mL	1 mL	2 mL	2 mL

*1% lidocaine unless specified.

INDEX